Legacies in Ethics and Medicine

Legacies in Ethics and Medicine

Chester R. Burns

Editor

Science History Publications
New York · 1977

Science History Publications
a division of
Neale Watson Academic Publications, Inc.
156 Fifth Avenue, New York 10010

R
724
L414

Library of Congress Cataloging in Publication Data
Main entry under title:

Legacies in ethics and medicine.

   Bibliography: p.
   1. Medical ethics--History--Addresses, essays,
lectures. I. Burns, Chester R.
R724.L414   174'.2'09   76-44908
ISBN 0-88202-166-4

Contents

Acknowledgements

We should like to express our appreciation to the following scholarly publications for granting us permission to reprint the articles in this volume: *The Bulletin of the History of Medicine* (The Johns Hopkins University Press), "The Hippocratic Oath: Translation and Interpretation," Supplement No. 1, 1943, "The Professional Ethics of the Greek Physician," *30*: 391-419, 1956, "Medical Ethics in Hippocratic Bone Surgery," *42*: 297-311, 1968, "An Ancient Poem on the Duties of a Physician," *7*: 315-323, 1939, "The Physician's Prayer Attributed to Moses Maimonides," *41*: 440-454, 1967, "Medical Ethics and Etiquette in the Early Middle Ages," *26*: 1-31, 1952, "The Hippocratic Oath in Elizabethan England," *4*: 201-219, 1936, "Samuel Sorbière and His Advice to a Young Physician," *24*: 255-287, 1950, "Bernard Mandeville, M.D., and Eighteenth Century Ethics," *45*: 430-443, 1971, "Cabot, Peabody, and the Care of the Patient," *24*: 462-481, 1950; *The Journal of the History of Medicine and Allied Sciences*, "The Ideal Doctor as Depicted in Ancient Hebrew Writings," *12*: 37-41, 1957, "Isaac Israeli's Fifty Admonitions to the Physician," *17*: 245-257, 1962; The University of Chicago Press, "A Study in Fourteenth Century Medical Deontology," in *Medieval and Historiographical Essays in Honor of James Westfall Thompson*, 1938; Robert E. Krieger Publications, "Thomas Percival: Medical Ethics or Medical Jurisprudence?" in *Medical Ethics*, Huntington, N.Y., 1975; The Wellcome Institute of the History of Medicine, "Reciprocity in the Development of Anglo-American Medical Ethics, 1765-1865," in *Proceedings of the XXIII International Congress of the History of Medicine*, vol. 1, London, 1974.

INTRODUCTION

CHESTER R. BURNS

As with *Legacies in Law and Medicine*,[1] this collection of essays is designed primarily for use in the classroom by teachers of history, philosophy, and religion. It is a convenient introduction to some principal legacies of ethics and medicine, especially those in Western culture. The following comments serve *only* as guideposts to the essays which follow. (When referring to the essays included in this volume, I shall place the author's last name in parentheses. The numbers enclosed in parentheses refer to the references listed at the end of this Introduction.)

The history of ethics and the history of medical ethics are distinctive, but it is not possible to understand the latter without an appreciation of the former. Every medical practitioner functions within a web of personal ideals and social norms which unquestionably affect many of his judgments. As professionals, however, physicians assume specialized roles in their communities, elaborating specifically professional norms which are not identical with personal or social ones. These professional ethics may, in turn, perfuse and mold the personal and group values of the society as a whole. The history of medical ethics is the history of these professional ideals and their associated values as they have been discovered and claimed from antiquity to the present day.

Antiquity. Religious beliefs and practices constitute one of the most important sources of value judgments about human behavior. Since religion and medicine were intertwined during the early centuries of human civilization, it is not surprising that religious ethics assumed a prominent place in concepts of professional ethics in medicine. These relationships between religious values and medical practices have been outstanding in the Jewish legacy.[2] The Talmud, the five books of Moses, and the Rabbinic literature have numerous passages that deal with physicians and medical practices (Margalith). Many of these involve references to a divine being, and some express eternal judgments about righteous or evil practitioners. Many specific practices, such as abortion, infanticide, suicide, treatment of prisoners, fees, castration, sterilization, visits to the sick, and truth-telling, are examined in this literature, but all within a framework of religious valuing. Supernatural assessments reign supreme: It appears unlikely that a physician could be good without being a devout Jew.

Hippocratic physicians of ancient Greece are usually given special recognition for their efforts to divest medicine of supernatural influences, especially those that might be involved in the causation of disease.[3] Yet, the author of the *Oath* ascribed to Hippocrates begins the declamation by invoking "Apollo Physician and Asclepius and Hygieia and Panacea and all the gods and goddesses" as his witnesses. In contrast to the Hebrew writings, however, it is not religion, but philosophy which provides a theoretical structure for the judgments contained in the Hippocratic *Oath*.

The *Oath's* prohibitions were not respected by all Greek physicians; nor did the citizens of ancient Greece expect their doctors to honor them. Suicide and infanticide were acceptable under certain circumstances. Those who wrote the *Oath* did not agree with these judgments, and forbade physicians to use poisons and abortifacients. The *Oath's* claims—both covenant and special rules about diet, poisons, abortifacients, and surgery—are best understood within a context of Pythagoreanism, a philosophy that included ideals of justice, forbearance, purity, and holiness (Edelstein, 1943).

Pythagoreanism was not the only philosophy which affected notions of professional ethics among Graeco-Roman physicians in antiquity (Edelstein, 1956). Gentlemanly virtues of the Aristotelian school are expressed in the treatise *On the Physician*. A doctor should be fair, prudent, and kind; he should not be vulgar or harsh. *Precepts* and *On Decorum*—other Hippocratic writings composed in Hellenistic times—reveal Stoic values of wisdom and rational choice. Emphasized are gentleness, kindliness, and charitableness, not purity or holiness. Ancient Greek religion had little, if any, moral import; and as the ideal of civic virtue became less tenable with the disappearance of city-states, medical practitioners could find important ideals primarily in the teachings of philosophers.[4]

Could these physicians differ as moralists and still be good practitioners? That is, were physicians *good* physicians because they were loyal disciples of Aristotelianism or Platonism or Stoicism? At least one physician of the first century A.D., Scribonius Largus, discovered specifically professional virtues in the Stoic humanism transmitted by Cicero. Yet, this fascinating linkage between Stoic ideals and professional virtues in medicine was not exclusive, as indicated by the other values expressed in the aforementioned deontological writings of Graeco-Roman medicine.

Furthermore, it would be erroneous to suppose that philosophical ethics were simply superimposed on the clinical judgments of medical craftsmen in antiquity. A careful analysis of some clinical writings reveals that Hippocratic physicians forged their professional norms within crucibles of daily practice (Michler). Surely, an ethos of adequate knowledge and skill coupled with rigorous self-assessment, including the admission of professional mistakes, did not emerge solely or primarily from speculations about human morality.

Yet, these professional judgments were seldom, if ever, strictly divorced from the religious and philosophical values current at the time of their expression. For example, the uniquely medical humanism of Scribonius, ideals of Pythagorean holiness and Stoic brotherhood, and, possibly, the language of Christian judgment appear in a poem about the duties of a physician, probably written in the second century, A.D. (Maas and Oliver).

The Medieval Era.   The evolution of professional ethics in medicine during the Middle Ages is linked to traditions of the Christian, Jewish, and Islamic religions. Precepts of the latter religion are abundantly evident in what was probably the earliest systematic treatise on medical ethics in the Arabic world: the *Adab al-tabib* or "Practical Ethics of the Physician" by Ishaq ibn ' Ali al-Ruhawi (Levey). The ethics of the pagan Greeks provided numerous conflicts for devout Muslim physicians, and the lofty ideals of the Greek philosophers and the Islamic prophets had to be tempered with concrete judgments arising out of bedside practices. Al-Ruhawi's view is remarkably comprehensive and eclectic. His efforts to discover realistic paths of action among conflicting cultural norms and perplexing circumstances of patient care are strikingly modern, although they occurred within the context of ninth-century Islam.[5]

Isaac Israeli, a contemporary of al-Ruhawi, practiced medicine in Egypt and Tunisia. His numerous medical works were translated into several languages and used extensively by medieval physicians. One of these writings was entitled "The Book of Admonitions to the Physicians" (Bar-Sela and Hoff). Although Isaac Israeli was acknowledged to be a great Jewish physician, his "admonitions" are notably secular. His precepts about thorough knowledge, attention to patients, and prompt response to their needs are quite modern; but reliance on ancient authorities and repeated praise of the healing power of nature remind us that his ethical standards were evolved during a lifetime that probably extended from 840 A.D. to 950 A.D.[6]

Religious ideals of the Jewish legacy were sustained forcefully in the provocative and sobering "'Daily Prayer of a Physician," attributed to Moses Maimonides (an outstanding physician-philosopher of the late twelfth century) but possibly written by an eighteenth-century physician to the Jewish Hospital in Berlin, Dr. Marcus Herz (Rosner).

In their search for professional ethics, Christian physicians, like their Islamic and Jewish colleagues, could not ignore the ideals of the Greek philosophers and attempted to reconcile them with religious values. In responding to ever-present conflicts, these practitioners could be pious and ascetic, on the one hand, and characteristically secular and earthy on the other (MacKinney). God was the ultimate healer; Christians were admonished to honor physicians as God's servants. In other writings, physicians were urged to be humble, modest, and chaste as well as affable, charming, and good conversationalists— these latter values hardly Christian ideals. Several medieval pronouncements dealt with educational requirements for future physicians. Others refer to standards about transactions between practitioners and patients. There are frequent references to the Hippocratic writings—*Oath, Law, Precepts, Decorum,* and *On the Physician.*

The assertions about proper methods for education suggest the growing importance of medieval universities in framing the quest for professional ideals. As fundamental sources of ideals, medieval physicians in the Latin West could ignore neither the Greek philosophical legacy nor the Church as an institution. But universities, guilds, and hospitals—institutions emerging during the medieval era—were profoundly changing the nature of medical ethics.

As the latter centuries of the medieval period evolved into the early centuries of the modern era, the Greek legacies (Hippocratic and Galenic) became preeminent, in medical ethics as well as medical science and practice. Physicians and surgeons of the fourteenth, fifteenth, and sixteenth centuries repeatedly acknowledged the deontological treatises of the Hippocratic writings, especially the *Oath.* But their acceptance of these ideals was not merely passive or imitative: They offered both comments about the Greek legacy and their own professional ideals in response to the conflicts and challenges of their day (Welborn).

The Modern Period. The Hippocratic legacy in medical ethics did not disappear with the decline of the Middle Ages. In fact, among the Hippocratic writings, the *Oath* was the most frequently printed in Elizabethan English (Larkey). Conditions had changed, however, and the Elizabethan authors, especially John Securis, did not hesitate to offer their own interpretations and additions to the classical *Oath*. Securis, for example, refers to the "common weale" and offers suggestions for some laws about medical practice.

Present throughout the ethical considerations of physicians in antiquity and the Middle Ages is a concern with proper physician-patient interactions;· but conspicuous by its absence is a focus on the community-at-large, or the public. The idea of a "public" or "society" is introduced during the modern period. The fairly widespread appearance of medical licensing by 1600 was, if nothing else, symbolic of the society's need for measures of public accountability. It is within this context that we can best understand the seventeenth-century exhortations of the French physician and philosopher, Samuel Sorbière (Pleadwell). His strong opposition to the public's indifference toward the medical profession indicates Sorbière's great need for public approval. At a time when credulity outpaced credibility, Sorbière advocated various techniques, including the finer points of rhetoric and oratory, to gain a patient's confidence. Although exhibiting religious devotion and a philosophic grasp, Sorbière's counsel is free of ethereal pieties and abstract ideals. His discussion of medical sects, his critique of undue reliance on urine examination and pulse-taking, his complaints about the inadequate compensation of physicians, his analysis of consultations, and his comments about the relationships of physicians and apothecaries usher us into the richly complex setting of modern medicine, where oaths, prayers, and occasional comments in medical and surgical texts seem, at worst, archaic and, at best, immature. For the modern physician must, as did Sorbière, fashion a philosophy of medicine congruent with the social realities of the day. Moreover, the modern physician has the dilemma of limiting his value judgments to medicine proper, or of extending them to the broader, more inclusive, problems of the society in which he offers his professional services and experiences his personal frustrations and satisfactions.

The paradoxes and conflicts of this predicament are well illustrated in the writings of an eighteenth-century London physician, Bernard Mandeville (Clark). Not only did Mandeville practice medicine without a license from the Royal College of Physicians, but he also plunged into the medical controversies of the day, not hesitating to offer normative judgments about relations between physicians and apothecaries, the lack of clinical teaching at Oxford and Cambridge, and the scientific improprieties of theoretical systems. But, his value assessments went far beyond medical practice. He offered a program for social reform in prisons and, writing anonymously, elaborated rigorous critiques of religious and educational institutions. As London physician and British citizen, he was—in all that the phrase implies—an eighteenth-century moralist.[7]

Thomas Percival, a general practitioner in Manchester, England, was also an eighteenth-century moralist. In contrast to Mandeville, however, Percival correlated his professional ethics with religious sentiments, philosophical abstractions, and legal rules (Burns, 1975). The result was the first comprehensive view of professional ethics in medicine, entitled *Medical Ethics, or a Code of Institutes and Precepts, Adapted to the Professional Conduct of Physicians and Surgeons,* and published in 1803. Percival spent nine years composing the 92 sections of his four-chapter book. His view of professional ethics is based on four fundamental dimensions of a medical practitioner's obligations: those to himself as a person, those to his practitioner colleagues, those to his patients, and those to the community as a whole. It is not possible to understand Percival fully without acknowledging and considering his belief in a significant relationship between law and ethics.[8]

During the nineteenth century, Percival's *Medical Ethics* was profoundly influential in the United States. Even the format of numbered sections was copied in the various codes adopted by American practitioners. By 1850, the exchange of professional ideals between Great Britain and the United States had become a two-way street, and the ideal of mutual obligations between physicians and patients, or profession and society, was being explored on both sides of the Atlantic (Burns, 1974).

During the nineteenth century, the hegemony of the code of ethics adopted by the American Medical Association was striking.[9] The majority of American physicians considered ethical problems only within the code's framework, and the adhesiveness of the British legacy was noteworthy, with some of Percival's own words still present in the revised code adopted in 1903. Innovation came later with the careers of two Boston physicians: Richard Clarke Cabot, who died in 1939, and Francis Peabody, who died prematurely in 1927 (Williams).

A study of these essays will reveal a nexus of relationships between important ethical and medical traditions in Western culture. They also suggest numerous possibilities for teachers and scholars who wish to explore uncharted historiographical territories.

References and Notes

1. Chester R. Burns, *Legacies in Law and Medicine.* New York: Science History Publications, 1976

2. For a more extensive review, see Immanuel Jakobovits, *Jewish Medical Ethics.* New York: Bloch, 1962; and "Medical ethics in the *Kitsur Shulchan Aruch,*" by Theodore F. Dagi in *Reports of the Institute Fellows 1973-74,* Institute on Human Values in Medicine, Society for Health and Human Values, 1974, pp. 67–79.

3. Chester R. Burns, "Diseases versus healths: some legacies in the philosophies of modern medical science," in *Evaluation and Explanation in the Biomedical Sciences,* edited by H.T. Engelhardt, Jr. and S. Spicker. Boston: Reidel Pub. Co., pp. 29–47.

4. See the other essays in Part Three of *Ancient Medicine Selected Papers of Ludwig Edelstein,* edited by Owsei Temkin and C. Lilian Temkin, Baltimore: The Johns Hopkins Press, 1967.

6

5. For a translation of al-Ruhawi's book, see Martin Levey, "Medical ethics of medieval Islam with special reference to al-Ruhawi's 'Practical ethics of the physician'," *Transactions of the American Philosophical Society*, Vol. 57, Part Three, 1967.

6. Another translation is offered by Saul Jarcho, "Guide for Physicians (Musar Harofim) by Isaac Judaeus (880?–932?)," *Bull. Hist. Med.* 1944, *15*:180–188.

7. For other details about the British legacy, see Robert Forbes, "A historical survey of medical ethics," *Brit. Med. J.*, 1935, *II*:137–140.

8. For another look at Percival, see Lester King, "The development of medical ethics," in *The Medical World of the 18th Century*. Chicago: University of Chicago Press, 1958, pp. 227–262.

9. Compare the codes offered as appendices in Chauncey Leake's edition of *Percival's Medical Ethics* reprinted by Robert Krieger in 1975; also see the first and last chapters of Donald Konold, *A History of American Medical Ethics 1847–1912*. Madison: The State Historical Society of Washington, 1962.

The Ideal Doctor as Depicted in Ancient Hebrew Writings

DAVID MARGALITH*

IN Talmudic sources one does not find any medical treatises or descriptions of physicians or their practices which had been written for their own sakes. Many of our great sages practised medicine and specialized in anatomy, physiology, epidemiology, and surgery since a thorough knowledge of these subjects was essential to answer ritual and judicial questions. However, in some places in the Talmud there is reflected the high moral standard ascribed by our sages to the medical profession and the strong demands made upon physicians. Here are a number of instances:

"My son, should you fall sick, place yourself in the hands of a doctor, for this is his calling and God has given him of His wisdom." (Ben Sira, 38.)[1]

". . . 'And he shall heal' [Exodus, 20, 19]—that is to say, the doctor has been allowed to attend to the sick (and one should not say 'The Almighty has inflicted the wound and shall the doctor be able to heal?')" (Rashi's [1040-1105] commentary—Berakhot 60; Baba Kama, 85.)[2]

Ben Sira says: "God has grown medicines from the soil and the wise man shall not abhor them. Therewith the doctor heals the wound, the chemist makes up the prescription." (Bereshit Rabba, 10.)[3]

". . . The Almighty has created healing substances to grow from the earth, and the wise man knows their functions." (Ben-Sira, 30.)[1]

". . . The Doctor who heals free of charge is worth nothing; the doctor who comes from afar [one who is not well acquainted with the patient and his disease] is like a blind man." (Baba Kama, 85.)[2]

* Tel Aviv, Israel.

[1] The book "The Wisdom of Yeshua (Jesus) Ben Sira" was written in the third century B.C. It was not included in the Holy Scriptures, but the Talmud quotes from it very often and bases its arguments upon it.

[2] Berachot, Baba Kama, Taanit, Sanhedrin etc. These are treatises in the Talmud Bavli (Babylonian). The Talmud was begun about 200 years B.C. and was completed in the sixth century A.D. There is also a Talmud Yerushalmi (of Jerusalem) which was compiled in Eretz Israel at about the same time.

[3] These are commentaries on the Pentateuch, chapter by chapter. They were compiled at the time of the Talmud.

". . . A doctor comes to a sick man and says to him: 'Do not drink cold drinks, and do not lie in a humid place, this you shall eat and that not . . .' But when a doctor sees that the patient is in mortal danger and will die anyhow, he should say to him and his family: 'Let him eat anything he wishes'; however, the man who can be cured should be taken good care of." (Shemot Rabba, 30, Vayikra Rabba, 33.)[4]

". . . Should a woman have a difficult delivery, the child is cut up in her womb and taken out limb by limb, for her life comes first. However, if most of the child has come out, it may not be harmed—for one life should not be sacrificed for another." (Ohalot, 7, 6.) In other words, so long as the child is as yet unborn, the mother's life should be saved and the baby's sacrificed; but when he is almost completely out in the world, he should not be touched, in accordance with the sublime maxim: 'One soul shall not be sacrificed for another.'

". . . Should a woman die in labour (on Sabbath), a knife shall be taken and her belly cut and the child taken out." ('Arakin, 7.)[5] The new interpretation here was firstly that the Sabbath was violated and the mother's body operated on in order to save the living child which had not yet been born, and secondly that mutilation of the corpse was no deterrent and it was operated on, for life (that of the unborn child) is sacred.

". . . He who goes out to be killed is given frankincense to drink to confuse his senses." (Sanhedrin, 43.)[6] This was merely a humane gesture, as explained by Rashi, "so that he may not worry, thus prolonging the suffering of being killed."

While explaining a certain sentence in the Scriptures (Deuteronomy, 32, 10—'He found him in a desert land, and in the waste howling wilderness; he led him about, he instructed him, he kept him as the apple of his eye'), the Zohar[7] quotes a wonderful description of the healing activities of a pious and benevolent doctor. In view of the interest in this extract we reproduce it here in translation:

"In connection with this sentence (Deuteronomy, 32, 10) it is written in the Book of Kratnae [some regard this name as a mis-

---

4 See note 3.
5 See note 2.
6 *Ibid.*
7 "The book of Zohar" is the basic work of Cabbala, which according to tradition is ascribed to Rabbi Shimon Bar Yohai (about 150 A.D.). There is, however, evidence that it was first published by Rabbi Moshe De Leon, a Cabbalist who lived in France in the fourteenth century.

nomer for Hippocrates] the Physician:[8] The wise doctor should take the following measures in attending to a patient who is the King's prisoner. He should pray for him to the Creator, since the doctor has found him 'in a desert land,' that is to say, suffering from diseases and a prisoner. What should the doctor do? He should analyse the causes and devise means of removing from the patient all things that may be harmful to him; he will bleed him to draw the 'bad blood' from his body; he will examine him in order to find out what has caused the disease and what will prevent its aggravation. He will then 'keep him as the apple of his eye'— he will take good care of the patient with the aid of such medicines and cures as are required. And he shall make no mistakes, for should he err but once, the Almighty will regard it as if he had shed blood and killed his patient; for the Almighty's wish is that even though a sick man be in prison he should nonetheless have someone to intercede for him and help him to secure his release.

"The Lord in Heaven passes sentence on all mortals—for life and death; some are punished by being maimed or penalised financially. He who has deserved corporal chastisement falls sick and is not cured until he has suffered the full measure of the punishment meted out to him. And a man who is punished financially and has disbursed the full amount imposed on him, is then cured and released from prison. The doctor should therefore see to it that the patient should pay the penalty and be freed.

"A man who has deserved to be flogged, is arrested and imprisoned until he has received a flogging all over his body and occasionally only on some parts of his body, or even one member only. Then he is freed. He who is sentenced to death may not escape this penalty even should he pay high ransom or all the money in the world. For this reason the wise doctor should make an effort on his behalf; if he can heal his body—well and good; if not, he should try to cure his spirit. Such a doctor will be rewarded by the Lord in this world and the next.

"Rabbi Elazar said: I have so far not heard of such a doctor or of that book. But once upon a time I was told by a certain Ishmaelite, who had it from his father, that in his father's time there lived a doctor who by just looking at a patient would be able to foretell whether the man would live or die. It was said about him that he was a saintly, god-fearing man, and when a poor patient came to him he would buy the medicines for him as well as any

---

[8] This is the only place in ancient writings where the physician Kratnae is mentioned.

other necessities. They used to say·of him that there was no other doctor like him in the world. And his prayers were even more effective than the work of his hands. It seems to me that the doctor referred to here is the one mentioned by that Ishmaelite. It is certain that he is in possession of that doctor's book, as he had inherited it from his father. All that is written in that book is based on secrets from the Torah; it contains many mysteries and wonderful medical tracts. He used to say, however, that only a god-fearing doctor may make use of these. Everything contained in that book was perfectly clear as it stipulated precisely what a pious man may and what he may not do.

"Rabbi Elazar said: I had this book with me for twelve months and I found in it sublime enlightenment. When I came across the mysteries in the book, I called the Jew named Rabbi Yossi Ben-Yehuda and gave the book to him. Some of the mystic cures I found in this book were based on secrets from the Torah, and I am convinced that they had been written in sanctity and prayer and repentence toward the Lord. The doctor had transmitted the secrets from the Torah and extracted from them medical secrets, the like of which I have never seen. And I said: Blessed be our God who imparts of His divine wisdom to human beings." (Zohar, part 3, 299.)

That was a portrait of the righteous, god-fearing doctor, to whom may be entrusted the body and soul of the sick man imprisoned by Divine Providence, so that he may save him from damnation.

Our sages were loud in their praise of a certain 'craftsman' (a blood-letter used to be called a craftsman) whose name was Abba Umana.[9] About him it is said: "Abba Umana daily received greetings from the Heavenly Assembly. But what were his good deeds that brought him such reward? This is what he used to do: When he was blood-letting he would seat the men apart and the women apart. And he had a special garment in which he kept a sharp horn for blood-letting. When a woman came to him to be bled, he would put that garment on her and she would wrap herself up, so that none should look at her (to prevent immodesty). Also he had a hidden place where his customers would put their coins. He who

---

[9] The name Abba Umana is apparently derived from the word "Uman" (craftsman), used in the Talmud for a blood-letter, and the title "Abba Umana" indicates that the man was an expert at blood-letting, e.g. ". . . the father of all such as handle the harp . . ." (Genesis, 4,21). For the word Umman (blood letter) see Preuss, J., *Biblisch talmudische Medizin* (Berlin, 1911), pp. 36-9; for Abba, see the same, pp. 38-9.

had one would place it there in payment for the blood-letting and he who had not was not shamed. And when a scholar happened to come to be bled, he would take no fee from him. Moreover, if he saw that a man had nothing to eat after the blood-letting, he would give him a coin and say to him: 'Go and eat.' " (Babylonian Talmud, Treatise Taadnit, 21.)[10]

These few excerpts paint a clear picture of the medical profession in its ideal form.

We have seen two model, god-fearing doctors who have reached the peak of life eternal: (i) the righteous Abba Umana, who was extremely strict about modest behaviour by men and women and was also very decent towards his patients in money matters so that a poor man should not be shamed; (ii) Kratnae, the divine doctor, who had been entrusted with the execution of verdicts pronounced by the Heavenly Court—monetary fines, physical disability, and death sentences. The doctor may never err, for he may pay with his life for any mistake. The sick prisoner is a trust placed in the doctor's hands by divine providence, and the doctor answers for the life of that prisoner. Indeed, the responsibility is tremendous.

Happy is the man who can stand up to such demands and can with a clear conscience compare himself with Kratnae and Abba Umana.

---

[10] See note 2.

THE HIPPOCRATIC OATH
TEXT, TRANSLATION AND INTERPRETATION
LUDWIG EDELSTEIN

INTRODUCTION

That for centuries the so-called Hippocratic Oath was the exemplar of medical etiquette and as such determined the professional attitude of generations of physicians, no one will doubt. Yet when it is asked what historical forces were instrumental in the formulation of this document, no answer can be given that is generally agreed upon. Uncertainty still prevails concerning the time when the Oath was composed and concerning the purpose for which it was intended. The dates proposed in modern debate vary from the 6th century B. C. to the 1st century A. D. As for the original intent of the manifesto, it is maintained that the Oath was administered in family guilds of physicians; or that it formed the statute of societies of artisans which perhaps were organized in secret; or that it was an ideal program designed without regard for any particular time or place.

In my opinion it is not necessary to resign oneself to leaving the issue undecided. If some data provided by the text itself are evaluated in their true import and are combined with others the proper meaning of which has previously been established, it seems possible to determine the origin of the Hippocratic Oath with a fair degree of certainty. At any rate, it is with this aim in mind that I propose to re-examine the document.

In so doing I shall scrutinize the Hippocratic text sentence by sentence—the treatise is short enough to allow completeness of interpretation—for it is only in this way that the adequacy or inadequacy of the thesis to be offered can be tested. Moreover, I shall give in full the testimony of ancient authors on which I depend in my inquiry. The material used is scattered and in some cases difficult of access, and it should be at hand if the cogency of the argument is to be judged. Such a method of investigation necessarily results in a certain copiousness, but this hardly needs justification in view of the importance of the Hippocratic Oath, both for the history of medicine and of ethics.

12

Ὄμνύω Ἀπόλλωνα ἰητρὸν καὶ Ἀσκληπιὸν καὶ Ὑγείαν καὶ Πανάκειαν
καὶ θεοὺς πάντας τε καὶ πάσας ἵστορας ποιεύμενος ἐπιτελέα ποιήσειν κατὰ
δύναμιν καὶ κρίσιν ἐμὴν ὅρκον τόνδε καὶ ξυγγραφὴν τήνδε·

5 ἡγήσασθαί τε τὸν διδάξαντά με τὴν τέχνην ταύτην ἴσα γενέτῃσιν
ἐμοῖσιν καὶ βίου κοινώσασθαι καὶ χρεῶν χρηίζοντι μετάδοσιν ποιήσασθαι
καὶ γένος τὸ ἐξ αὐτοῦ ἀδελφεοῖς ἴσον ἐπικρινέειν ἄρρεσι καὶ διδάξειν τὴν
τέχνην ταύτην, ἢν χρηίζωσι μανθάνειν, ἄνευ μισθοῦ καὶ ξυγγραφῆς, παραγγελίης τε καὶ ἀκροήσιος καὶ τῆς λοιπῆς ἁπάσης μαθήσιος μετάδοσιν
10 ποιήσασθαι υἱοῖσί τε ἐμοῖσι καὶ τοῖσι τοῦ ἐμὲ διδάξαντος καὶ μαθηταῖσι
συγγεγραμμένοις τε καὶ ὡρκισμένοις νόμῳ ἰητρικῷ, ἄλλῳ δὲ οὐδενί.

διαιτήμασί τε χρήσομαι ἐπ' ὠφελείῃ καμνόντων κατὰ δύναμιν καὶ κρίσιν
ἐμήν· ἐπὶ δηλήσει δὲ καὶ ἀδικίῃ εἴρξειν.

οὐ δώσω δὲ οὐδὲ φάρμακον οὐδενὶ αἰτηθεὶς θανάσιμον οὐδὲ ὑφηγήσομαι
15 ξυμβουλίην τοιήνδε· ὁμοίως δὲ οὐδὲ γυναικὶ πεσσὸν φθόριον δώσω. ἁγνῶς
δὲ καὶ ὁσίως διατηρήσω βίον ἐμὸν καὶ τέχνην ἐμήν.

οὐ τεμέω δὲ οὐδὲ μὴν λιθιῶντας, ἐκχωρήσω δὲ ἐργάτῃσιν ἀνδράσιν
πρήξιος τῆσδε.

ἐς οἰκίας δὲ ὁκόσας ἂν ἐσίω, ἐσελεύσομαι ἐπ' ὠφελείῃ καμνόντων ἐκτὸς
20 ἐὼν πάσης ἀδικίης ἑκουσίης καὶ φθορίης τῆς τε ἄλλης καὶ ἀφροδισίων
ἔργων ἐπί τε γυναικείων σωμάτων καὶ ἀνδρείων ἐλευθέρων τε καὶ δούλων.

ἃ δ' ἂν ἐν θεραπείῃ ἢ ἴδω ἢ ἀκούσω ἢ καὶ ἄνευ θεραπηίης κατὰ βίον
ἀνθρώπων, ἃ μὴ χρή ποτε ἐκλαλέεσθαι ἔξω, σιγήσομαι ἄρρητα ἡγεύμενος
εἶναι τὰ τοιαῦτα.

25 ὅρκον μὲν οὖν μοι τόνδε ἐπιτελέα ποιέοντι καὶ μὴ ξυγχέοντι εἴη ἐπαύ-
ρασθαι καὶ βίου καὶ τέχνης δοξαζομένῳ παρὰ πᾶσιν ἀνθρώποις ἐς τὸν
αἰεὶ χρόνον, παραβαίνοντι δὲ καὶ ἐπιορκοῦντι τἀναντία τουτέων.

Titulus: ἱπποκράτους ὅρκος M V R U *Mg.* ā′ V   2 ὄμνυμι R U   3 ἅπαντας V τε]
om. V   *Supra* ἴστορας *scr.* μάρτυρας U, *m. rec.* R   ποίησιν V   4 συγγραφήν *supra scr.*
ξ V, *supra add.* συμφωνίαν U, *m. rec.* R   5 τε] V, δὲ M R U, μὲν *Littré*   ἴσα γενέτῃσιν]
ἴσα καὶ γενέτοισιν R U   6 ἐμοῖσι V R U   χρέους V, χρέος? *Diels*   χρήζοντι V   7 καὶ
γένος — ποιήσασθαι (10) *om.* V   αὐτοῦ] *Ermerins*, ἑωυτέου M R, ὡυτέου U   ἀδελφοῖς U
ἀποκρινέειν U, *sed corr.*   8 *Supra* ξυγγραφῆς *scr.* συμφωνίας U, *m. rec.* R   8-9 *Supra*
παραγγελίης *scr.* παρακλῆ *m. rec.* R, παρακλήσεως U   10 τοῖσι] *in Mg. transiens* U
11 *supra* συγγεγραμμένοις *scr.* συμφωνίαν δοῦσι R   τε] *euan.* V   ὡρκιζομένοις M, *sed corr.*
13 *Supra* δηλήσει *scr.* βλάβῃ U   14 *supra* ὑφηγήσομαι *scr.* ὑποβαλῶ *m. rec.,* *mg.* ὑπο-
θήσομαι συμβουλεύσω R   15 φθόριον δώσω πεσσόν R U   16 ἐμόν] τὸν ἐμὸν R U   ἐμήν]
τὴν ἐμήν R U   17 *post* δὲ *lac. statuit Diels*   ἀνδράσιν] M, ἀνδράσι V R U   18 πρήξεος
V   19 ἐς] V, εἰς M R U   καμνόντων] κα- *in ras.* U   21 ἀνδρείων] V M², ἀνδρίων M,
ἀνδρώων R U   22 pr. ἢ *om.* V   θεραπηίης V   23 ἐκκαλέεσθαι U   24 τὰ τοιαῦτα εἶναι V
25 ποιέοντι] -εο- *in ras mai.* U   26 εἰς M R U   *In fine:* ὅρκος M V

I **swear** by Apollo Physician and Asclepius and Hygieia **and** Panaceia and all the gods and goddesses, making them my witnesses, that I will fulfil according to my ability and judgment this oath **and** this covenant:

To hold him who has taught me this art as equal to my parents and to live my life in partnership with him, and if he is in need of money to give him a share of mine, and to regard his offspring as equal to my brothers in male lineage and to teach them this art—if they desire to learn it—without fee and covenant; to give a share of precepts and oral instruction and all the other learning to my sons and to the sons of him who has instructed me and to pupils who have signed the covenant and have taken an oath according to the medical law, but to no one else.

I will apply dietetic measures for the benefit of the sick according to my ability and judgment; I will keep them from harm and injustice.

I will neither give a deadly drug to anybody if asked for it, nor will I make a suggestion to this effect. Similarly I will not give to a woman an abortive remedy. In purity and holiness I will guard my life and my art.

I will not use the knife, not even on sufferers from stone, but will withdraw in favor of such men as are engaged in this work.

Whatever houses I may visit, I will come for the benefit of the sick, remaining free of all intentional injustice, of all mischief and in particular of sexual relations with both female and male persons, be they free or slaves.

What I may see or hear in the course of the treatment or even outside of the treatment in regard to the life of men, which on no account one must spread abroad, I will keep to myself holding such things shameful to be spoken about.

If I fulfil this oath and do not violate it, may it be granted to me to enjoy life and art, being honored with fame among all men for all time to come; if I transgress it and swear falsely, may the opposite of all this be my lot.

The Hippocratic Oath clearly falls into two parts. The first speci-
fies the duties of the pupil towards his teacher and his teacher's
family and the pupil's obligations in transmitting medical knowledge.[1]
The second gives a number of rules to be observed in the treatment
of diseases, a short summary of medical ethics as it were.[2] Most
scholars consider these two sections to be only superficially connected
or at least determined by different moral standards.[3] Be this as it
may, the two parts certainly diverge in their subject matter, and,
for the purpose of analyzing their content, it is advantageous first to
discuss them separately and then to ask how they are related to each
other. Again for the sake of convenience, I shall deal with the so-
called ethical code first, the main question being whether the historical
setting in which these rules of conduct were conceived can be ferreted
out.

Modern interpreters are wont to see in the ethical provisions of
the Oath the expression of certain general principles the recognition
of which is demanded by human decency or by the responsibilities
inherent in the physician's art. In this sense timeless validity is
usually attributed to the moral law here established.[4] At best such
an evaluation is qualified by the admission that the Oath represents
only the ancient ideal of the physician. Justice is enjoined upon him,
it is said, in contrast to charity that motivates the Christian doctor,
and in contrast to duty towards the community that determines the
doctor of today.[5] Even if such characterizations were correct, it

[1] Cf. above, pp. 2, 5-11.   [2] Cf. above, pp. 2, 12-24.
[3] Cf. e. g. W. H. S. Jones, *The Doctor's Oath*, 1924, p. 56; K. Deichgräber, Die
ärztliche Standesethik des hippokratischen Eides, *Quellen u. Studien z. Geschichte
d. Naturwissenschaften u. d. Medizin*, III, 1932, p. 34. Cf. also below, p. 50.
[4] Cf. e. g. Jones, *op. cit.*, p. 46: " Custom and convenience, to say nothing of the
human conscience, would sooner or later lay down most of the rules of conduct
comprised in *Oath* . . ."; cf. also p. 50: " . . . the appeal to his (*sc.* the Greek
doctor's) better feelings." Cf. also O. Körner, *Der Eid des Hippokrates*, 1921,
p. 20: " Alle diese Gelöbnisse dienen allein dem Wohle der Kranken und keinen
Sonderinteressen der Ärzte. Erschöpfend umfassen sie in grossen Zügen, was der
Arzt dem Kranken schuldet."
[5] Cf. Deichgräber, *op. cit.*, pp. 38 ff.; esp. pp. 41 ff. (" Die Idee des δίκαιος ἰατρός
ist in den Bestimmungen des Eides Gestalt geworden, wenn man so will, die Idee
des apollinischen Arztes " [p. 42]).

would not be superfluous to ask when and where this supposedly general attitude towards medicine and its tasks was codified. Besides, it is only by uncovering the specific ethical agents which brought about this formulation that the origin of the Oath can be ascertained.

Unfortunately, most of the statements contained in the document are worded in rather general terms; they are vague in their commending of justice, of purity and holiness, concepts which in themselves do not imply any distinct meaning but may be understood in various ways. Yet there are two stipulations that have a more definite character and seem to point to the basic beliefs underlying the whole program which is here evolved: the rules concerning the application of poison and of abortive remedies. Their interpretation should therefore provide a clue for a historical identification of the views embodied in the Oath of Hippocrates.

I

THE ETHICAL CODE

A

Rules concerning Poison and Abortion

" I will neither give a deadly drug to anybody if asked for it, nor will I make a suggestion to this effect. Similarly I will not give to a woman an abortive remedy. In purity and holiness I will guard my life and my art " — such is the vow made.[1] It concerns the physician not so much in his capacity as the healer of diseases but rather in that of the pharmacist who is in possession of the drugs which he prescribes. Poison is a drug and so is the pessary.[2] The physician agrees not to deliver either one to his patient. The term used in both instances is the same; just as he will not *give* the pessary to a woman who comes to seek his help, he will not *give* poison to anyone who is under his care.[3]

Why regulations concerning cases of abortion are introduced into the document is immediately understandable. Under ancient conditions the physician was often presented with the problem as to whether he should give an abortive remedy.[4] But what about the physician's supplying poison? Did he so frequently have occasion to

[1] Cf. above, pp. 2, 14-16.

[2] E. Littré, *Œuvres complètes d'Hippocrate*, IV, 1844, pp. 622 ff., has shown that this clause presupposes a state of affairs in which the physician was his own apothecary. This he was even in those centuries in which pharmacies existed, cf. *e. g.* Galen, *Opera*, ed. C. G. Kühn, XIV, 1827, pp. 5 ff. For the pessary, a " Stäbchen . . . mit bestimmten φάρμακα bestrichen," cf. Deichgräber, *op. cit.*, n. 10.

[3] As far as I am aware, Littré was the first to suggest another meaning of the sentence in question. He says, *op. cit.*, IV, p. 630, n. 12, in commenting on δώσω— the word I have translated by *give*—: " Les traducteurs rendent δώσω par *propinabo* (*sc.* in the first stipulation) ; mais δώσω, qui, un peu plus bas (*sc.* in the second instance), est joint à πεσσός, et qui là ne peut se rendre par *administrer*, montre que dans les deux cas il s'agit d'une substance malfaisante remise à des tiers. . . ." Littré seems to have believed that no physician could possibly give a pessary to his patient directly. But as C. Daremberg, *Œuvres choisis d'Hippocrate*[2], 1855, p. 9, later pointed out, ancient physicians did do so, and it is in connection with the Hippocratic Oath that it was discussed whether this was right; cf. below, pp. 11 f. Littré's reasoning for his interpretation then is not valid.

[4] For abortion as a general practice in antiquity, cf. below, p. 10.

17

give poison that it seemed worth while to ordain what he should do in such instances? What exactly is the situation referred to in the Oath?

All modern interpreters assume that the interdiction of the supplying of poisons means that the physician is charged not to assist his patient in a suicide which he might contemplate. Some interpreters claim that here the physician is also, or even primarily, asked to refrain from any criminal attempt on his patient's life. Cases of poisoning, they say, were very frequent in antiquity; the law, though of course it threatened punishment for murder, was of little avail because the lack of proper scientific methods made it impossible to ascertain whether poison had been administered or not. As a means of strengthening civil jurisdiction, therefore, a clause was introduced into the ancient medical code which today would be entirely out of place.[5] I shall not argue that the Greeks could hardly have been aware of that inability to cope with the situation under discussion which resulted from their ignorance of *post-mortem* examinations and modern chemistry. As a matter of fact they were convinced that they were quite capable of detecting such a crime as poisoning and the criminal who had perpetrated it.[6] More important, if the prohibition were instigated by the wish of society to defend itself against a pernicious assault, then the rules given would be concerned not with the doctor's attitude towards his patient but towards a third party. For the patient himself certainly would not ask his doctor for the poison with which he is to be murdered, and yet the physician vows not to give poison when asked to do so. There is no evidence, however, that the Oath refers to anybody except patient and physi-

---

[5] Cf. Littré, *op. cit.*, IV, pp. 622 ff.; Deichgräber, *op. cit.*, p. 36 (Deichgräber apparently accepts Littré's conception of the motive as well as his explanation). It is often overlooked that Littré admits the probability that suicide is also referred to here, but cf. *op. cit.*, IV, p. 630, n. 12. Jones, *op. cit.*, p. 50, is the only one who seems to exclude the latter possibility.

[6] Cf. L. Lewin, *Die Gifte in der Weltgeschichte,* 1920, pp. 37 ff., where ancient methods of determining cases of poisoning are discussed. Besides, torture of those who were suspected was an excellent substitute for scientific inquiry into the case, cf. Apuleius, *Metamorphoses,* X, 10. Note moreover the harshness of Plato, *Laws,* XI, 932 e ff., in dealing with such a crime, especially when committed by a doctor. As understood by most interpreters the stipulation of the *Oath* would be a useless duplication of the existing laws.

cian.[7] The words in question, then, can mean only that the doctor promises not to supply his patient with poison if asked by him to do so nor to suggest that he take it. It is the prevention of suicide, not of murder, that is here implied.[8]

But was suicide an instance to be reckoned with in medical practice? Could the doctor ever advise such an act to his patient? In antiquity this was indeed the case. If the sick felt that their pains had become intolerable, if no help could be expected, they often put an end to their own lives. This fact is repeatedly attested and not only in general terms; even the diseases are specified which in the opinion of the ancients gave justification for a voluntary death.[9]

[7] Cf. above, p. 6, n. 3. Littré is well aware of the fact that his interpretation necessitates a reference to a third person (*op. cit.*, IV, p. 623-24); cf. also J. E. Pétrequin, *Chirurgie d'Hippocrate*, I, 1877, p. 185. Deichgräber, *loc. cit.*, and Jones, *loc. cit.*, do not discuss at all the problem as to whom this stipulation refers. Nor have the modern interpreters pondered over the difficulty that on their assumption, according to which the clause concerns suicide as well as murder, the statement is logically incoherent; for in one instance the patient would be referred to, in the other somebody outside the physician's practice.

[8] Cf. Daremberg, *op. cit.*, p. 9: "... l'ensemble de la phrase ne me laisse aucun doute sur cette interprétation." The old Latin and Arabic translations of the *Oath* reproduced by Jones, *op. cit.*, p. 35; p. 31, seem to presuppose the same meaning. (It is hardly necessary to add that in regard to the issue at stake one cannot possibly draw any conclusion from an undated pharmacological poem whose dependence on the Hippocratic *Oath* cannot be proved, as Deichgräber himself admits, *op. cit.*, p. 36, n. 33.) Most important: Scribonius Largus urges that the physician should not murder anyone, not even his enemy (p. 2, l. 19 ff. Helmreich). In confirmation of such a postulate he quotes the Hippocratic *Oath* in the following way: "Hippocrates, conditor nostrae professionis, initia disciplinae ab iureiurando tradidit, in quo sanctum est, ne praegnati quidem medicamentum, quo conceptum excutitur, aut detur aut demonstretur a quoquam medico, longe praeformans animos discentium ad humanitatem. qui enim nefas existimaverit spem dubiam hominis laedere, quanto scelestius perfecto iam nocere iudicabit" (p. 2, l. 27–p. 3, l. 2)? It would be meaningless for Scribonius to argue in such a complicated and indirect manner, if the *Oath* outlined a criminal assault *expressis verbis*.

[9] Cf. *e. g.* Aristotle, *E. E.*, 1229 b 39: "... οὔτ' εἰ φεύγοντες τὸ πονεῖν, ὅπερ πολλοὶ ποιοῦσιν, οὐδὲ τῶν τοιούτων οὐδεὶς ἀνδρεῖος, καθάπερ καὶ Ἀγάθων φησί· 'φαῦλοι βροτῶν γὰρ τοῦ πονεῖν ἡσσώμενοι/θανεῖν ἐρῶσιν.' ὥσπερ καὶ τὸν Χείρωνα μυθολογοῦσιν οἱ ποιηταὶ διὰ τὴν ἀπὸ τοῦ ἕλκους ὀδύνην εὔξασθαι ἀποθανεῖν ἀθάνατον ὄντα. The reference to Chiron and his disease makes it certain that the term τὸ πονεῖν means "to suffer bodily pains," cf. also below pp. 14 f. Cf. also Pliny, *Nat. Hist.*, XX, 199: "Sic scimus interemptum P. Licini Caecinae praetorii viri patrem in Hispania Bavili, cum valetudo inpetibilis odium vitae fecisset; item plerosque alios." For the diseases in question cf. Pliny, *Nat. Hist.*, XXV, 23: "Qui (*sc.* morbi) gravis-

Moreover, the taking of poison was the most usual means of committing suicide, and the patient was likely to demand the poison from
his physician who was in possession of deadly drugs and knew those
which brought about an easy and painless end.[10] On the other hand,
such a resolution naturally was not taken without due deliberation,
except perhaps in a few cases of great distress or mental strain.
The sick wished to be sure that further treatment would be of no
avail, and to render this verdict was the physician's task. The
patient, therefore, consulted with him, or urged his friends to speak
to the doctor. If the latter, in such a consultation, confirmed the
seriousness or hopelessness of the case, he suggested directly or
indirectly that the patient commit suicide.[11]

Of course, I do not mean to claim that everybody whose illness
had become desperate thought of ending his own life. Even if human
aid was no longer effectual, recourse to the gods was still possible,
and men did seek succor in the sanctuaries; even if the pain was

simi ex his sint, discernere stultitiae prope videri possit, cum suus cuique ac praesens
quisque atrocissimus videatur. et de hoc tamen iudicavere aevi experimenta,
asperrimi cruciatus esse calculorum a stillicidio vesicae, proximum stomachi, tertium
eorum, quae in capite doleant, non ob alios fere morte conscita."

[10] For poison commonly used in suicide, cf. Lewin, *op. cit.*, p. 139; p. 65. For
instances where poison is demanded from the physician, cf. *e. g. Scriptores Historiae
Augustae, Vita Hadriani*, 24, 13; Tacitus, *Annals*, XV, 64; Apuleius, *Metamorphoses*, X, 9. Even Theophrastus, *Hist. Plant.*, IX, 16, 8, speaks of men who
invented especially efficacious and painless poisons for suicide; since he says that
these people were also versed in all other branches of medicine it is not necessary
to understand with Littré, *op. cit.*, IV, p. 622, that they were merely vendors of
drugs. They may just as well have been physicians.

[11] Cf. Pliny, *Epistulae*, I, xxii, 7 ff.: "Mirareris, si interesses, qua patientia
hanc ipsam valitudinem toleret, ut dolori resistat, ut sitim differat, ut incredibilem
febrium ardorem inmotus opertusque transmittat. nuper me paucosque mecum quos
maxime diligit advocavit rogavitque ut medicos consuleremus de summa valitudinis,
ut, si esset insuperabilis, sponte exiret e vita, si tantum difficilis et longa, resisteret
maneretque: dandum enim precibus uxoris, dandum filiae lacrimis, dandum etiam
nobis amicis ne spes nostras, si modo non essent inanes, voluntaria morte desereret.
id ego arduum in primis et praecipua laude dignum puto. nam impetu quodam et
instinctu procurrere ad mortem commune cum multis, deliberare vero et causas
eius expendere, utque suaserit ratio, vitae mortisque consilium vel suscipere vel
ponere ingentis est animi. et medici quidem secunda nobis pollicentur." This
passage, the importance of which is rightly stressed by A. W. Mair, *Encyclopaedia
of Religion and Ethics, s.v.* suicide, XII, pp. 31-32, certainly is tinged with Stoic
feeling. But there is no reason to doubt that earlier generations were as cautious
and responsible in making their decisions as were the Romans.

excruciating and relief was to be had neither from human nor from divine physicians, men could, and did go on living in spite of all their suffering.[12] Yet the fact remains that throughout antiquity many people preferred voluntary death to endless agony. This form of "euthanasia" was an everyday reality.[13] Consequently it is quite understandable that the Oath deals with the attitude which the physician should take in regard to the possible suicide of his patient. From a practical point of view it was no less important to tell the ancient doctor what to do when faced with such a situation than it was to advise him about cases of abortion.[14]

The relevance of the "pharmacological rules" for a medical oath having been established, one may now ask why the Oath forbids the physician to assist in suicide or in abortion. Apparently these prohibitions did not echo the general feeling of the public. Suicide was not censured in antiquity.[15] Abortion was practiced in Greek times no less than in the Roman era, and it was resorted to without scruple. Small wonder! In a world in which it was held justifiable to expose children immediately after birth, it would hardly seem objectionable to destroy the embryo.[16] Why then should the physician not give a helping hand to those of his patients who wanted to end their own lives or to those who did not wish to have offspring?

[12] For the seeking of religious help in hopeless cases, cf. L. Edelstein, Greek Medicine in its Relation to Religion and Magic, *Bulletin of the History of Medicine,* V, 1937, pp. 238 ff. For instances of rejection of suicide cf. below p. 14.

[13] Strangely enough none of the interpreters of the *Oath* has pointed to this fact. Deichgräber, the only one to mention the problem of euthanasia, *op. cit.,* p. 36, even denies that it had any importance for the ancients. The writers on suicide, on the other hand, though they refer to voluntary death on account of illness, do not mention the *Oath,* cf. *e. g.* R. Hirzel, Der Selbstmord, *Archiv f. Religionswissenschaft,* XI, 1908, pp. 75 ff.; 243 ff.; 417 ff.; *E. R. E., s. v.* suicide, XII, pp. 26 b ff.

[14] In my opinion it is the neglect of the question of euthanasia that gave currency to the belief that in the *Oath* not only suicide but also manslaughter are forbidden (cf. Deichgräber, *op. cit.,* p. 36: "*Da* das Euthanasieproblem, an das der moderne Mensch denken könnte, in der Antike unbekannt ist, *kann* es sich hier *nur* um den Giftmord und als einen besonderen Fall, den durch Gift herbeigeführten Selbstmord sowie um die Beihilfe zu beidem handeln." [Italics mine.]).

[15] Cf. above, pp. 8 ff., and below, pp. 13 ff.

[16] Cf. in general A. E. Crawley, *E. R. E., s. v.* foeticide, VI, pp. 54 b ff. For the parental power over children of which exposure after birth and destruction of the embryo are the consequences, cf. Wilamowitz, *Staat u. Gesellschaft der Griechen, Die Kultur der Gegenwart,* II, IV, 1², 1923, p. 36.

For a moment one might harbor the idea that the interdiction of poison and of abortive remedies was simply the outgrowth of medical ethics. After all, medicine is the art of healing, of preserving life. Should the physician assist in bringing about death?[17] I do not propose to discuss this issue in general terms. It suffices here to state that in antiquity many physicians actually gave their patients the poison for which they were asked. Apparently *qua* physicians they felt no compunction about doing so.[18] Although in later centuries some refused to participate in an attempt on men's lives, because, as they said, it was unfitting for their sect "to be responsible for anyone's death or destruction,"[19] it is not reported that they ever employed the same reasoning in cases of self-murder.[20] As for abortions, many physicians prescribed and gave abortive remedies. Medical writings of all periods mention the means for the destruction of the embryo and the occasions where they are to be employed.[21]

[17] It is permissible to say that this is the most commonly accepted explanation of the rules, cf. *e. g.* Körner, *op. cit.*, p. 12: "Seine· (*sc.* the physician's) höchste Aufgabe ist Heilen, und sein schlimmstes Verbrechen wäre also Töten oder Vorschubleisten zu Mord, Selbstmord und Kindesabtreibung."

[18] Cf. *e. g.* Tacitus, *Annals*, XV, 64; cf. also Apuleius, *Metamorphoses*, X, 9, where the physician is approached for poison by a slave, and since he becomes suspicious, gives him a harmless drug only. But he is not astonished about the demand made, nor does he refuse it on general grounds. This can easily be explained, for those suffering from incurable diseases were doomed to die anyhow; the only issue was, whether they should be condemned to an unnecessarily protracted suffering. Moreover, death seemed desirable to the sick, and even the Hippocratic maxim "to help, or at least not to do harm" (*Epidemiae*, I, 11, *Hippocratis Opera*, ed. H. Kuehlewein, I, 1894, p. 190) could not restrain the physician when he was face to face with those who believed that they would be helped rather than harmed by annihilation.

[19] Cf. Apuleius, *Metamorphoses*, X, 11; note that these are the words of the same physician who before (X, 9, cf. preceding note) did not reject the giving of poison to a suicide.

[20] This assertion, of course, is not refuted by the fact that in Oxyrhynchus Papyrus 437 (III, 77, 3rd century A. D.) the giving of poison is rejected as incompatible with the art by a quotation from the *Oath*; cf. Deichgräber, *op. cit.*, n. 42. Through this document the interdiction of poison became part of medical ethics; that does not mean, however, that originally it was the outgrowth of medical considerations.

[21] Cf. R. Hähnel, Der künstliche Abortus im Altertum, *Archiv f. Geschichte d. Medizin*, XXIX, 1937, pp. 224 ff. J. Ilberg, Zur gynäkologischen Ethik der Griechen, *Archiv f. Religionswissenschaft*, XIII, 1910, pp. 12 ff., holds that the Greek physicians did not apply abortive remedies; but this thesis is untenable in

In later centuries some physicians rejected abortion under all circumstances; they supported their decision with a reference to the prohibition in the Hippocratic Oath and added that it was the duty of the doctor to preserve the products of nature. Soranus, the greatest of the ancient gynaecologists, had little patience with these colleagues of his. In agreement with many other physicians he contended that it was necessary to think of the life of the mother first, and he resorted to abortion whenever it seemed necessary, much as he deprecated it if performed for no other reason than the wish to preserve beauty or to hide the consequences of adultery.[22] In short, the strict attitude upheld by the Oath was not uncontested even from the medical point of view. In antiquity it was not generally considered a violation of medical ethics to do what the Oath forbade. An ancient doctor who accepted the rules laid down by "Hippocrates" was by no means in agreement with the opinion of all his fellow physicians; on the contrary, he adhered to a dogma which was much stricter than that embraced by many, if not by most of his colleagues. Simple reflection on the duties of the physician, on the task of medicine alone, under these circumstances, can hardly have led to the formulation and adoption of the "pharmacological stipulations."

In my opinion, the Oath itself points to other, more fundamental considerations that must have been instrumental in outlining the prohibitions under discussion. For the physician, when forswearing the use of poison and of abortive remedies, adds: "In purity and in holiness I will guard my life and my art."[23] It might be possible to construe purity as a quality insisted upon by the craftsman who is conscious of the obligations of his art. The demand for holiness,

---

view of the facts now conveniently surveyed by R. Hähnel, *loc. cit.*; cf. also Deichgräber, *op. cit.*, n. 37; P. Diepgen, *Die Frauenheilkunde der Alten Welt*, 1937, p. 301.

[22] Cf. Soranus, ed. J. Ilberg, *C. M. G.*, IV, 1927, p. 45, 8 ff. Incidentally the passage in Soranus proves that the rejection of abortion as advocated in the *Oath* is laid down without qualification (contrary to the assumption made by F. J. Dölger, *Antike u. Christentum*, IV, 1934, p. 8).

[23] Cf. above, pp. 2, 15-16. It is interesting to note that Körner who sees in these stipulations the expression of medical ethics (cf. above p. 4, n. 4) translates ἁγνῶς δὲ καὶ ὁσίως with "ohne Fehl und unbescholten" (*op. cit.*, p. 5), a translation which in no way does justice to the meaning of the words. All other interpreters in their rendering rightly reflect the notions of holiness and purity.

however, can hardly be understood as resulting from practical thinking or technical responsibility. Holiness belongs to another realm of
values and is indicative of standards of a different, a more elevated
character.

Yet certainly not such purity and holiness are meant as might
accrue to men from obedience to civil law or common religion.
Ancient jurisdiction did not discriminate against suicide; it did not
attach any disgrace to it, provided that there was sufficient reason for
such an act. And self-murder as a relief from illness was regarded
as justifiable, so much so that in some states it was an institution
duly legalized by the authorities.[24] Nor did Greek or Roman law
protect the unborn child. If, in certain cities, abortion was prose-
cuted, it was because the father's right to his offspring had been
violated by the mother's action.[25] Ancient religion did not proscribe
suicide. It did not know of any eternal punishment for those who
voluntarily ended their lives.[26] Likewise it remained indifferent to

[24] Cf. Hirzel, *op. cit.*, pp. 264 ff.; *E. R. E., loc. cit.* The special regulations for
the burial of a suicide in Athens (Aristotle, *N. E.*, 1138 a 9 ff.) have been rightly
explained by Hirzel, *ibid.*, p. 264; 271, as directed against those who committed
suicide when still able to bear arms; the same is true of Rome (*ibid.*, p. 266).
This fact has been overlooked by Deichgräber, *op. cit.*, p. 36, n. 35. Note moreover
that not even these people were deprived of burial. For city regulations concerning
the delivery of poisons to suicides, cf. *E. R. E., loc. cit.*, pp. 28 ff. Temporary
legislation against suicide (cf. Hirzel, *ibid.*, p. 275) indicative of the frequency of
such occurrences was never directed against suicide on account of illness. Thebes
was the only city where, according to late evidence, suicide was forbidden (cf.
Hirzel, *ibid.*, p. 268); for the explanation of this fact, cf. below, p. 18, n. 44.

[25] For lawsuits based on the father's claim to his children, cf. *e. g.* Lysias, *Fr.*
X, p. 333 [Thalheim], and Cicero, *Pro Cluentio*, XI, 32 (for more material,
especially for the Roman centuries, cf. Dölger, *op. cit.*, pp. 37 ff.). Even Dölger,
ibid., p. 13, admits that in these cases the wish to protect the life of the embryo is
not involved, though he is inclined to believe that the Greeks at least knew of laws
against abortion. But the so-called laws of Solon and Lycurgus, quoted only in a
Ps. Galenic book of unknown date and origin (*An animal sit id quod in utero est*
XIX, p. 179 K.; cf. K. Kalbfleisch, *Abh. Berl. Akad.*, 1895, p. 11, n. 1), to which
Dölger refers, *ibid.*, pp. 10 ff. (cf. also W. Aly, *R. E.*, III A, p. 963), cannot prove
this thesis. They are late inventions, determined by the thought of the Christian
era. Dölger himself, *ibid.*, p. 14, admits such a falsification in the case of Musonius,
Fr. XVa, p. 77H, the only other passage which in general terms speaks of laws
against abortion.

[26] This has been shown conclusively by Hirzel, *op. cit.*, pp. 76 ff.; p. 276; on
later changes under the influence of Jewish-Christian ideas, cf. *ibid.*, p. 277, and
below, p. 17, n. 40. In *E. R. E.*, XII, pp. 30 b ff., after an elaborate proof that

foeticide. Its tenets did not include the dogma of an immortal soul for which men must render account to their creator.[27] Law and religion then left the physician free to do whatever seemed best to him.

From all these considerations it follows that a specific philosophical conviction must have dictated the rules laid down in the Oath. Is it possible to determine this particular philosophy? To take the problem of suicide first: Platonists, Cynics and Stoics can be eliminated at once. They held suicide permissible for the diseased. Some of these philosophers even extolled such an act as the greatest triumph of men over fate.[28] Aristotle, on the other hand, claimed that it was cowardly to give in to bodily pain, and Epicurus admonished men not to be subdued by illness.[29] But does that mean that the Oath is determined by Aristotelian or Epicurean ideas? I shall not insist that it is hard to imagine a physician resisting the adjurations of his patients if he has nothing but Aristotle's or Epicurus' exhortations to courage to quote to them and to himself. It is more important to stress the fact that the Aristotelian and Epicurean opposition to suicide did not involve moral censure. If men decided to take their lives, they were within their rights as sovereign masters of themselves. The Aristotelian and Epicurean schools condoned suicide. Later on the Aristotelians even gave up their leader's teaching, and under the onslaught of the Stoic attack withdrew their disapproval

according to the evidence available suicide was not stigmatized by ancient religious dogma, it is nevertheless assumed that popular religious feeling opposed it. This is due to a non-permissible identification of popular religion with the tenets of one particular sect (the Orphics), cf. below p. 15, n. 33.

[27] Cf. Dölger, *op. cit.*, pp. 15 ff. Here again as in the case of laws against abortion the first indication of its rejection on religious grounds is found in the 1st century A. D. Cf. O. Weinreich, Stiftung u. Kultsatzungen eines Privatheiligtums in Philadelphia in Lydien, *S. B. Heidelb.*, 1919.

[28] For Plato, cf. *Laws*, IX, 873c, and Hirzel, *op. cit.*, p. 279, n. 1; for the Cynics, cf. Hirzel, *ibid.*, pp. 279-80; for the Stoics, cf. especially *Stoicorum Veterum Fragmenta*, ed. H. v. Arnim, III, 1923, pp. 187 ff., and in general E. Benz, Das Todesproblem in der stoischen Philosophie, *Tübinger Beiträge z. Altertumswissenschaft*, VII, 1929, pp. 54 ff. The Cyrenaics too permitted suicide, cf. Hirzel, *op. cit.*, p. 422.

[29] For Aristotle, cf. *N. E.*, 1116 a 12 ff.; for Epicurus, cf. *Fr.* 138 [Usener]. It is debatable whether Epicurus opposed suicide at all, cf. Diogenes Laertius, X, 119, and A. Kochalsky, *Das Leben u. die Lehre des Epikur*, 1914, n. 111; in general Hirzel, *op. cit.*, p. 422; p. 282.

of self-murder.[30] At any rate, Aristotelianism and Epicureanism do not explain a rejection of suicide which apparently is based on a moral creed and a belief in the divine.

Pythagoreanism, then, remains the only philosophical dogma that can possibly account for the attitude advocated in the Hippocratic Oath. For indeed among all Greek thinkers the Pythagoreans alone outlawed suicide and did so without qualification. The Platonic Socrates can adduce no other witness than the Pythagorean Philolaus for the view that men, whatever their fate, are not allowed to take their own lives. And even in later centuries the Pythagorean school is the only one represented as absolutely opposed to suicide.[31] Moreover, for the Pythagorean, suicide was a sin against god who had allocated to man his position in life as a post to be held and to be defended. Punishment threatened those who did not obey the divine command to live; it was considered neither lawful nor holy to seek release, "to bestow this blessing upon oneself." [32] Any physician who accepts such a dogma naturally must abstain from assisting in suicide or even from suggesting it. Otherwise he would be guilty of a crime, he no less than his patient, and in this moral and religious conviction the doctor can well find the courage to remain deaf to his patient's insistence, to his sufferings, and even to the clamor of the world which disagrees almost unanimously with the stand taken by him. It seems safe to state this much: the fact that in the Hippocratic Oath the physician is enjoined to refrain from aiding or advising suicide points to an influence of Pythagorean doctrines.[33]

[30] Cf. in general Hirzel, op. cit., p. 422. For the later Aristotelians, cf. R. Walzer, Magna Moralia und aristotelische Ethik, Neue Philologische Untersuchungen, VII, 1929, p. 192.·

[31] Cf. Phaedo, 61 d ff., and Hirzel, op. cit., p. 278, who is right in saying that this concept is so emphatically formulated because it is expressed here for the first time. Note that the stipulation is laid down even for those οἷς βέλτιον τεθνάναι ἢ ζῆν (62a). For later Pythagoreans, cf. Athenaeus, IV, 157 C (Euxitheus).

[32] Cf. Phaedo, 61 d: τὸ μὴ θεμιτὸν εἶναι ἑαυτὸν βιάζεσθαι . . . 62 a: μὴ ὅσιον αὐτοὺς ἑαυτοὺς εὖ ποιεῖν . . . 62 b: ὁ μὲν οὖν ἐν ἀπορρήτοις λεγόμενος περὶ αὐτῶν λόγος, ὡς ἔν τινι φρουρᾷ ἐσμεν οἱ ἄνθρωποι καὶ οὐ δεῖ δὴ ἑαυτὸν ἐκ ταύτης λύειν οὐδ' ἀποδιδράσκειν . . .

[33] I say Pythagorean doctrines. How far this dogma is influenced by Orphism or even dependent upon it, is not for me to decide. J. Burnet, E. R. E., s. v. Pythagoras and Pythagoreanism, X, 526 a-b, holds that Philolaus' view as represented by Plato is different from Orphic beliefs and characterizes as Pythagorean

In my opinion the same can be asserted of the rule forbidding abortion and rejecting it without qualification. Most of the Greek philosophers even commended abortion. For Plato, foeticide is one of the regular institutions of the ideal state. Whenever the parents are beyond that age which he thinks best for the begetting of children, the embryo should be destroyed.[34] Aristotle reckons abortion the best procedure to keep the population within the limits which he considers essential for a well-ordered community.[35]

To be sure, one limitation apparently is recognized by ancient philosophers. Aristotle advocates that abortion should be performed before the foetus has attained animal life; after that time he no longer considers abortion compatible with holiness.[36] But such a restriction is based on the biological notion that the embryo from a certain time on partakes in animal life. Other philosophers and scientists, in fact most of them, including the Platonists and the Stoics, denied that such was the case. Animation, they thought, began at the moment of birth. Therefore, in their opinion, abortion must have been permissible throughout pregnancy.[37]

It was different with the Pythagoreans. They held that the embryo was an animate being from the moment of conception. That they did so is expressly attested by a writer of the 3rd century A. D.[38]

the "higher side" of this teaching, that is, its moral implications. But cf. also I. M. Linforth, *The Arts of Orpheus*, 1941, esp. pp. 168 ff. At any rate, one cannot claim on the basis of the words ἐν ἀπορρήτοις which Plato uses that the rejection of suicide is Orphic rather than Pythagorean (contrary to S. Reinach, Ἄωροι βιαιοθάνατοι, *Archiv f. Religionswissenschaft*, IX, 1906, p. 318). For the present purpose the expression "Pythagorean doctrines" seems justified by the fact that the teaching under discussion is directly ascribed to the Pythagoreans by Plato and other writers; cf. below, pp. 18 f.

[34] Cf. *Republic*, V, 461 c; *Laws*, V, 740 d, and for the interpretation of the latter passage, Diepgen, *op. cit.*, p. 297.

[35] Cf. Aristotle, *Politics*, VII, 1335 b 20 ff.

[36] Cf. Aristotle, *Politics*, VII, 1335 b 25: τὸ γὰρ ὅσιον καὶ τὸ μὴ διωρισμένον τῇ αἰσθήσει καὶ τῷ ζῆν ἔσται. Cf. also Dölger, *op. cit.*, pp. 7 ff.

[37] Cf. *Stoicorum Veterum Fragmenta*, II, p. 213 [Arnim], and also Herophilus (H. Diels, *Doxographi Graeci*, 1929, V, 15, p. 426). Concerning the Platonists and Neo-Platonists who denied animation of the embryo because the soul enters the body from without, cf. Kalbfleisch, *op. cit.*, pp. 5 ff.

[38] Cf. Ps. Galen, Πρὸς Γαῦρον περὶ τοῦ πῶς ἐμψυχοῦται τὰ ἔμβρυα, p. 34, 20 [Kalbfleisch]: εἰ δὲ δυνάμει ζῷον ὡς τὸ δεδεγμένον τὴν ἕξιν ἢ μᾶλλον ζῷον ἐνεργείᾳ ἦν τὸ ἔμβρυον, δύσκολον μὲν τὸν καιρὸν ἀφορίσαι τῆς εἰσκρίσεως καὶ πολύ γε τὸ ἀπίθανον ἕξει καὶ πλασματῶδες ὁποῖος ἂν εἶναι ἀφορισθῇ, τοῦ μὲν ὅταν καταβληθῇ τὸ σπέρμα τὸν

The same can be concluded from the Pythagorean system of physiology as it was outlined in the Hellenistic period by Alexander Polyhistor: the germ is a clot of brain containing hot vapors within it, and soul and sensation are supposed to originate from this vapor. Similar views were previously accepted by Philolaus in the 4th century B. C.[39] Consequently, for the Pythagoreans, abortion, whenever practiced, meant destruction of a living being. Granted that the righteousness of abortion depends on whether the embryo is animate or not, the Pythagoreans could not but reject abortion unconditionally.[40]

Furthermore, abortion was irreconcilable with their ethical beliefs no less than with their scientific views. In their ascetic rigorism, in their strictness concerning sexual matters and regarding matrimony in particular, they went farther than any other sect. They banned extramarital relations. Even in matrimony coitus was held justifiable only for the purpose of producing offspring.[41] Besides, children

καιρὸν τοῦτον ἀποδιδόντος ὡς ἂν μηδ' οἵου τε ὄντος ἐν τῇ μήτρᾳ γονίμως κρατηθῆναι μήτι γε ψυχῆς ἔξωθεν τῇ εἰσκρίσει ἑαυτῆς τὴν σύμφυσιν ἀπεργασαμένης—κἀνταῦθα πολὺς ὁ Νουμήνιος καὶ οἱ τὰς Πυθαγόρου ὑπονοίας ἐξηγούμενοι . . . The author of the book is Porphyry, cf. Kalbfleisch, ibid.; p. 25.

[39] Cf. Diogenes Laertius, VIII, 28-9. Kalbfleisch, op. cit., p. 80 ad p. 34, 26 (cf. E. Zeller, Die Philosophie d. Griechen, III, 2³, 1881, pp. 89 f.; p. 96) referred to this passage as a parallel to the Galenic statement. The tradition which Diogenes follows is ascribed to the early Peripatos by Diels (H. Diels–W. Kranz, Die Fragmente d. Vorsokratiker, 1934⁵, 58 B 1a). For the similarity of such views with theories of Philolaus (44 A 27 [Diels-Kranz]), cf. in general M. Wellmann, Hermes, LIV, 1919, pp. 232 ff.

[40] Deichgräber, op. cit., p. 37, n. 38, has stated that opposition to abortion is in line with certain philosophical ideas, without saying, however, which ideas these are. As his only reference he quotes Phocylides, ll. 184-5. But this poem was written by a Hellenistic Jew at the beginning of the Christian era, cf. W. Christ–W. Schmid, Geschichte d. griechischen Literatur, II⁶, 1920, pp. 621 f. Concerning the general importance of the agreement between Pythagorean and Jewish-Christian theories, cf. Dölger, op. cit., p. 23, who refers to Philo and Josephus, cf. also below, pp. 63 f.

[41] Cf. in general 58 D 8, pp. 476, 7 ff.; 477, 7 ff. [Diels-Kranz] (from Aristoxenus), and Zeller, op. cit., III, 1, p. 143, n. 3; cf. ibid. I, 1⁵, p. 462, n. 2. Cf. especially p. 476, 4 [Diels-Kranz]: ὑπελάμβανον δ', ὡς ἔοικεν, ἐκεῖνοι οἱ ἄνδρες περιαιρεῖν μὲν δεῖν τάς τε παρὰ φύσιν γεννήσεις καὶ τὰς μεθ' ὕβρεως γιγνομένας, καταλιμπάνειν δὲ τῶν κατὰ φύσιν τε καὶ μετὰ σωφροσύνης γινομένων τὰς ἐπὶ τεκνοποιίᾳ σώφρονί τε καὶ νομίμῳ γινομένας. It is sometimes claimed that Aristoxenus' report is reminiscent of Platonic ethics, cf. E. Rohde, Kleine Schriften, II, 1901, p. 162. Yet in regard to

to them were more than future members of a community or citizens of a state. It was considered man's duty to beget children so as to leave behind in his own place another worshipper of the gods.[42] With such convictions how could the Pythagoreans ever allow abortive remedies to be applied? How could they fail to condemn practices of this kind, so common among their compatriots?[43]

It stands to reason, then, that the Hippocratic Oath, in its abortion-clause no less than in its prohibition of suicide, echoes Pythagorean doctrines. In no other stratum of Greek opinion were such views held or proposed in the same spirit of uncompromising austerity.[44] When the physician, after having foresworn ever to give poison or abortive remedies, adds: " In purity and holiness I will guard my life and my art," it must be the purity and holiness of the " Pythagorean way of life "[45] to which he dedicates himself.

B

The General Rules of the Ethical Code

The question now arises whether what is true of certain of the ethical clauses of the Hippocratic Oath is true of all of them, in other words, whether the whole medical code is in agreement with Pythagorean philosophy. By this latter term I mean Pythagoreanism as it was understood in the 4th century B. C. It is to this form of the dogma that the rules discussed so far were related, and it seems fair

the matter under discussion Plato's views certainly were more lax than those of the Pythagoreans, cf. *Laws*, VIII, 841 d, and above, p. 16.

[42] Cf. 58 C 4, p. 465, 5 [Diels-Kranz]: . . . ὅτι δεῖ τεκνοποιεῖσθαι ἕνεκα τοῦ καταλιπεῖν ἕτερον ἀνθ' ἑαυτοῦ θεῶν θεραπευτήν; cf. also *ibid.*, p. 464, 22. These statements are considered by Diels to be part of the old Pythagorean *Symbola*. Plato, *Laws*, VI, 773 e; 776 b, agrees with the point of view of the Pythagoreans, much as he deviates from it in other passages.

[43] Reinach, *op. cit.*, p. 321, on the evidence of a very late Orphic fragment, claims that it was the Orphics who favored rejection of abortion. But his argument is no more cogent in this respect than it is in regard to suicide, cf. above, p. 15, n. 33.

[44] It seems worth pointing out that both stipulations of the *Oath* show some affinity with ideas credited especially to Philolaus, cf. above, p. 15; p. 17, n. 39, and below, p. 57. This philosopher lived for some time in Thebes. It is therefore hardly by chance that this city alone in late sources is said to have had laws against suicide, cf. above, p. 13, n. 24. It seems probable that the well-known theory of the famous philosopher was projected into the legislation of Thebes.

[45] Cf. Plato, *Republic*, X, 600 b: . . . Πυθαγόρειον τρόπον . . . τοῦ βίου.

to assume that the rest of the stipulations, if at all influenced by Pythagorean thinking, correspond to the same concept of Pythagoreanism. At any rate, wherever I shall speak of Pythagorean doctrines without qualification, it is neither the teachings of the "historical" Pythagoras, nor those of the later so-called Neo-Pythagoreans which I have in mind, but rather those theories and beliefs which writers of the 4th century B. C., men like Plato, Aristotle and their pupils, attributed to Pythagoras and his followers.[46]

To start, then, with the analysis of that section of the ethical code which deals with the treatment of diseases proper:[47] here mention is made of diet, drugs and cutting. In a more technical language, medicine is viewed as comprising dietetics, pharmacology and surgery. Consequently those matters are discussed which seem most important for the attitude of the physician within these three departments of his art.[48] Now a division of medicine into these branches is not unusual and in itself is not indicative of any particular medical or philosophical school. But, according to Aristoxenus, the Pythagoreans were among those who accepted this particular classification of medicine; moreover, the sequence of the various parts of the

[46] For the very complex Pythagoras problem, cf. e. g. F. Ueberweg- K. Praechter, *Die Philosophie des Altertums*[12], 1926, pp. 61 ff. That the various forms of Pythagoreanism, especially the earliest doctrine and that of the 4th century B. C., must be sharply distinguished admits of no doubt after the studies of E. Frank, *Plato u. d. sogenannten Pythagoreer*, 1923. To him I am also indebted for his advice in many a controversial matter discussed in this paper.

[47] The ethical code can be divided into two parts of which the first (cf. above, p. 2, 12-18) outlines rules for the healing of diseases, whereas the second (cf. above, p. 2, 19-24) regulates the physician's behavior in all matters indirectly connected with the treatment, such as his relations to the patient, to the patient's family, and so forth.

[48] Cf. e. g. Münzer, *Münchener Medizinische Wochenschrift*, 1919, p. 309; Körner, *op. cit.*, p. 7. Concerning poison and abortive remedies as drugs, cf. above, p. 6. The οὐ τεμέω-clause, whatever its meaning (cf. below, pp. 24 ff.), certainly refers to surgical procedure. Deichgräber, *op. cit.*, p. 31, translates διαιτήματα with "Verordnungen" and adds, n. 24: "... eigentlich handelt es sich ... um diätetische Verordnungen." There is no reason for taking the word to mean anything but "diätetische Verordnungen"; moreover, whatever may be understood by this term, the application of drugs cannot be covered by it, cf. below, p. 23. Therefore Körner, *op. cit.*, p. 11, is not right in saying: "... Diät ... es ist also das gesamte Heilverfahren gemeint;" he himself admits that διαιτήματα does not include drugs.

healing art in the Pythagorean doctrine is the same as it is in the Hippocratic Oath, dietetics coming first, pharmacology next, surgery last.[49]

In detail, the physician is asked to use dietetic means to the advantage of his patients as his judgment and capacity permit; moreover he is enjoined to keep them from mischief and injustice.[50] That the doctor's dietetic prescriptions should be given to help the patient is an obvious truth. It is the goal of all good craftsmanship to seek the best for the object with which the craftsman is concerned. Every ancient physician would have subscribed to such a formulation.[51] It suffices to say that the Pythagorean physicians did not feel differently, for this school acknowledged the useful and the advantageous as second among the aims of human endeavor.[52]

But what exactly is meant by the promise to keep the patient from mischief and injustice? Can this really imply, as some scholars have

[49] Littré, op. cit., IV, p. 622, says that such a division is known only since the time of Herophilus, cf. Celsus, I, 1; cf. also below, p. 29. As a matter of fact, it is attributed to the Pythagoreans by Aristoxenus, cf. 58 D 1, p. 467, 5 ff. [Diels-Kranz]. Since this passage is fundamental for the interpretation of Pythagorean medicine, and the most extensive one preserved, I shall give it here in full: τῆς δὲ ἰατρικῆς μάλιστα μὲν ἀποδέχεσθαι τὸ διαιτητικὸν εἶδος καὶ εἶναι ἀκριβεστάτους ἐν τούτῳ· καὶ πειρᾶσθαι πρῶτον μὲν καταμανθάνειν σημεῖα συμμετρίας ποτῶν τε καὶ σίτων καὶ ἀναπαύσεως. ἔπειτα περὶ αὐτῆς τῆς κατασκευῆς τῶν προσφερομένων σχεδὸν πρώτους ἐπιχειρῆσαί τε πραγματεύεσθαι καὶ διορίζειν. ἅψασθαι δὲ [χρὴ] καὶ καταπλασμάτων ἐπὶ πλείω τοὺς Πυθαγορείους τῶν ἔμπροσθεν, τὰ δὲ περὶ τὰς φαρμακείας ἧττον δοκιμάζειν, αὐτῶν δὲ τούτων τοῖς πρὸς τὰς ἑλκώσεις μάλιστα χρῆσθαι, ⟨τὰ δὲ⟩ περὶ τὰς τομάς τε καὶ καύσεις ἥκιστα πάντων ἀποδέχεσθαι.

[50] Cf. above, p. 2, 12-13. Littré, op. cit., IV, p. 631, says: "Je m'abstiendrai de tout mal et de toute injustice;" the same meaning is given by F. Adams, The Genuine Works of Hippocrates, II, 1886, p. 279, and also by Jones, op. cit., p. 9. But εἴρξειν is transitive; it cannot possibly refer to the physician himself, cf. Daremberg, op. cit., p. 8, n. 6, with regard to Littré's translation: "Le text se refuse absolument à ce sens." With Daremberg agree Deichgräber, op. cit., p. 31, and Körner, op. cit., p. 11. The latter quite rightly points out that in Littré's interpretation the words are a mere duplication of what is said later on, cf. below, p. 32.

[51] Cf. e. g. Ps. Hippocrates, Epidemiae, I, 11, quoted above p. 11, n. 18, where the aim of medicine is defined as "to help or not to harm."

[52] For the Pythagoreans, cf. p. 474, 36 ff. [Diels-Kranz] (Aristoxenus). The συμφέρον and ὠφέλιμον were second in rank to the καλόν and εὔσχημον. It is worth noting that in later Pythagorean tradition Pythagoras himself is said to have come into this world for the benefit (εἰς ὠφέλειαν) of mankind, and to have philosophized and acted to this end (ἐπ' ὠφελείᾳ), cf. Iamblichus, De Vita Pythagorica, 30; 162; 222.

suggested, that the physician shall enforce his treatment even against the resistance or indifference of his patient's family?[53] It is true, interference of others may occur and the physician may have to contend with it, but this happens rarely, too seldom indeed to have been considered in the medical code. Moreover, while mischief may be done to the sick by his friends, why should he suffer injustice from those who wish him well?[54] And why should this danger be any greater in regard to the dietetic treatment of diseases for which case alone mention is made of it, than it would be in regard to everything else the physician may prescribe or do? No, it can scarcely be protection from the wrong done by others that the physician vows to give to his patients. But since it can neither be protection from the wrong which he himself may do,[55] one must conclude that he promises to guard his patients against the evil which they may suffer through themselves. That men by nature are liable to inflict upon themselves injustice and mischief, and that this tendency becomes apparent in all matters concerned with their regimen, this is indeed an axiom of Pythagorean dietetics.[56]

The Pythagoreans defined all bodily appetites as propensities of the soul, as a craving for the presence or absence of certain things. Most of these appetites they considered as acquired or created by

[53] Cf. Körner, *op. cit.*, p. 11: "Der Arzt soll es (*sc.* the treatment) auch durchsetzen gegenüber Gleichgültigkeit oder Widerspenstigkeit der Umgebung des Kranken. Nur so kann es verstanden werden, wenn der Schwörende im Anschluss an die Anordnung des Heilverfahrens verspricht, Gefährdung und Schädigung vom Kranken abzuwehren." Daremberg, *op. cit.*, p. 8, n. 6, compares the statement with the Hippocratic ὠφελεῖν ἢ μὴ βλάπτειν (cf. above, p. 20, n. 51), but here it is certainly the physician himself who is supposed not to do any harm, and yet, as Daremberg has shown (cf. above, p. 20, n. 51), this is not what is meant in the *Oath.* The other interpreters are silent about the implications of the words in question.

[54] Körner, *loc. cit.*, very significantly translates δήλησις and ἀδικίη with "Gefährdung und Schädigung," terms which do not bring out the full impact of the Greek words.

[55] Cf. above p. 20, n. 50.

[56] In order to gain a picture of Pythagorean medicine the evidence must be put together bit by bit. Modern literature on the subject is scarce. The outline given by I. Schumacher, *Antike Medizin*, I, 1940, pp. 34 ff., proves unsatisfactory because here the sources are not properly evaluated. Of great importance are the study of the doctrine of κάθαρσις by E. Howald, *Hermes*, LIV, 1919, pp. 203 ff., and the discussion of some of the fragments by A. E. Taylor, *A Commentary on Plato's Timaeus*, 1928, pp. 629 ff.

men themselves, and therefore they thought human desires were to be watched closely and to be scrutinized severely. As a natural process they acknowledged only that the body should take in an appropriate amount of food and should be cleansed again appropriately after it had been filled. To overload oneself with superfluous food and drink was regarded as an acquired inclination of the soul.[57]

But unfortunately all bodily passions have the tendency to increase indefinitely. Of themselves they become "idle, irreverent, harmful and licentious,"[58] as one can readily see in those who are in the position to live according to their wishes. In order to live right from early youth on, one must learn to hold in contempt those things that are "idle and superfluous."[59] It is necessary, therefore, to select the nourishment of the body with great caution, to determine its quality and quantity most carefully, a supreme wisdom entrusted to the physicians.[60]

This is the Pythagorean doctrine concerning the regimen of the healthy. It is clear, I think, that in such a theory bodily and psychic factors are blended in a peculiar way. At the same time there is a moral element involved: unhealthy desire is uncontrolled desire; a decision is to be made between those appetites which ought to be satisfied and those which ought to be disregarded. Moreover, the Pythagorean teaching, in a strange manner, insists on negative instances. Not that alone which one does is important; that which one does not do, or is not allowed to do, carries just as much consequence. Right living is brought about not only, not even primarily, through positive actions, but rather through avoidance of those steps that are dangerous, through the repression of insatiable desires which if left to themselves would cause damage.[61]

The same consideration for body and soul, the same combination

---

[57] Cf. 58 D 8, p. 474, 40-p. 475, 8 [Diels-Kranz] (from Aristoxenus).

[58] Ibid., p. 475, 14-17: μάλιστα δ' εἶναι κατανοῆσαι τάς τε ματαίους καὶ τὰς βλαβερὰς καὶ τὰς περιέργους καὶ τὰς ὑβριστικὰς τῶν ἐπιθυμιῶν παρὰ τῶν ἐν ἐξουσίαις ἀναστρεφομένων γινομένας.

[59] Ibid., p. 475, 11: . . . ἀφέξονται δὲ τῶν ματαίων τε καὶ περιέργων ἐπιθυμιῶν . . . .

[60] Cf. ibid., p. 475, 29-33; for ancient theories concerning the dietetics of the healthy in general, cf. L. Edelstein, Die Antike, VII, 1931, pp. 255 ff.

[61] A late Pythagorean poem still defines the right measure to be applied in matters concerning health, the μέτρον, as ὃ μή σ' ἀνιήσει, that which will not harm you (Carmen Aureum, l. 34); for the date of this poem, cf. below p. 33, n. 105.

of precepts and prohibitions seems to be characteristic of the Pythagorean treatment of diseases. Most illnesses, in the opinion of these philosophers, are due to opulent living; too much food is consumed which cannot be digested properly, and thus extravagance destroys the body, just as it destroys wealth.[62] If health, the retention of the form, changes into disease, the destruction of the form, the body needs purification through medicine, just as the sick soul needs purification through music.[63] The physician in such a case must give assistance by changing the patient's regimen. He must use dietetical means, as the Hippocratic Oath says.[64] In choosing them he will be intent on his patient's benefit according to the best of his judgment and ability. Whatever he prescribes, as a true follower of Pythagoras he will remember one fundamental truth: everything that is given to the body creates a certain disposition of the soul. Men in general, though they are aware of the fact that some things, such as wine, may suddenly bring about a striking change in a person's behavior, do not apprehend that every kind of food or drink causes a certain mental habit, slight as the variations may be. But the physician

[62] Cf. Diodorus, X, 7, 1: ὅτι παρεκάλει τὴν λιτότητα ζηλοῦν· τὴν γὰρ πολυτέλειαν ἅμα τάς τε οὐσίας τῶν ἀνθρώπων διαφθείρειν καὶ τὰ σώματα. Aristoxenus expresses the same idea by speaking of human beings as a ποικιλώτατον . . . γένος κατὰ τὸ τῶν ἐπιθυμιῶν πλῆθος (p. 475, 18-19 [Diels-Kranz]). A similar view is ascribed to Pythagoras himself by Apollonius, cf. Iamblichus, De Vita Pythagorica, 218; cf. also Rohde, op. cit., p. 164. I owe this reference to Schumacher, op. cit., p. 56.

[63] Cf. 58 C 3, p. 463, 26 [Diels-Kranz]: ὑγίειαν τὴν τοῦ εἴδους διαμονήν, νόσον τὴν τούτου φθοράν (from Aristotle). This concept can be elaborated by comparing the definition of health as harmony, the proper attunement of the body, ibid., p. 451, 11 (early Peripatetic tradition), and by referring to Alcmaeon's definition of health as ἰσονομία of the qualities, and of disease as μοναρχία of one quality (24 B4 [Diels-Kranz]; note also the expression φθοροποιόν). For medicine as κάθαρσις cf. ibid., 58 D 1, p. 468, 19 ff.: ὅτι οἱ Πυθαγορικοί, ὡς ἔφη Ἀριστόξενος, καθάρσει ἐχρῶντο τοῦ μὲν σώματος διὰ τῆς ἰατρικῆς, τῆς δὲ ψυχῆς διὰ τῆς μουσικῆς; cf. Howald, op. cit., p. 203.

[64] That in these instances the prescription of diet is the correct way of treatment follows from the alleged cause of the diseases, cf. above, pp. 21 f. This is also confirmed by the fact that dietetics was the principal treatment given by the Pythagoreans, as Aristoxenus says, cf. below, p. 29. The methods outlined in the Platonic Timaeus, a Pythagorean dialogue if there is any, are identical. Plato uses almost the same words: διὸ παιδαγωγεῖν δεῖ διαίταις . . . (89 c); Littré, op. cit., IV, p. 622, also referred to this passage in explanation of the Hippocratic δίαιται; cf. Körner, op: cit., p. 11.

knows that—his art primarily consists in this knowledge.[65] Consequently, he must see to it that the soul of the sick, through a wrong
diet, does not fall into "idle, irreverent, harmful and licentious passions." Since he acts according to this principle when assisting the
healthy,[66] he must certainly do likewise when treating the sick. Or
in the words of the Hippocratic Oath: the physician must protect
his patient from the mischief and injustice which he may inflict
upon himself if his diet is not properly chosen.[67] He must be a
physician of the soul no less than of the body; he must not overlook
the moral implications of his actions, nor even the negative indices
to be watched; for the regimen followed by a person concerns both
his bodily and his psychic constitution.[68]

The rules concerning dietetics, then, agree with Pythagoreanism,
in fact they acquire meaning only if seen in the light of Pythagorean
teaching. That the pharmacological precepts, the stipulations concerning poison and abortion, are Pythagorean in origin has already
been demonstrated.[69] It remains to be shown that the laws laid down
for surgery, too, are most easily understandable on the theory that
they are founded on Pythagorean doctrine.

The physician vows: "I will not use the knife either on sufferers
from stone, but I will give place to such as are craftsmen therein";
this at least is the most common rendering of the words in question.[70] Supposing that it be correct, what should be the reason for

[65] Cf. p. 475, 25-33 [Diels-Kranz]: διὸ δὴ καὶ μεγάλης σοφίας ⟨δεῖσθαι⟩ τὸ κατανοῆ-
σαί τε καὶ συνιδεῖν, ποίοις τε καὶ πόσοις δεῖ χρῆσθαι πρὸς τὴν τροφήν. εἶναι δὲ ταύτην
τὴν ἐπιστήμην τὸ μὲν ἐξ ἀρχῆς Ἀπόλλωνός τε καὶ Παιῶνος, ὕστερον δὲ τῶν περὶ τὸν
Ἀσκληπιόν (from Aristoxenus).

[66] Cf. above, pp. 21 f.

[67] Mischief (δήλησις) obviously is identical with what Aristoxenus calls βλαβεραὶ
ἐπιθυμίαι; injustice (ἀδικία) is a concept that is implied by ὑβριστικαὶ ἐπιθυμίαι;
cf. above, p. 22.

[68] Note that Plato in the Timaeus, 87 d, says that nothing is more dangerous
than the ἀμετρία . . . ψυχῆς . . . πρὸς σῶμα; later on he states that most of the
so-called physicians are deceived in their treatment because they seek the cause of
the disease in the body, whereas in reality it is to be found in the soul (88 a).

[69] Cf. above p. 18. What the Pythagoreans understood by pharmacology and
how they made use of it can be concluded from Aristoxenus' statement, quoted
above, p. 20, n. 49. For more details cf. below, pp. 29 f.

[70] For the text, cf. above, p. 2, 17-18; for the translation, cf. Jones, op. cit., p. 11
(but cf. below, p. 28, n. 84); Littré, op. cit., IV, p. 631; Daremberg, op. cit., p. 5;

the prohibition here pronounced? The treatment of stone-diseases by operation, in Greek medicine, seems to have been an old-established procedure; at any rate, since the rise of Alexandrian medicine, such an operation was performed throughout the centuries.[71] Why then is it forbidden in the Oath?

From the Renaissance down to the 19th century there was only one answer to this question: the Oath in the clause concerning lithotomy intends to draw a line between the practice of internal medicine and that of surgery. This separation, it was added, is introduced because surgery was held to be beneath the dignity of the physician.[72] With finer historical judgment, Littré rejected this generally accepted view. He pointed out that the ancient practitioner was a surgeon as well as a physician and considered the interpretation current before his time to be influenced by modern prejudices; but he had to admit that if this were so the statement seemed to defy explanation.[73] Indeed if the words in question do not have the meaning usually presumed, what else could they signify?

Littré with great hesitation and caution intimated that the stumbling block could perhaps be removed by the assumption that the Oath does not refer to lithotomy at all, but to castration. Some modern scholars have accepted this suggestion. For moral reasons

Pétrequin, *op. cit.*, I, p. 187; J. Hirschberg, *Vorlesungen über hippokratische Heilkunde*, 1922, p. 27; Körner, *op. cit.*, p. 12.

[71] Littré, *op. cit.*, IV, pp. 615 ff., has argued very convincingly that the operation must have been known since an early period because in Ps. Hippocrates, *De Morbis*, I, 6, diagnosis of the disease by means of a catheter is referred to as part of good craftsmanship. From Celsus, VII, 26, it follows that in his time great improvements in technique were made. Meges and Ammonius whom he mentions probably lived in the 1st century A. D.; cf. Hirschberg, *op. cit.*, p. 31; but the operation was certainly performed before; cf. Littré's interpretation of the passage, *op. cit.*, I, p. 342. For lithotomy in late centuries, cf. Ps. Galen, *Introductio* (Galen, XIV, p. 787 K.). Hirschberg, *op. cit.*, p. 32, believes that the Alexandrian physicians were the first to practice lithotomy, but this assumption he derives from the interdiction of this operation in the Hippocratic *Oath* which he considers a very old document (cf. *ibid.*, p. 27). Such an argumentation, of course, is not cogent, since it is precisely the date of the *Oath* which has not been established so far.

[72] Cf. *e. g.* Th. Zwinger, *Hippocratis Opera*, 1579, p. 59. Cf. also I. Cornarius, *Hippocratis Opera*, 1558, p. 8; P. Memmius and J. Fabricius in their commentaries on the *Oath*, published in 1577 and 1614 respectively. Cf. in general Körner, *op. cit.*, pp. 14 ff.; but cf. also below, p. 27, n. 80.

[73] Cf. Littré, *op. cit.*, IV, pp. 616-17.

they have said the physician abhorred such a treatment.[74] I shall not repeat the argument that has been brought forward before: to reject castration on moral grounds and yet to leave it to others would be " like compounding a felony, if not something worse." [75] Although from a linguistic point of view it is not impossible to understand the text as referring to castration, such a rendering is not consistent with the subject matter. For it is not attested that the ancients ever thought of applying castration as treatment of stone-diseases.[76] The sentence under discussion, therefore, must concern lithotomy, not castration.

Now some scholars, recognizing the fact that the Oath refers to lithotomy, contend that impotence was likely to result from the operation and that the physician recoiled from this risk—" it was against his liking"; "a higher concept of his profession" is supposed to have determined his renunciation of operative treatment by which he lost a good source of making money.[77] But such an inter-

[74] Cf. Littré, *op. cit.*, IV, p. 620 (with reference to R. Moreau, a physician of the 17th century; cf. *ibid.*, p. 618); Th. Gomperz, *Griechische Denker*, I⁴, 1922, p. 231; in general S. Nittis, The Hippocratic Oath in reference to lithotomy, A new interpretation with historical notes on castration, *Bulletin of the History of Medicine*, VII, 1939, pp. 719 ff.

[75] Cf. Jones, *op. cit.*, p. 48; cf. also Körner, *op. cit.*, pp. 12 ff. Nittis being aware of the difficulties pointed out by Jones and Körner tries to evade them by translating ἐκχωρήσω etc. by " I will keep apart from men engaging in this deed" (*op. cit.*, p. 721). He thinks that this might be the meaning of the verb ἐκχωρήσω, but he is unable to adduce any evidence for such a usage: the meaning of χωρέω of course does not prove anything in regard to that of ἐκχωρέω, and ἀποστήσομαι to which Nittis refers as a parallel has exactly the sense of ἐκχωρέω as it is usually taken. How inappropriate Nittis' rendering is, one can easily conclude from an old variant of the *Oath*: οὔτ᾽ ἐμοῖσι δὲ οὔτ᾽ ἄλλοισι ἐκχωρήσω . . . (Jones, *op. cit.*, p. 19).

[76] Nittis who has carefully investigated the history of castration comes to the following conclusion (*op. cit.*, p. 728): " Castration . . . was . . . probably practiced for the cure and prevention of diseases. Lithiasis is not mentioned directly by any writer as one of the diseases preventable by castration . . . ." In view of the fact that castration cannot be meant here, it is unnecessary to discuss the many emendations proposed to facilitate this interpretation, cf. Hirschberg, *op. cit.*, p. 29. To rectify an assertion which has frequently been made, I wish to mention at least that ancient physicians are known to have practiced castration for purposes other than medical, cf. Littré, *op. cit.*, IV, pp. 618 ff.

[77] Cf. Hirschberg, *op. cit.*, p. 30: " Eine solche Operation ging der Gilde gegen den Strich." As he says, Wilamowitz and Diels accepted his view. So does Deichgräber, *op. cit.*, p. 37, who writes: " Auch hier erhebt sich der Eid über die Sphäre der gewöhnlichen Handelsweise zu einer höheren Auffassung und wieder wird dem praktischen Arzte eine Erwerbsquelle verschlossen."

pretation can hardly be correct. To emphasize it once more: if the physician for moral reasons refuses to undertake the operation, he cannot possibly say in the same breath that he "will give place to such as are craftsmen therein." [78] The author of the Oath in other instances does not shrink from forbidding unconditionally what is held immoral or objectionable: when prohibiting the use of poison and of abortive remedies he does not say that the application of these drugs should be left to somebody else. The concession made in regard to lithotomy proves beyond doubt that the operation as such is not condemned: the performance of lithotomy, though not considered the business of the physician, is left to others for whom apparently it is judged legitimate.[79]

If this is true it seems to follow that lithotomy was to be given into the hands of specialists who were better able to do the job, that the Oath requires the physician to keep strictly within the limits of his own knowledge and recognize the superior skill of others who in some instances could be of greater help to his patients.[80] Such an explanation again leads into great difficulties. To be sure, specialization in certain operations or diseases of certain organs was known in antiquity. The stone-disease may have been one of these illnesses; lithotomy may have been practiced by craftsmen who were experts in this specific operation.[81] But lithotomy as performed in antiquity was not a more daring operation than many another which the general practitioner undertook without hesitation. Why then should the physician acknowledge his own limitations in this par-

---

[78] Cf. above, p. 24.

[79] Incidentally, it is not attested that in the opinion of the ancients lithotomy could injure the procreative faculty, cf. Hirschberg's discussion of the medical aspect of the problem, *op. cit.*, pp. 30 ff., especially the passages from Celsus and Paulus of Aegina, *ibid.*, p. 32.

[80] Cf. Körner, *op. cit.*, pp. 15 ff. A very similar interpretation has been proposed by J. H. Meibom, *Hippocratis Jus Jurandum*, 1643, p. 163.

[81] The question of specialists in antiquity has been widely discussed. That from Alexandrian times on medicine became specialized can hardly be doubted. In Rome specialization in certain diseases reached a climax. Nothing definite is known about the classical period. In spite of Cicero's emphatic statement that Hippocrates still mastered the whole range of medical knowledge (*De Oratore*, III, 33) it is hard to believe that in the Hippocratic period specialization was unknown (contrary to Littré, *op. cit.*, IV, p. 615, n. 1, who follows A. Andreae, *Zur ältesten Geschichte der Augenheilkunde*, 1841); the material is too scanty to admit a decision of the issue.

ticular case?[82] If moderation on his part is the general issue, why is he not asked to forego the treatment of all diseases for which the ancients had specialists? It is true, a distinction is made in the Oath between that which the physician should do and that which he should leave to others. But this division is recommended only in regard to lithotomy, and it has to be understood with reference to this particular instance.

There is no way out of the dilemma! The words must mean what in the opinion of all early interpreters they seemed to mean: lithotomy is here excluded because the performance of operations is held to be incompatible with the physician's craft, and by the one example given the Oath intends to exclude surgery in general from the field of the physician. It is possible that originally more operations were named as forbidden, that these references are missing only in the preserved text. But such a hypothesis cannot be verified.[83] It is more probable, however, that the statement as it stands is intact but in itself carries broader implications. For instead of translating "I will not use the knife either on sufferers from stone," it is equally well possible to translate "I will not use the knife, not even on sufferers from stone."[84] This would signify that the physician

---

[82] For operations performed by general practitioners, cf. Littré, *op. cit.,* IV, p. 617. That other operations made were more dangerous than lithotomy (contrary to Körner, *op. cit.,* p. 15) has been emphasized by Hirschberg, *op. cit.,* p. 30, who also stresses the fact that the ancient writers do not speak of an especially high mortality rate in this instance.

[83] Körner, *op. cit.,* n. 16, mentions the possibility of a lacuna after οὐ τεμέω δὲ; cf. also *C. M. G.,* I, 1, p. 4, 19: post δὲ lacunam statuit Diels (though for other reasons; cf. Hirschberg, *op. cit.,* p. 30). Deichgräber, *op. cit.,* n. 11, considers such an assumption unnecessary.

[84] Jones is the only one who has strongly emphasized the possibility of such a rendering. Moreover he has stressed the great difference in meaning that the two translations involve (*op. cit.,* pp. 46-47; cf. also *ibid.,* p. 11, n. 1, and Hippocrates, I, pp. 293 ff. [Loeb]) ; cf. also Nittis, *op. cit.,* p. 720, who goes so far as to say that the usual translation of the words is grammatically incorrect. I am not sure that in this respect he is right, but I do prefer the other rendering. Deichgräber, *op. cit.,* n. 11, says of the crucial words: " οὐδὲ verstärkt die Negation wie Z. 15 (*sc.* after οὐ δώσω δὲ); μήν beteuert, wie oft gerade in Eidschwüren und Versprechen." But in the passage quoted by Deichgräber, οὐδὲ is used, not οὐδὲ μήν; this fact is indicative of a difference in meaning. For οὐδὲ μήν in the sense of intensification (not even), cf. Kühner-Gerth, *Griechische Grammatik,* II, 2, § 502, 4 b, p. 137. Cf. also the old Latin translation (Jones, *op. cit.,* p. 37) : non incidam autem neque lapiditatem patientes; another translation (*op. cit.,* p. 35) corresponds to the rendering of most modern interpreters.

directly renounces operative surgery altogether. He will not resort
to it even in the case of that disease which more than any other,
according to the testimony of the ancients, drove men to suicide.[85]
The prohibition could not be formulated in more emphatic and
solemn words.

Whatever rendering is chosen, the statement under discussion
enjoins a separation of medicine and surgery. Driven back to this
interpretation which no doubt is drastically at variance with reality,
one feels almost inclined to say with Littré that such an explanation
must be rejected, and that consequently the motive for the interdiction of lithotomy in the Oath remains obscure.[86] Yet this seems
to be too rash a conclusion. It is true that the depreciation of surgery was foreign to ancient physicians in general.[87] It is likewise
true, however, that one medical sect valued surgery less highly than
dietetics and pharmacology, I mean the Pythagorean physicians.
As Aristoxenus says, they believed "most of all" in dietetics; they
applied poultices more liberally than did their predecessors, but
"thought less" of the efficacy of drugs; "they believed least of all
in using the knife and in cauterizing." [88] In other words, according
to Aristoxenus, the Pythagoreans attributed different values to the
various branches of medicine, and in their classification operative
surgery together with cauterization was ranked lowest. If one remembers that in Aristoxenus' opinion the Pythagoreans explained
most diseases as the result of unreasonable living,[89] one is at first
inclined to conclude that they were mainly interested in dietetics

[85] Cf. above, p. 8, n. 9, finis.

[86] Cf. Littré, *op. cit.*, p. 617. It is of course impossible to say with Jones, *op. cit.*,
p. 48, or K. Sprengel, *Apologie des Hippokrates*, I, p. 77 (cf. Littré, *op. cit.*, I,
p. 342), that the words in question are a later addition. If this statement were
missing, surgery would not be referred to at all in the *Oath*.

[87] Cf. *e. g.* Littré, *op. cit.*, IV, p. 617. A separation of surgery from internal
medicine can be traced at best to Galen's time (cf. Galen, X, pp. 454-55 K.; Jones,
op. cit., p. 48), that is, in the sense that physicians refused to practice surgery
because they held it beneath their dignity. The study and teaching of the various
branches of medicine had become specialized long before, cf. Celsus, *Introductio*,
9; cf. also above, p. 27, n. 81.

[88] Cf. 58 D 1 [Diels-Kranz] (quoted above, p. 20, n. 49); cf. Porphyry, *Vita
Pythagorae*, 22: φυγαδευτέον πάσῃ μηχανῇ καὶ περικοπτέον πυρὶ καὶ σιδήρῳ καὶ
μηχαναῖς παντοίαις ἀπὸ μὲν σώματος νόσον . . . (Aristoxenus = *Fr.* 8 [Müller]).

[89] Cf. above, pp. 20 ff.

and pharmacology, because these were the more appropriate means of treatment. Still this can hardly be the whole truth. For Plato in the *Timaeus*, when outlining the Pythagorean treatment of diseases, does not mention cutting or cauterizing at all, though he agrees with Aristoxenus in placing the importance of pharmacology after that of dietetics.[90] Evidently, then, there must have been Pythagoreans who refused to apply any surgical means of treatment which were otherwise so universally used in Greek medicine. This inference from the Platonic *Timaeus* seems quite certain though no express statement to this effect is preserved.[91]

It is most likely that Aristoxenus' report is one of his typical attempts to reconcile the rigorous Pythagorean attitude with the demands of common sense and the exigencies of daily life: such compromises he introduces in many instances where other sources attest the uncompromising attitude of the Pythagoreans.[92] Seen

[90] Cf. *Timaeus*, 87 c ff.; esp. 89 d.

[91] Note how in contrast to the passage in the *Timaeus*, Plato in the *Republic*, III, 405 c ff., defines medicine as the art which should deal with drugs or cauterization and cutting, whereas the pedagogics of dietetic medicine is rejected (406 d). It can hardly be by chance that Plato omits a reference to cutting and cauterization in the *Timaeus*. In K. Sprengel– I. Rosenbaum, *Versuch einer pragmatischen Geschichte der Arzneikunde*, I, 1846, p. 251, it is said: "Der schneidenden und brennenden Werkzeuge enthielt er (*sc.* Pythagoras) sich gänzlich," but the only testimony adduced is the fragment of Aristoxenus (cf. above, p. 20, n. 49). J. F. K. Hecker, *Geschichte der Heilkunde*, I, 1822, p. 77, claims that: ". . . die Pythagorische Arzneikunst sich viel mit äusseren Mitteln beschäftigte, von der kühnern Chirurgie aber ganz entfernt blieb." He does not give any proof for this assertion. The more recent books on Pythagorean medicine do not discuss the problem at all. For the modern it may be difficult to imagine a medical art without surgery in the strict sense of the word (the treatment of fractures and so forth is of course not curtailed by the prohibition of operative surgery). Yet in antiquity popular opposition to "cutting and cauterization" was strong indeed. Cf. *e. g.* Plato, *Gorgias*, 456 b, and the parallels collected in Stallbaum's commentary *ad locum*. The attitude of the ancients never changed in this respect; cf. the most impressive statement of Scribonius Largus, *Compositiones*, p. 2, ll. 3 ff. [Helmreich]: ". . . siquidem verum est antiquos herbis ac radicibus earum corporis vitia curasse, quia timidum genus mortalium inter initia non facile se ferro ignique committebat. quod etiam nunc plerique faciunt, ne dicam omnes, et nisi magna conpulsi necessitate speque ipsius salutis non patiuntur sibi fieri, quae sane vix sunt toleranda."

[92] Note *e. g.* Aristoxenus' denial of the contention that Pythagoras refrained from all bloody sacrifices, p. 101, 13 ff. [Diels-Kranz], or his claim that he did not reject beans as nourishment, *ibid.*, p. 101, 19 ff., whereas others see in this prohibition a means of purification, *ibid.*, p. 463, 10 (Aristotle), p. 451, 15 ff. (early

from this angle, the stipulation of the Oath appears as another compromise, more lenient and at the same time more rigid than that reported by Aristoxenus: the use of cauterization obviously is allowed, operative surgery is completely eliminated. On the other hand, the Pythagorean physician will allow others to help his patient in his extremity. The stipulation against operating is valid only for him who has dedicated himself to a holy life. The Pythagoreans recognized that men in general could not observe any elaborate rules of purity; in this fact they saw no argument against that which they considered right for themselves. To give place to another craftsman, especially in such instances where the patient might fall prey to a sinful temptation,[93] certainly was a duty demanded by philanthropy, by commiseration with those who suffered.[94]

But why should the Pythagorean have avoided the use of the knife? The answer can only be a conjecture: he who believed that bloody sacrifices should not be offered to the gods and saw in them a defilement of divine purity could well believe that he himself would be defiled in his purity and holiness by using the knife in bloody operations.[95] However that may be, it is only in connection with

Peripatos). P. Corssen, *Rheinisches Museum*, LXVII, 1912, p. 258, intimated that Aristoxenus in his interpretation of Pythagorean philosophy is inclined to make the doctrine appear less rigid than it is portrayed by others. Cf. moreover Ueberweg-Praechter, *op. cit.*, p. 64.

[93] Cf. above, p. 8, n. 9; p. 15.

[94] Already in Peripatetic attacks on the Pythagorean way of life the question was raised how a state could be governed in which everybody followed the Pythagorean taboos. The answer was that these purity-observances were not meant to be valid for everybody; cf. Porphyry, *De Abstinentia*, I, and J. Bernays, *Theophrastos' Schrift über Frömmigkeit*, 1866, p. 13. Moreover, the Pythagorean ideal of government is that of an aristocracy with proportionally divided rights and duties, cf. M. Pohlenz, *Aus Platos Werdezeit*, 1913, p. 154, n. 1 (Dicaearchus).

[95] There is no need for an elaborate discussion of the Pythagorean rejection of bloody sacrifices in which their insistence on purity manifested itself most clearly, cf. *e. g.* Diogenes Laertius, VIII, 13, and in general Bernays, who quite rightly speaks of the " Pythagoreische Blutscheu " (*op. cit.*, p. 33) ; cf. also the Pythagorean objections to the drinking of wine " the blood of the earth," Corssen, *op. cit.*, pp. 246 ff. (Androcydes). For the concept of defilement, cf. such expressions as Plato, *Laws*, VI, 782 c: τοὺς τῶν θεῶν βωμοὺς αἵματι μιαίνειν; cf. also Bernays, *op. cit.*, p. 130. For purification rites in regard to the knife that is used in bloody sacrifices, cf. Bernays, *op. cit.*, p. 91. Note that Aristoxenus, according to whom surgery, though valued least, was nevertheless practiced by the Pythagoreans, denies that they offered only bloodless gifts to the gods; cf. above, p. 30, n. 92.

Pythagorean medicine that the injunction of the Hippocratic Oath, according to which operative surgery was forbidden to the physician, acquires any meaning and plausibility at all. The rules given in regard to surgery no less than those concerning dietetics and pharmacology are Pythagorean in character.[96]

Those stipulations of the Oath which deal with the medical treatment proper are finally followed by two more general provisions bearing on medical ethics in the strict sense of the word. The behavior of the physician towards his patient and the patient's family is regulated; reticence is imposed upon him in regard to whatever he may see or hear. Is it really true that in non-medical literature no parallels can be found to these postulates?[97] In my opinion these ethical rules, too, in their specific wording are understandable only in connection with Pythagorean doctrine.

As for the first vow, he who swears the Oath promises to come, into whatever house he enters, to help the sick, refraining from injustice and mischief, especially from all sexual incontinence.[98] That the physician should act for the sole purpose of assisting his patient, is a demand that seems self-evident. It certainly is as compatible with any ethical standard to which a doctor may subscribe, as it is with Pythagorean ethics.[99] It may seem equally natural that the physician is bidden to refrain from all injustice and mischief. Yet, the appropriateness of the statement does not imply that it is not in need of further explanation, be it in regard to its meaning or its motivation.[100]

Those who believe that only medical parallels can be adduced for

[96] Cf. above, pp. 19 f., where it is shown that even the sequence of dietetics, pharmacology and surgery, as given in the *Oath*, corresponds to the sequence of these branches of medicine in the report of Aristoxenus.

[97] Cf. Deichgräber, *op. cit.*, p. 37: "Während sich die drei ersten Bestimmungen (*sc.* concerning dietetics, pharmacology, and surgery) mit ausserhalb der medizinischen Kreise und des medizinischen Bereiches geltenden Maximen vergleichen lassen, ist für diese Beschränkungen eine derartige Gegenüberstellung nicht möglich. Nur ein Vergleich mit den sonst in der hippokratischen Pflichtenlehre geltenden Anschauungen lässt sich durchführen . . ." (cf. however below, p. 33, n. 104). The other interpreters do not attempt at all to give an explanation of these rules.

[98] Cf. above, p. 2, 19-21.

[99] For the ὠφέλιμον and its rôle in Pythagoreanism, cf. above, p. 20, n. 52.

[100] Cf. Körner, *op. cit.*, p. 16, who in his interpretation of the *Oath* simply says: "Das nun folgende Gelöbnis bedarf keiner Erklärung."

44

the stipulations of the Oath point to seemingly similar utterances in one of the so-called Hippocratic writings, the book "On the Physician." [101] Here it is stated that in his relations with the sick the doctor ought to be just, for the patients have no small dealings with their physician. They put themselves into his hands, and the physician comes in contact with women and maidens and with very precious possessions indeed; so toward all these self-control should be used.[102] I do not wish to raise the issue, whether justice is here commended for utilitarian rather than moral reasons. Nor do I emphasize the fact that only if it had a moral bent could this assertion be likened to the Oath.[103] In refutation of the argument of modern interpreters it is enough to say that the parallel referred to is by far less comprehensive and less rigorous than the statement which it is supposed to explain. The Oath, unlike the Hippocratic treatise "On the Physician," does not speak only of the avoidance of injustice, it also excludes mischief. Moreover, the Oath enjoins continence in regard to women and men alike; it stresses that the same continence must be observed towards free-born people and slaves, features that are entirely missing in the other passage.[104] A more satisfactory interpretation of the words in question, therefore, must be sought.

Now a plea for justice and continence may of course be derived from many ancient philosophical systems. As for justice, the Platonists and the Aristotelians praised its dignity no less than did the Pythagoreans.[105] But so much it is safe to claim: that the physician

[101] Cf. Deichgräber, op. cit., p. 38; but cf. also Daremberg, op. cit., p. 57.

[102] Cf. C. M. G., I, 1, p. 20, 18 ff. In my paraphrase of the very difficult passage I have partly followed Jones' translation, Hippocrates, II, p. 313 [Loeb].

[103] For the idealistic point of view consistently observed in the Oath, cf. above, p. 27, and below, p. 50. As a matter of fact the author of Περὶ ἰητροῦ is an utilitarian, cf. below, p. 37, n. 119.

[104] That this is so, is also admitted by Deichgräber, op. cit., p. 38, who adds that the attitude taken in the Oath is in agreement with that taken by certain philosophers, but he does not say who they are.

[105] For Plato and Aristotle, cf. below, p. 35, n. 112, for the Pythagoreans in general, cf. Zeller, op. cit., I, 1, p. 390. I admit that the ultimate principles of Pythagorean ethics are not well known, but this much one may venture to say: justice played an important rôle in their system. Otherwise, why should justice determine men's relation to the gods and to all other creatures in the world (cf. 58 C 4, p. 464, 8 [Diels-Kranz]; Diogenes Laertius, VIII, 23; Iamblichus, De Vita Pythagorica, 168)? Why should Pythagoras have said of salt that it should be brought to table to remind us of what is just—for salt preserves whatever it

is required to abstain from all intentional injustice and mischief—
such a formulation savors of the famous Pythagorean sayings by
which injustice and mischief are proscribed, even if committed
against animals and plants.[106] And indeed, to blend the concept of
justice with that of forbearance is characteristic of the Pythagoreans.
They abhorred violence; only if provoked by injustice would they
resort to force. In this recoiling from aggression the asceticism of
Pythagorean ethics culminated.[107] Moreover, the consequences drawn
in the Oath from the ethical standards there imposed are in strict
keeping with those principles which the Pythagoreans enforced upon
their followers. Their views on sexual matters were severer than
those of all other ancient philosophers. They alone judged sexual
relations in terms of justice, meaning thereby not that which is
forbidden or allowed by law : for the husband to be unfaithful to his
wife was considered to be unjust toward her.[108] The Pythagoreans
upheld the equality of men and women. They alone condemned
sodomy.[109] Besides, in the performance of moral duties, they did not

seasons, and it arises from the purest sources, sun and sea (cf. 58 C 3, p. 463, 27
[Diels-Kranz]) ? Cf. also *Carmen Aureum*, ll. 13-16. But I do not wish to lay too
much emphasis on this source, since it is of relatively late date (usually ascribed
to the first century B. C. or A. D., cf. Ueberweg-Prächter, *op. cit.*, p. 518).
Hierocles in his commentary on the *Carmen Aureum, Fragmenta Philosophorum
Graecorum*, ed. F. G. A. Mullach, I, 1883, p. 433, goes so far as to claim that
justice was the principal virtue of the Pythagoreans. But this is a late Neo-Platonic
re-interpretation.

[106] Cf. Diogenes Laertius, VIII, 23 (from Androcydes, cf. Corssen, *op. cit.*,
p. 258) : φυτὸν ἥμερον μήτε φθίνειν μήτε σίνεσθαι, αλλὰ μηδὲ ζῷον ὃ μὴ βλάπτει
ἀνθρώπους. In other passages the words used are even more reminiscent of the
phraseology of the *Oath*, cf. Iamblichus, *De Vita Pythagorica*, 168: μήτε ἀδικεῖν
. . . μήτε φονεύειν; ibid., 99: μήτε βλάπτειν μήτε φθείρειν.

[107] The renunciation of violence is a natural consequence of the Pythagorean
concept of purity and holiness. I do not think that such an ideal is to be found in
any other ethical system of the ancients. Zeller rightly ascribes to the Pythagoreans
" Gerechtigkeit und Sanftmut gegen alle Menschen," *op. cit.*, I, 1, p. 462.

[108] Cf. Ps. Aristotle, *Oeconomica*, I, 4: . . . ὑφηγεῖται δὲ [δ] καὶ ὁ κοινὸς νόμος,
καθάπερ οἱ Πυθαγόρειοι λέγουσιν, ὥσπερ ἱκέτιν καὶ ἀφ' ἑστίας ἠγμένην ὡς ἥκιστα δεῖν
[δοκεῖν] ἀδικεῖν· ἀδικία δὲ ἀνδρὸς αἱ θύραζε συνουσίαι γιγνόμεναι. Cf. also Diodorus,
X, 9, 3 ; 4; Iamblichus, *De Vita Pythagorica*, 132, and in general, above, pp. 17 f.;
cf. also Zeller, *op. cit.*, I, 1, p. 462, n. 2. How foreign such reflections are to common
Greek thought becomes apparent from Aristotle who considers adultery unjust, if
committed for gain's sake; otherwise he calls it self-indulgence, *N. E.*, 1130 a 24 ff.

[109] Concerning women in the Pythagorean school, cf. Iamblichus, *De Vita
Pythagorica*, 267 ; cf. Zeller, *op. cit.*, I, 1, p. 314, n. 4. As for the γεννήσεις παρὰ

discriminate between social ranks. In that respect free-born people and slaves, for the Pythagoreans, were on equal footing.[110] Everything, then, that the Oath stipulates in regard to sexual continence agrees with the tenets of Pythagorean ethics, in fact with the ideals of these philosophers alone.

Finally, as a Pythagorean postulate the clause takes on a peculiar significance for the physician. It is justice first of all that is required from him. This virtue, to the average people, meant to live in accordance with the laws of the state.[111] To Plato, wherever he does not speak of justice in his own peculiar usage as the perfect working of the human soul in all its functions, justice was mainly a civic virtue. Aristotle tried to establish justice as a political virtue, and as one that applies to contracts and dealings in the law-courts.[112] All these aspects are also inherent in the Pythagorean concept of justice, and they certainly are of some concern for the physician. While in his direct dealings with men, in his personal contact with them and their households, it may be of less importance whether generally speaking he is a law-abiding citizen, it makes a great difference indeed, whether he is an honest man or not. It is in this sense, that even the author of the Hippocratic book " On the Phy-

φύσιν, rejected by the Pythagoreans, cf. p. 476, 4-5 [Diels-Kranz], quoted above, p. 17, n. 41. Even Plato, *Laws*, VII, 841 d, does not go as far as the Pythagoreans. For the usual Greek point of view, cf. Aristotle, *N. E.*, 1148 b 29 ff.

[110] For the Pythagorean attitude towards slaves, cf. E. Zeller–W. Nestle, *Grundriss d. Geschichte d. griech. Philosophie*[13], 1928, p. 40; but they speak only of " humane Behandlung." It would be more adequate, however, to speak of equality, though there is no express statement to this effect among the Pythagorean testimonies, cf. J. Burckhardt, *Vorträge*, 1919, p. 193. As Aristoxenus says, p. 471, 8 f. [Diels-Kranz], the true Pythagorean will not punish anybody in anger, be he slave or free. Moreover, according to Aristotle, *N. E.*, 1132 b 22, the Pythagoreans define justice as reciprocity without qualification; cf. Zeller, *op. cit.*, I, 1, p. 390, n. 1. Aristotle adds that reciprocity fits neither distributive nor rectificatory justice, meaning thereby that punishment must differ in regard to the official status of the offender. In the *Magna Moralia*, 1194 a 28, the Pythagorean definition of justice is rejected because it cannot hold good in relation to all persons, " for the same thing is not just for a domestic as for a freeman." Obviously, then, the Pythagoreans did not believe that justice should be administered differently in the case of slaves. They believed in the equality of all human beings.

[111] Cf. Aristotle, *N. E.*, V, ch. 1, where also the proverbial saying is quoted: " In justice is every virtue comprehended," 1129 b 29-30.

[112] For Plato, cf. especially *Republic*, IV, 441 c ff., and *Laws*, VI, 757 a ff.; in general cf. Zeller, *op. cit.*, II, 1[4], pp. 884-86. For Aristotle, cf. *N. E.*, V, chs. 2 ff.

sician " counsels the doctor not to infringe upon the possessions of others with whom he is doing business.[113] But such justice, essential as it may be for good morals, is not all that the Pythagorean ideal of justice implies. To the adherents of this dogma, justice was the social virtue par excellence. As Aristoxenus reports,[114] they believed that "in any relation with others" some kind of justice is involved. "In all intercourse" it is possible to take "a well-timed and an ill-timed attitude." In order to do what is proper, one must differentiate according to circumstances. Speech and actions necessarily vary depending on the particular situation and the persons concerned. From the right decision result timeliness, appropriateness, and fitness of behavior, and it is justice that reveals itself in good manners.[115] Interpreted in the light of Pythagorean teaching, then, the recommendation of justice epitomizes all duties of the physician towards his patient in the contacts of daily life, all he should do or say in the course of his practice; it gives the rules of medical deportment in a nutshell.[116]

Last but not least: the promise of silence. The physician accepts

[113] Cf. above, p. 33.

[114] 58 D 5, p. 470, 1 ff. [Diels-Kranz] : ἐπεὶ δὲ καὶ ἐν τῇ πρὸς ἕτερον χρείᾳ ἔστι τις δικαιοσύνη, καὶ ταύτης τοιοῦτόν τινα τρόπον λέγεται ὑπὸ τῶν Πυθαγορείων παραδίδοσθαι. εἶναι γὰρ κατὰ τὰς ὁμιλίας τὸν μὲν εὔκαιρον, τὸν δὲ ἄκαιρον, . . . ἔστι γάρ τι ὁμιλίας εἶδος, ὃ φαίνεται νεωτέρῳ μὲν πρὸς νεώτερον οὐκ ἄκαιρον εἶναι, πρὸς δὲ τὸν πρεσβύτερον ἄκαιρον. . . . τὸν αὐτὸν δ' εἶναι λόγον καὶ περὶ τῶν ἄλλων παθῶν τε καὶ πράξεων καὶ διαθέσεων καὶ ὁμιλιῶν καὶ ἐντεύξεων. . . . ἀκόλουθα δὲ εἶναι καὶ σχεδὸν τοιαῦτα, οἷα συμπαρέπεσθαι τῇ τοῦ καιροῦ φύσει τήν τε ὀνομαζομένην ὥραν καὶ τὸ πρέπον καὶ τὸ ἁρμόττον, καὶ εἴ τι ἄλλο τυγχάνει τούτοις ὁμοιογενὲς ὄν.

[115] Such a concept of justice seems entirely different from what Greek philosophers in general understand by justice. Aristotle, N. E., 1126 b 36 ff., for instance discusses under temperance that which the Pythagoreans call justice. On the other hand, the Pythagorean definition of justice in part overlaps with the common one in so far as the law also touches upon conduct, cf. Aristotle, N. E., V, ch. 1, and above, p. 35. In Aristoxenus' representation Pythagorean ethics often approximates the tenets of popular reflection, cf. Zeller, op. cit., I, 1, p. 460, and above, p. 30, n. 92.

[116] Deichgräber, who was the first to emphasize the importance which the concept of justice has in the Oath (op. cit., pp. 37; 41 ff.), goes so far as to say that the Oath embodies the ideal of the just physician (cf. above, p. 4, n. 5). This in my opinion is an exaggeration because the Oath combines the ideal of justice with that of forbearance (cf. above, p. 34) ; moreover, holiness and purity are also insisted upon (cf. above, p. 18). Justice then, important as it is, is not the only standard which is here applied to human actions. Cf. also below, p. 38, n. 123.

the obligation to keep to himself all that he sees or hears during the treatment; he also swears not to divulge whatever comes to his knowledge outside of his medical activity in the life of men.[117] The latter phrase in particular has always seemed strange. It is so far-reaching in scope that it can hardly be explained by professional considerations alone.[118] To be sure, other medical writings also advise the physician to be reticent. The motive in doing so is the concern for the physician's renommée which might suffer if he is a prattler.[119] But the Oath demands silence in regard to that "which on no account one must spread abroad." It insists on secrecy not as a precaution but as a duty.[120] In the same way silence about things which are not to be communicated to others was considered a moral obligation by the Pythagoreans. They did not tell everything to everybody. They did not indiscriminately impart their knowledge to others. They expected the scientist to be reticent and ready to listen.[121] They observed silence even in daily life. That they were taciturn beyond all other men no less than the fact that they were

---

[117] Cf. above, p. 2, 22-24.

[118] Cf. Jones, op. cit., p. 50.

[119] Cf. Hippocrates, Περὶ ἰητροῦ, C. M. G., I, 1, p. 20, 9: τὰ δὲ περὶ τὴν ψυχὴν σώφρονα, μὴ μόνον τῷ σιγᾶν . . . μέγιστα γὰρ ἔχει πρὸς δόξαν ἀγαθά. Deichgräber, op. cit., p. 37, refers to this passage; he himself admits that the statement serves merely utilitarian purposes.

[120] Incidentally, Körner, op. cit., p. 6, translates ἃ μὴ χρή ποτε ἐκλαλέεσθαι ἔξω by "wenn es nicht in die Öffentlichkeit gebracht werden muss," and in his interpretation, ibid., p. 17, states that this clause means that the physician should keep to himself everything except that which it is his duty to bring to public attention. In other words, Körner finds in the Oath a distinction between that which the physician owes to his patient and that which he owes to the community. Apart from the fact that the physician's obligations towards the state are nowhere mentioned in the document, such an interpretation is not warranted by the words. ἔξω is not "Öffentlichkeit" but simply "outside." Moreover, the text gives no indication as to what the physician should say, but only as to what he should keep to himself. Cf. also next note.

[121] Cf. Diogenes Laertius, VIII, 15 (Aristoxenus): μὴ εἶναι πρὸς πάντας πάντα ῥητά. Cf. 58 D 1, p. 467, 4 [Diels-Kranz]: σιωπηλοὺς δὲ εἶναι καὶ ἀκουστικοὺς . . . (from Aristoxenus after introductory remarks about the sciences accepted by the Pythagoreans [music, medicine, mantics]); cf. also below, pp. 46 f., concerning the transmission of knowledge in the Pythagorean school. Later, the ability to be reticent, in Pythagorean education, was considered the strongest proof of self-continence, the sign by which to distinguish good from bad pupils. Compare ἃ μὴ χρή in the Oath with Iamblichus, De Vita Pythagorica, 71: καὶ τὴν σιωπὴν καὶ τὴν λαλιὰν παρὰ τὸ δέον (from Apollonius [?]; cf. Rohde, op. cit., p. 137).

frugal in their habits made them the object of ridicule in ancient comedy.[122] Certainly if the doctor who promises not to talk about anything that he may see or hear is to be placed in any philosophical school, it must be the Pythagorean.

To sum up the results of the analysis of the ethical code: the provisions concerning the application of poison and of abortive remedies, in their inflexibility, intimated that the second part of the Oath is influenced by Pythagorean ideas. The interpretation of the other medical and ethical stipulations showed that they, too, are tinged by Pythagorean theories.[123] All statements can be understood only, or at any rate they can be understood best, as adaptations of Pythagorean teaching to the specific task of the physician. Even from a formal point of view, these rules are reminiscent of Pythagoreanism: just as in the Oath the doctor is told what to do and what not to do, so the Pythagorean oral instruction indicated what to do and what not to do.[124] Far from being the expression of the common Greek attitude towards medicine or of the natural duties of the physician, the ethical code rather reflects opinions which were peculiarly those of a small and isolated group.

[122] Cf. the fragment from Alexis, p. 479, 36 [Diels-Kranz]; cf. also, *ibid.*, p. 466, 20: γλώσσης πρὸ τῶν ἄλλων κράτει θεοῖς ἑπόμενος (old *Symbolon*), and *ibid.*, p. 97, 33 (Isocrates, *Busiris*, 29); in general cf. Zeller, *op. cit.*, III, 2, p. 80, n. 1. I need hardly refer to the proverbial *Silentium Pythagoricum*.

[123] Deichgräber, taking Apollo as the symbol of purity and justice, has characterized the morality advocated in the *Oath* as Apolline ethics, but this term as he uses it, is an invention *ad hoc* (*op. cit.*, p. 42: . . . " wenn man so will, die Idee des apollinischen Arztes "). To be sure, the Delphic religion promoted a certain ethical attitude, but the little that is known about it concerns men's relation to God and Fate rather than to his fellow men, cf. E. Howald, *Ethik des Altertums, Handbuch der Philosophie*, 1926, p. 11. An ethics as it is found in the Hippocratic *Oath* was a historical reality only in Pythagoreanism. That in some respects this philosophical system itself was influenced by Delphic concepts is possible; the ancients thought so themselves, cf. Diogenes Laertius, VIII, 8 (Aristoxenus). But such an agreement between Delphi and Pythagorean philosophy does not cover all those detailed injunctions in which the *Oath* coincides with the Pythagorean system.

[124] Cf. p. 464, 4 [Diels-Kranz]: Ἀκούσματα . . . τρία εἴδη . . . τὰ δὲ τί δεῖ πράττειν ἢ μὴ πράττειν. Deichgräber, *op. cit.*, p. 41, contends that the *Oath* " nur negative Bestimmungen enthält." Although the negative formulations are more numerous in the *Oath*, one cannot overlook the most emphatic positive statements concerning the physician's purity and holiness (cf. above, p. 2, 15-16), and concerning his promise to bring help to his patient (cf. above, p. 2, 12; 19).

II

THE COVENANT

The ethical code by the acceptance of which the physician gives a higher sanction to his practical endeavor is preceded by a solemn agreement concerning medical education. The pupil promises to regard his teacher as equal to his parents, to share his life with him, to support him with money if he should be in need of it. Next he vows to hold his teacher's children as equals to his brothers and to teach them the art without fee and covenant if they should wish to learn it. Finally he takes upon himself the obligation to impart precepts, oral instruction and all the other learning to his own sons, to those of his teacher and to pupils who have signed the covenant and have taken an oath according to the medical law, to all these, but to no one else.[1]

Whatever the precise purport of the single terms and phrases used in this covenant, so much is immediately clear in regard to its general meaning and is commonly admitted: the teacher here is made the adopted father of the pupil, the teacher's family becomes the pupil's adopted family. In other words, the covenant establishes between teacher and pupil the closest and most sacred relationship that can be imagined between men, and it does so for no other apparent reason than that the pupil is being instructed in the art.

In explaining this stipulation modern interpreters usually allege that in Greece, in early centuries, medicine like all the other arts was passed on from father to son in closed family guilds. When at a certain time these organizations began to receive outsiders into their midst, they are said to have demanded from them full participation in the responsibilities of the "real" children. Consequently those who wished to be admitted to all the privileges and rights of the family had to become its members through adoption. The Hippocratic covenant, then, it is claimed, is an engagement which was signed by newcomers joining one of the medical artisan families, and it was probably the family of the Asclepiads in which this formula held good.[2]

[1] Cf. above, p. 2, 5-11.
[2] Cf. *e. g.* Littré, *op. cit.,* IV, pp. 611 ff.; I, pp. 341 ff.; Daremberg, *op. cit.,* p. 2; for later proponents of this view, cf. Jones, *op. cit.,* p. 44.

The evidence for such a theory, in my opinion, is insufficient. Galen is the only ancient author who asserts that the Asclepiads, after having been for generations the sole possessors of medicine, later shared their knowledge with people not belonging to their clan. And even he says that these outsiders were men whom the family esteemed "on account of their virtue"; he does not contend that they were made members of the family or forced to accept any obligations.[3] It is hardly by chance, therefore, that Galen himself does not refer to the Hippocratic Oath as bearing out the truth of his story. In any case, his words cannot be adduced as corroborative proof for the assumptions of modern scholars. Nor does it increase the strength of the modern argument if Galen's testimony is combined with that of Plato, according to whom "physicians taught their sons medicine and . . . Hippocrates taught outside pupils for a fee."[4] Though Plato says this, it still does not follow that the outsiders became the adopted children of their masters. On the contrary, who will believe that the young Athenian aristocrat Hippocrates of whom Plato speaks would have considered paying a fee to the great Hippocrates for instruction, had that meant that he should enter the family of the Coan physician![5]

If thus the usual interpretation of the Hippocratic covenant is unsupported by external testimony, it is equally unfounded as far as the wording of the text is concerned. For the covenant itself does not refer to a family guild of physicians. It speaks only of the pupil and the teacher, leaving open the question whether the latter is the son of a physician, the member of a clan of doctors, or not.[6] In view

[3] Cf. Galen, *Opera*, II, pp. 280 ff. K. The most important words are: . . . καὶ τοῖς ἔξω τοῦ γένους ἔδοξε καλὸν (!) εἶναι μεταδιδόναι τῆς τέχνης . . . ἤδη γὰρ τελέοις ἀνδράσιν, οὓς ἐτίμησαν ἀρετῆς ἕνεκα, ἐκοινώνουν τῆς τέχνης.

[4] Cf. Jones, *op. cit.*, p. 56; the Platonic passages referred to are *Laws*, IV, 720 b; *Protagoras*, 311 b. Substantially the same considerations are to be found in Littré, *op. cit.*, IV, pp. 611 ff., and in most authors who take the covenant as a document indicative of the state of family organizations.

[5] Cf. *Protagoras*, 311 b. Hirschberg, *op. cit.*, p. 28, seems the only one to admit that Plato does not give evidence for the *Oath*. For he emphasizes that in Plato's time the regulations found in the Hippocratic covenant—which he considers early— did no longer exist.

[6] As far as I know Jones has been the first to stress this fact. Cf. Jones, *Hippocrates*, I, p. 293: "Some scholars regard the *Oath* as the test required by the Asclepiad Guild. The document, however, does not contain a single word

of this fact it does not help to concede, as some scholars have done, that adoptions of outsiders into artisan families are hardly known from any other source, and yet to maintain that the Hippocratic covenant only confirms what must be presumed anyhow on the basis of generally valid laws of economic development. In all civilizations, it is stated, crafts were first restricted to family guilds; eventually these organizations became mere trade unions accessible to all; in a transitory period between these two stages the families adopted outsiders as "quasi-children."[7] I am not prepared to discuss the correctness of these so-called economic laws, nor do I wish to judge whether they are applicable to the Greek situation. The Hippocratic covenant at all events neither confirms such a theory, nor can it be explained by it; for there is no indication in the text that the document is concerned with family interests or family politics.[8]

Yet, if through the covenant the pupil is not received into a family guild, if he is made rather the adopted son of his teacher—was such a relationship common among the Greeks of any period? Some scholars answer this question in the affirmative. In the time preceding that of the Sophists, they say, the teacher generally was esteemed as the "spiritual father" of his pupil.[9] But this assertion

which supports this contention. It binds the student to his master and his master's family, not to a guild or corporation." Cf. also *The Doctor's Oath*, p. 56: "a private agreement between master and apprentice." Nevertheless Jones accepts the general view (*ibid.*, p. 44) that the covenant has something to do with the Asclepiad guild; but cf. also below, p. 47, n. 28.

[7] Cf. Deichgräber, *op. cit.*, pp. 32 ff. He says, p. 32: ". . . eine Idee, wie wir sie vielleicht im griechischen Vereinswesen hier und dort voraussetzen dürfen, aus antiken Nachrichten aber kaum kennen." As a matter of fact, even E. Ziebarth, *Das griechische Vereinswesen*, 1896, p. 96, to whom Deichgräber refers, apparently in explanation of his "vielleicht" and "kaum" (n. 18), knows of no other testimony than the Hippocratic *Oath*. Concerning Galen, II, p. 280, cf. above, p. 40. Plato, *Republic*, X, 599 c and *Fragmenta Historicorum Graecorum*, ed. G. Müller, II, 1848, p. 263, passages which Ziebarth quotes in addition, do not yield anything concerning the problem of adoption.

[8] I should mention that in consequence of the usual interpretation of the covenant different ethical standards have to be presupposed for the two sections of the *Oath* (cf. above, p. 4). To use the characterization of Deichgräber who has most strongly brought out this discrepancy (*op. cit.*, p. 38; p. 42): the first part shows a business point of view, whereas the second is determined by Apolline concepts of purity. Concerning this problem, cf. also above, p. 38, n. 123, and below, pp. 50 ff.

[9] Cf. E. Hoffmann, Kulturphilosophisches bei den Vorsokratikern, *Neue Jahr-*

can be made only if the Hippocratic covenant is taken as the basis for speculations and generalizations which are not warranted by any additional evidence. Granted that the covenant is determined by a concept of spiritual kinship between teacher and pupil, it is nowhere attested that the same idea prevailed in all schools and guilds of the pre-classical era, or in any of them for that matter.[10] Surely, it is not permissible to conclude from the covenant that the lack of such evidence in regard to other than medical teaching in the 6th and early 5th centuries is merely fortuitous. For it is uncertain when the Hippocratic Oath was composed, and the document which itself needs explanation and identification cannot possibly serve as the starting point for theorizing about otherwise unknown circumstances.[11] There is no reason, then, to assume that the adoption of the pupil by the teacher was a common characteristic of archaic education. Nor is such a practice known to have been customary in ancient scientific or practical training at any other time.[12]

bücher f. Wissenschaft u. Jugendbildung, V, 1929, pp. 19-20. This article, in spite of its importance, is strangely neglected in the literature on the Oath.

[10] Hoffmann, loc. cit., says: "Über andere als ärztliche Schulen haben wir aus jener Zeit leider nur Legenden, aber diese Legenden sagen uns ganz Ähnliches. In dem Bunde der Pythagoreer z. B. war die Treue unter den Schülern des Meisters wie die Treue zwischen Brüdern: Damon und Phintias. Die geistigen Söhne des Meisters sind eben Brüder." Hoffmann himself, then, admits that these stories portray situations only distantly related to those of the Oath, for he speaks only of "similarity." Note, moreover, that the legend of Damon and Phintias to which alone Hoffmann refers in proof of his statement concerns events taking place in the 4th century B. C., in the time of Dionysius of Syracuse; cf. p. 472, 1 ff. [Diels-Kranz]. In view of the uncertainty in regard to the history of the old Pythagorean school (cf. above, pp. 18 f.), it is impossible simply to reconstruct conditions of the 6th century on the evidence of the 4th century. Finally, even if the old Pythagorean society was a fraternity and was based on a spiritual kinship with the master, Pythagoras would not necessarily be the direct teacher of his pupils as is the master of the covenant; he would be the teacher and father of all Pythagoreans, even of those who lived long after him, because he was the founder of the school. In how far the covenant is determined also by a concept of spiritual kinship between teacher and pupil will be discussed below, p. 57, n. 10.

[11] For the divergent assumptions concerning the date of the Oath, cf. below, pp. 55 ff. Hoffmann's thesis which presupposes the pre-Sophistic origin of the Oath without adducing any proof can be characterized only as ignotum per ignotius.

[12] S. Nittis, The Authorship and Probable Date of the Hippocratic Oath, Bulletin of the History of Medicine, VIII, 1940, pp. 1012 ff., who takes the covenant as the statute of a medical fraternity around 420 B. C., comparable to that of other

There is one particular historical setting, however, one particular province of Greek pedagogics where a counterpart of the Hippocratic covenant can be found: the Pythagoreans of the 4th century apparently were wont to honor those by whom they had been instructed as their fathers by adoption. So Epaminondas is said to have done; and in Epaminondas' time it was told of Pythagoras himself that he had revered his teacher as a son reveres his father.[13] If the Hippocratic covenant is viewed against the background of such testimony, the specific form in which the pupil is here bound to his teacher is no longer an unexplainable and isolated phenomenon. Compared with Pythagorean concepts of teaching and learning as they were evolved in the 4th century B. C., the vow of the medical student assumes definite historical meaning.[14]

This result seems to imply that the covenant as a whole must be influenced by Pythagorean philosophy. The agreement between the Hippocratic treatise and the Pythagorean reports concerns so unusual a circumstance that they are most unlikely to be independent of each other. Nor is it probable that the Pythagoreans derived their pattern of instruction from a medical manifesto that in the range of medical education and indeed of general education is without parallel.[15] Nevertheless one should hesitate to claim Pythagorean origin for the covenant by reason of one feature only, even if it be the main feature of this document.[16] But as matters stand, all the other demands enjoined upon the pupil may likewise be explained

fraternal societies of this time and later centuries, has not succeeded in finding one instance where in such organizations the pupil was adopted by the teacher.

[13] Cf. Diodorus, X, 11, 2: καὶ πατὴρ αὐτοῦ (sc. of Epaminondas) θεὸς ἐγένετο δι' εὔνοιαν (sc. his teacher Lysis); cf. Plutarch, De Genio Socratis, ch. 13, 583 C: . . . πατὴρ . . . ἐπιγραφείς. That the expression does not indicate a particular attachment of Epaminondas to Lysis is evident from what Diodorus, X, 3, 4, says about Pythagoras' relation to his teacher, Pherecydes: ὡσανεί τις υἱὸς πατέρα (Aristoxenus, cf. p. 44, 34 [Diels-Kranz]). Aristoxenus, too, relates of Epaminondas, p. 104, 3 [Diels-Kranz]: καὶ πατέρα τὸν Λῦσιν ἐκάλεσεν (for the source of this passage, cf. ibid., p. 103, n. 13). In these passages which Hoffmann apparently overlooked the father-son relation is expressly attested, and it is supposed to exist between the pupil and his teacher, just as in the Hippocratic Oath.

[14] Hoffmann, then, was fundamentally right in his suggestion that the Hippocratic Oath and Pythagorean doctrine are related, though the details of his argument are erroneous.

[15] Cf. above, p. 42.   [16] Cf. above, p. 39.

only in connection with Pythagorean views and customs, or at least they are compatible with them.

To take those duties first which the pupil acknowledges in regard to his mentor: he is asked to share his life with his teacher and to support him with money if need be.[17] This statement usually is considered an extravagant exaggeration that cannot be taken at its face value. Or, to avoid the stumbling block of excessive and improbable magnanimity, the words are said really to signify that the pupil should share with his master his livelihood, not his life, and if need be support him with money. Such an interpretation, however, itself falls prey to the objection that it gives to certain terms an unusual sense and makes the two stipulations of which the sentence consists meaningless repetitions.[18] In the light of what is known about the Pythagoreans the words chosen ring true. That the Pythagorean pupil shared his money with his teacher if necessary, one may readily believe. To support his father was the son's duty, even according to common law. This obligation was the more binding for the Pythagorean who was taught to honor his parents above all others.[19] But the Pythagorean also came to his teacher's assistance in all the vicissitudes of life, wherever and whenever he was needed: he tended

[17] Cf. above, p. 2, 5-6.

[18] For the former view, cf. e. g. Jones, *Hippocrates*, I, p. 292: " Indeed, such clauses could never be enforced; if they could have been, and if a physician had one or two rich pupils, his financial position would have been enviable." *Ibid.*, p. 295: " These (sc. clauses) might well contain promises to the teacher couched in extravagant language if taken literally, but which were intended to be interpreted in the spirit rather than in the letter." For the reinterpretation of the text, cf. e. g. Jones, *The Doctor's Oath*, p. 9: " To make him partner in my livelihood, and when he is in need of money to share mine with him "; Deichgräber, *op. cit.*, p. 31: " Mit ihm den Unterhalt zu teilen und ihn mitzuversorgen, falls er Not leidet." If pupil and teacher share their livelihood, how can the one be in need without the other being in need also? Or how could the one support the other in such a case? For βίος in the sense in which I have translated it, cf. the *Oath* itself, above, p. 2, 16; 26. Incidentally, Deichgräber, *op. cit.*, n. 7, rightly rejects as unwarranted Ziebarth's interpretation, *op. cit.*, p. 97, according to which the second part of the sentence is supposed to mean that if need be the pupil has to pay the teacher's debts.

[19] For the Pythagorean insistence on the reverence to be paid to parents, cf. Diogenes Laertius, VIII, 23: ἀνθρώπων δὲ μάλιστα τοὺς γονέας (sc. τιμᾶν); cf. p. 469, 12 ff. [Diels-Kranz] (Aristoxenus). In addition, one must remember that, according to Pythagorean doctrine, even friends shared everything, if one of them had lost his property, cf. below, p. 46, n. 25.

him in illness; he procured burial for him. All this is admiringly reported of Pythagoras himself.[20] The Pythagorean pupil was indeed supposed to share his life with his master, as the son does with his father. He did much more than advance money to him in case of an emergency.[21]

Next, the Hippocratic covenant admonishes the pupil to regard his teacher's offspring as his brothers, and without fee and covenant to teach them his art if they wish to learn it.[22] That the teacher's children should be the pupil's brothers naturally follows from the fact that the disciple acknowledges his master as his father. Thus the teacher's sons and his pupils become one flesh and blood.[23] But the preference shown for the interest of the members of the family, the unselfishness commended in the relationship to them, the confi-

[20] Cf. Diodorus, X, 3, 4, and above, p. 43, n. 13. The same story is told by Iamblichus, *De Vita Pythagorica*, 183-84, who concludes with the following words: οὕτω περὶ πολλοῦ τὴν περὶ τὸν διδάσκαλον ἐποιεῖτο σπουδήν. This statement is perhaps taken from Nicomachus, cf. Rohde, *op. cit.*, p. 159, but the story itself is older, as is clear from Diodorus and also from Aristoxenus, cf. above, p. 43, n. 13. For the Pythagorean emphasis on the importance of an appropriate burial, cf. Plutarch, *De Genio Socratis*, 585 E.

[21] The importance which such a life companionship had for the Pythagoreans in general is evident also from the name later given to them: κοινόβιοι, Iamblichus, *De Vita Pythagorica*, 29; cf. also the term συμβίωσις as characteristic of the relationship between the brothers, *ibid.*, 81.

[22] Cf. above, p. 2, 7-8. Concerning the exact meaning of the term "covenant," συγγραφή, cf. below, p. 47, n. 29. Deichgräber, *op. cit.*, n. 9, is certainly right in rejecting the interpretation "Schuldschein" as opposed to "barer Lohn" (μισθός) proposed by Th. Meyer-Steineg–W. Schonack, *Hippokrates, Über Aufgaben u. Pflichten d. Arztes, Kleine Texte*, 1913, nr. 120. Such a meaning of the word is not attested.

[23] Note that the pupil is asked to consider his teacher's children (γένος τὸ ἐξ αὐτοῦ) as his "male brothers" (ἀδελφοὶ ἄρρενες). Jones, *op. cit.*, p. 9, translates "brothers"; he thinks that the word ἄρρενες is "quite otiose" (*ibid.*, p. 43, n. 1). Deichgräber, *op. cit.*, p. 31, translates "männliche Geschwister." Earlier interpretations are collected and rejected by Daremberg, *op. cit.*, p. 6, n. 3. Daremberg himself translates "propres frères," *ibid.*, p. 5. Yet in Greek law the rights of kin differ as to male and female lineage, the former preceding the latter; cf. W. Erdmann, *Die Ehe im alten Griechenland*, 1934, pp. 117 ff.; pp. 125-6. ἀδελφοὶ ἄρρενες therefore probably means "brothers of male lineage" (for ἄρρενες in this sense, cf. e. g. Isaeus, VII, 20). Thus the relationship between adopted and real children is made as close as possible. Note that in *Carmen Aureum*, l. 4 (quoted below, p. 46, n. 25) the ἄγχιστ' ἐγγεγαῶτες are mentioned after the parents. They constitute the so-called ἀγχιστεία which is contrasted with the relatives of female lineage even in the late laws of Charondas, cf. Diodorus, XII, 15, 2, and Erdmann, *op. cit.*, p. 134, n. 62.

dence put in their reliability without any insistence on formal guarantees—all these features are characteristic of Pythagorean ethics.[24] The Pythagoreans were admonished to turn to their brothers first, and to make friends with them before all others outside the family. Moreover, all Pythagoreans considered themselves brothers and were believed, like brothers, to have divided their earthly goods among themselves. Their unquestioned belief in their brothers' trustworthiness did not falter even in the face of death.[25] Under these circumstances, how could the Pythagorean do other than teach his adopted brothers without fee the knowledge which he had acquired? What assurances could he expect or ask of them before he instructed them in the art that he had learned from their father?

Finally, the fact that in the Hippocratic covenant teaching is divided into precepts, oral instruction and the other learning,[26] is best understood as a Pythagorean classification. The precepts of Pythagoras, handed down from one generation to the other, were greatly renowned throughout the centuries. "Oral instruction" and "learning" were the two categories under which Aristoxenus listed all that was "taught and said" in Pythagorean circles, and all that the members of the school tried "to learn and remember."[27]

[24] That the form of a "Hausgemeinschaft" which is envisaged in the Hippocratic covenant is also typically Pythagorean will be shown below, pp. 57 f.

[25] For the seeking of their brothers' friendship, cf. Sotion, *Fragmenta Philosophorum Graecorum*, II, p. 47 [Mullach]: οἱ ἀδελφοὺς παρέντες καὶ ἄλλους φίλους ζητοῦντες παραπλήσιοι τοῖς τὴν ἑαυτῶν γῆν ἐῶσι, τὴν δὲ ἀλλοτρίαν γεωργοῦσιν (Sotion is a Neo-Pythagorean of the 1st century A. D.; cf. F. Susemihl, *Geschichte der Griechischen Literatur*, II, 1892, p. 332, n. 459); cf. *Carmen Aureum*, 1. 4: σούς τε γονεῖς τίμα, τούς τ' ἄγχιστ' ἐγγεγαῶτας; but the statements seem to echo old tradition, cf. the insistence on family relations, Diogenes Laertius, VIII, 23, quoted above, p. 44, n. 19; cf. also below, pp. 57 f. For the Pythagorean communism, cf. Diodorus, X, 3, 5: ὅτι ἐπειδάν τινες τῶν συνήθων ἐκ τῆς οὐσίας ἐκπέσοιεν, διῃροῦντο τὰ χρήματα αὐτῶν ὡς πρὸς ἀδελφούς. Cf. also Aristoxenus, p. 472, 16 ff. [Diels-Kranz], and Diogenes Laertius, VIII, 10; Gellius, *Noctes Atticae*, I, 9, 12. For the Pythagorean willingness to respond unhesitatingly to every demand made by one of their brothers, cf. the famous story of Phintias and Damon, Aristoxenus, p. 472, 1 ff. [Diels-Kranz]. Note especially ἡ προσποίητος πίστις (ibid., p. 472, 7), and ἔφη οὖν ὁ Διονύσιος θαυμάσαι τε καὶ ἐρωτῆσαι, εἰ ἔστιν ὁ ἄνθρωπος οὗτος, ὅστις ὑπομενεῖ θανάτου γενέσθαι ἐγγυητής (ibid., p. 472, 19).

[26] Cf. above, p. 2, 8-11.

[27] The terms used in the covenant are: παραγγελίη, ἀκρόησις, ἡ λοιπὴ μάθησις. For the first of these, cf. Aristoxenus, p. 477, 13 [Diels-Kranz]: παραγγέλματα (sc. of Pythagoras). For the second and third, cf. μαθήσεις καὶ ἀκροάσεις, Aristoxenus,

58

That knowledge, according to the covenant, is to be imparted to a closed circle of selected people alone, most assuredly is in agreement with those principles on which the transmission of Pythagorean doctrine was based. The Pythagoreans differed from all other philosophical sects in that they did not divulge their teaching to everybody.[28] They carefully examined those who wished to join them. It is attested even that they exacted an oath from the pupil who was to be admitted, just as the Hippocratic treatise speaks of outsiders who sign the covenant and take an oath before they are allowed to participate in the course of studies.[29]

To sum up: not only the main feature of the covenant, the father-

ibid., p. 467, 18. The exact meaning of these words is difficult to ascertain. Παραγγέλματα are maxims, perhaps similar to what in other reports are called ἀκούσματα, short practical rules without rational explanation, cf. p. 463, 33 [Diels-Kranz]; ἀκροάσεις probably are lectures; and μάθησις should comprise all other studies, whether theoretical or practical. Similarly the terms may also be used in the Hippocratic covenant. Cf. also next note. Whatever the correct explanation may be, one need not agree with Jones' statement, *op. cit.*, p. 43, n. 1: "... I feel sure that all scholars will consider the division of instruction into παραγγελίη, ἀκρόησις, and ἡ λοιπή μάθησις curious and unusual."

[28] Cf. Diogenes Laertius, VIII, 15, quoted above, p. 37, n. 121 (Aristoxenus), and in general Zeller, *op. cit.*, I, 1, pp. 315 ff. On account of the restriction of teaching demanded in the covenant one cannot explain παραγγελίη, ἀκρόησις, μάθησις (cf. preceding note) by parallels taken from non-Pythagorean schools of philosophy, or from other Hippocratic writings (cf. *e. g.* Daremberg, *op. cit.*, p. 7, n. 5; Jones, *op. cit.*, p. 9, n. 2). For these schools were open to everybody, and ἀκρόησις in Ps. Hippocrates, Παραγγελίαι, ch. XII, means "lecture before a crowd," just as the Παραγγελίαι themselves with which Jones compares the παραγγελίη of the covenant (*op. cit.*, p. 9, n. 2) formed a published book available to every reader. Incidentally, Jones, *op. cit.*, p. 45, refers to the Pythagoreans who, he says, perhaps held meetings from which outsiders were excluded. But he does not make use of this parallel for the interpretation of the *Oath*.

[29] For the Pythagorean Oath. cf. below, pp. 53 f. The covenant refers to pupils who are συγγεγραμμένοι τε καὶ ὡρκισμένοι νόμῳ ἰητρικῷ; Jones, *op. cit.*, p. 9, translates: "who have signed the indenture and sworn obedience to the physician's Law." But Deichgräber's rendering, *op. cit.*, p. 31: "vertraglich verpflichtet und vereidigt nach ärztlichem Brauch" seems more correct. The ξυγγραφή referred to here obviously is the same from which the teacher's children are exempted, cf. above, p. 45; but it is hardly identical with the covenant which the *Oath* contains, cf. below, p. 49. Nittis, *op. cit.*, p. 1019, says that the phrase implies that "others (*sc.* those who were not sons of physicians) had to qualify by a test, enrollment in the society, which naturally meant meeting the financial obligations of the association, taking the *Oath* and the payment of tuition." Not only does the covenant not concern societies, but as far as I can see, ξυγγραφή never has the meaning given to it by Nittis.

son relationship between teacher and pupil, but also all the detailed stipulations concerning the duties of the pupil can be paralleled by doctrines peculiar to the followers of Pythagoras.[30] If related to Pythagoreanism, the specific formulas used in the covenant acquire meaning and definiteness. What otherwise appears exaggerated, or strange, or even fictitious, thus becomes the adequate expression of a real situation. Since the rules proposed show no affinity with any other Greek educational theory or practice, it seems permissible to claim that the Hippocratic covenant is inspired by Pythagorean doctrine.

[30] As far as I am aware, my interpretation has covered all the points mentioned in the covenant, except the payment of a teaching-fee by the outside student,. a regulation to be inferred from the fact that fees are remitted to the children of the master (cf. above, p. 45). The evidence available does not indicate, whether the Pythagoreans took money for instruction. But even Hippocrates taught medicine for a fee (cf. Plato, *Protagoras*, 311 b), and many philosophers charged money for their courses.

III

THE UNITY OF THE DOCUMENT

Covenant and ethical code, the two parts of which the so-called Hippocratic Oath consists, in the preserved text form a unity. Without any marked transition the first section is followed by the second.[1] Is there any reason for believing that the two have not always belonged together?

It seems certain that the obligations laid down in the covenant and in the ethical code are assumed by the physician simultaneously, that is, at the moment of his entering the medical profession as a practitioner in his own right. The promise to help the teacher and the stipulation concerning the teaching to be given to others point to the fact that he who takes the Oath has become an independent craftsman.[2] In the same way the rules regarding the practitioner's behavior are best understandable if imposed upon the doctor who is now starting out on his career. For as long as the pupil is still under the supervision of his teacher, his actions of necessity are regulated by his master's orders. In short, covenant and ethical code are signed together, not by the beginner but rather by the student who has completed his course.[3]

---

[1] It should be noted, however, that the covenant is given in infinitives, whereas the code is given in the first person. That this difference in style is an indication of archaic speech Deichgräber, *op. cit.*, p. 30, n. 3, has assumed but has not proved; that it is indicative of an original independence of the two sections is quite possible. Perhaps the covenant originally was used in various fields of instruction and was only taken over into the medical manifesto; if that were so, it would be easier to understand why the covenant refers to " the art " instead of to medicine. This, no doubt, would be a better explanation of this strange fact than the one given by Jones, *op. cit.*, pp. 50-51, who says that the physician " here called his profession, with glorious arrogance, ' the art '." Incidentally, the juxtaposition of aorist and future tenses which Jones blames as incorrect, *op. cit.*, p. 7; p. 43, n. 1, is not an uncommon usage, cf. Kühner-Gerth, *Griechische Grammatik*, II, 1, § 389, p. 195 A 7, esp. p. 197 *finis*.

[2] Moreover, as Deichgräber has rightly pointed out, *op. cit.*, p. 32, the covenant mentions another oath, apparently sworn before instruction begins.

[3] Cf. Deichgräber, *op. cit.*, p. 32: " . . . der Schwörende, offenbar ein Schüler, der nach Abschluss der Ausbildung in die Praxis geht, ..." Jones, *op. cit.*, p. 44; pp. 56 ff., seems to be of the same opinion, but he characterizes the covenant as an agreement between pupil and teacher, while he calls the ethical code an

Moreover the two parts are a spiritual unity. For it is not true, contrary to what is sometimes claimed, that the covenant exhibits a realistic business attitude, whereas the ethical code is determined by a lofty and exalted standard of conduct.[4] The agreement concerning teaching and the rules of professional behavior both reflect the same idealistic outlook on human affairs, they are steeped in Pythagorean doctrine. The same can be said of the preamble and the peroration by which the document is introduced and concluded as one coherent formula.

In the invocation, Apollo the physician, Asclepius and his children, and all the gods and goddesses are made witnesses of the vow to be taken.[5] That all the divine powers are called upon is the usual form in which an ancient oath, at least an oath of some importance, is pronounced, for this makes the protestation all the more solemn.[6] That Apollo the physician and his son Asclepius are named in particular is quite appropriate for a medical oath. It is also in agreement with Pythagorean views that a member of the medical profession should invoke these deities. According to Aristoxenus, the art of selecting the right food and drink for the human regimen, in the belief of the Pythagoreans, had first been practiced by Apollo and Paeon, while later it was taken over by the physicians, the sons of Asclepius. The Pythagorean doctor, the healer of diseases by diet, then, must have revered precisely the gods whom the Oath addresses.[7]

obligation toward the society of physicians. There is no reason for such a distinction, cf. below, pp. 61-62. It is true, as O. Temkin suggests, that because in ancient medicine the apprentice assisted his master in his practice (cf. *e. g.* Ps. Hippocrates, *Prorrhetikon*, II, IX, p. 20 L.), the ethical rules might apply to the student. Cf. also C. Singer, *A Short History of Medicine*, 1928, p. 17. Yet for the reasons just given it seems more likely that the *Oath* was administered after the teaching had ended and the pupil became responsible for his own actions.

[4] Cf. Deichgräber, *op. cit.*, p. 34; p. 38. Deichgräber fails to explain how statements of so different an ethos should ever have become a unity. Jones, who also sharply distinguishes the two parts, seems not to find any difference in regard to the ethical standards though in his opinion the covenant is somewhat at variance with the code, cf. especially, *op. cit.*, p. 43.

[5] Cf. above, p. 2, 2-4.

[6] Cf. E. Ziebarth, *De iure iurando*, 1892, pp. 17 ff.; Deichgräber, *op. cit.*, n. 13.

[7] Cf. p. 475, 32 f. [Diels-Kranz] (quoted above, p. 24, n. 65). Apollo the physician, as the *Oath* has it, obviously is Apollo and Paeon of whom Aristoxenus speaks; the two were often merged into one deity of medicine; cf. H. Usener, *Götternamen*, 1896, pp. 153 ff. Note that contrary to Deichgräber, *op. cit.*, p. 42, Apollo here is

That Asclepius' divine children, Panaceia and Hygieia, are called upon in addition is not astounding. The names of all the members of the divine medical family come naturally to the mind of the believer in Apollo and Asclepius when he takes upon himself those obligations that will guide his future life as a physician.[8]

Having invoked the gods as witnesses and having bound himself to live in purity and holiness, justice and forbearance, he who swears asks that he may enjoy his life and art in fame if the vow is kept inviolate; if it is not carried out, the opposite shall befall him.[9] Does this peroration indicate that in his very heart the physician is motivated not by ethical standards but rather by the wish to attain success? Is it his reputation that he wants to see enhanced by all his actions and that he forswears in case of his failure to fulfil his obligations?[10] This can hardly be the meaning of the words in question. For it is not fame or a good name among his clients for which the juror prays, it is fame for all time among all men, it is immortal fame that is here implored or renounced.[11] Such a wish one cannot reasonably call aspiring to a good reputation in the interest of business, though a good reputation was of great practical

not necessarily the Delphic god, the god of purity. The Delphic Apollo renounces medicine in favor of his son Asclepius, cf. Wilamowitz, *Der Glaube der Hellenen*, II, 1932, p. 35. Nor is he commonly regarded as patron of the physicians (Deichgräber, *ibid.*); statements to this effect, such as Callimachus, *Hymnus in Apollinem*, II, 45-6, are very rare. But for the Pythagoreans who reformed medicine according to their concept of purity and who introduced music into medicine (cf. p. 467, 13-15 [Diels-Kranz]), the Delphic Apollo may indeed have been identical with the god of medicine.

[8] For Hygieia and Panaceia as daughters of Asclepius, cf. *e. g. Paean Erythraeus in Aesculapium*, ed. I. U. Powell, *Collectanea Alexandrina*, 1925, p. 136.

[9] Cf. above, p. 2, 25-27. That the prayer for divine blessing is coupled with an execration is typical for a solemn oath; cf. R. Hirzel, *Der Eid*, 1902, p. 138; cf. also H. Schöne, *Sokrates*, I, 1913, p. 127; Deichgräber, *op. cit.*, n. 14. It should also be emphasized that it is usual to invoke the gods at the beginning, while at the end only the consequences that will ensue in this world are mentioned; cf. Hirzel, *op. cit.*, p. 69.

[10] Cf. Deichgräber, *op. cit.*, pp. 35-36, who sees in the wish for fame the confirmation of his opinion that even here the utilitarian point of view is not set aside. The physician's regard for his reputation, he thinks, is only tempered by his concern for what is right, *ibid.*, p. 41.

[11] Cf. above, p. 2, 26-27: δοξαζομένῳ παρὰ πᾶσιν ἀνθρώποις ἐς τὸν ἀεὶ χρόνον. The expression is as tautological as the words of Plato, *Symposium*, 208 c: κλέος ἐς τὸν ἀεὶ χρόνον ἀθάνατον καταθέσθαι.

importance for the ancient doctor.[12] Rather is this prayer characteristic of the Greek love for glory, of the ancient belief in eternal fame on this earth as a stimulus to all good deeds. No less a man than Solon, in exactly the words of the Oath, asks for renown among all future generations in recompense for what he has done and written. In the same vein Plato acknowledges that the craving for undying fame is the real motive of all great achievements.[13]

That such an insistence on glory is in the opinion of the Greeks entirely compatible with an idealistic attitude can be proved by many instances. Even the earliest philosopher who upheld a philanthropic and moral belief against the philosophy of success saw in glory the righteous aim of human actions.[14] Nor did the Pythagoreans shun this goal. Aristoxenus reports that they were opposed only to such glory as consists in the approbation of the many, but thought it foolish to despise all fame.[15] It is for this reason that glory, though sometimes deprecated by the Pythagoreans and grouped together with the vices, in other instances is extolled as praiseworthy.[16] Most important: the Pythagoreans, too, were striving for that glory which

[12] I am the last to deny the significance which the physician's regard for reputation had in ancient medicine; cf. L. Edelstein, *Problemata*, IV, 1931, chap. III. But the attitude outlined in the *Oath* is enjoined in opposition to the realities and exigencies of daily life; here an attempt is made to better existing conditions, to remedy the rather deplorable state of affairs, cf. below, p. 59.

[13] Cf. Solon, I, 3-4: ὄλβον μοι πρὸς θεῶν μακάρων δότε καὶ πρὸς ἁπάντων/ ἀνθρώπων αἰεὶ δόξαν ἔχειν ἀγαθήν. Plato, *Symposium*, 208 c ff.; cf. also Pindar, *Isthmiae*, IV, 12; and in general J. Burkhardt, *Griechische Kulturgeschichte*, ed. J. Oeri, IV³, pp. 233 ff. (for the heroic time, *ibid.*, p. 17).

[14] I am thinking of the so-called *Anonymus Iamblichi*, 89 [Diels-Kranz]; cf. especially II, p. 402, 19-20 [Diels-Kranz]; cf. in general W. Capelle, *Die Griechische Philosophie*, II, 1, p. 24 (Göschen nr. 858) and also R. Roller, *Untersuchungen zum Anonymus Iamblichi*, Diss. Tübingen, 1931. Cf. below p. 53, n. 18.

[15] Cf. p. 473, 32 ff. [Diels-Kranz]: ἀνόητον μὲν εἶναι καὶ τὸ πάσῃ καὶ παντὸς δόξῃ προσέχειν . . . ἀνόητον δ' εἶναι καὶ πάσης ὑπολήψεώς τε καὶ δόξης καταφρονεῖν. (In the index of Kranz this passage is said to deal with δόξα in the sense of "opinion"; but δόξα παρὰ τῶν πολλῶν, lines 33-4, clearly is "fame"; note also the connection in which the passage is quoted by Iamblichus). A very similar statement is found in Iamblichus, *Protrepticus*, ch. 6, p. 40, 7 [Pistelli]; cf. also Iamblichus, *De Vita Pythagorica*, 72 (Apollonius), cf. Rohde, *op. cit.*, p. 137.

[16] Cf. such passages as p. 471, 23 [Diels-Kranz] (φιλοτιμία, ἐπιθυμία, ὀργή), or Iamblichus, *De Vita Pythagorica*, 69 (δόξα, πλοῦτος); cf. also *ibid.*, 188; 226. On the other hand, cf. *ibid.*, 223: . . . τὴν σωτηρίαν τῆς ἐννόμου δόξης, δι' ἣν αὐτός τε μόνα τὰ δοκοῦντα ἑαυτῷ ἔπραττε . . . .

makes a man's name live for all time to come. Pythagoras himself was said to have exhorted his pupils to philosophical endeavor by stating that "education stays with men unto death, and for some it brings immortal fame even after death."[17] No doubt, the Pythagoreans approved of the desire for fame. The physician who prays for glory does not violate the code of Pythagorean ethics.[18]

Yet one may object: even granted that the content of the invocation and the peroration seems to be Pythagorean, were the followers of Pythagoras allowed to take an oath, to swear in the names of the gods? Certainly some Pythagorean sources stipulate that one should not swear by the gods, but should rather make oneself the witness of one's own words.[19] Still this hardly means that the Pythagoreans intended to ban all oaths and all invocations of divine witnesses. No Greek could ever have gone that far.[20] It is true, "Pythagoras" tried to remedy the notorious Greek predilection for making oaths. Yet the aim of the Pythagoreans was the restriction, not the abolition of vows. As Diodorus expressly states, in the opinion of the school, an oath should be sworn only on rare occasions.[21] Even the

[17] Cf. Iamblichus, *De Vita Pythagorica*, 42: . . . τῆς δὲ παιδείας καθάπερ οἱ καλοὶ κἀγαθοὶ τῶν ἀνδρῶν μέχρι θανάτου παραμενούσης, ἐνίοις ὒὲ καὶ μετὰ τὴν τελευτὴν ἀθάνατον δόξαν περιποιούσης (from Timaeus through Apollonius [cf. Rohde, *op. cit.*, p. 134; P. Corssen, *Sokrates*, I, 1913, pp. 199 ff.]; "aus . . . Bruchstücken ächter Tradition" [Rohde, *ibid.*]).

[18] Burckhardt, *Griechische Kulturgeschichte*, IV, p. 166; *Vorträge*, p. 198, holds that Pythagoras was the only philosopher who opposed the Greek craving for glory. But Porphyry, *Vita Pythagorae*, 32: φιλοτιμίαν φεύγειν καὶ φιλοδοξίαν (from Diogenes), the only passage quoted by Burckhardt, must be interpreted in the light of the testimony of Aristoxenus referred to above, p. 52, n. 15. In addition it should be noted that the idealistic ethical system to which I have alluded (cf. above, p. 52, n. 14) is known only from Iamblichus who integrates these passages into his *Protrepticus* as the final incentive to the study of philosophy. The name of the author whom he follows is unknown (cf. II, p. 400, n. 1 [Diels-Kranz]). Could he have been a Pythagorean?

[19] Cf. Diogenes Laertius, VIII, 22: μηδ' ὀμνύναι θεούς· ἀσκεῖν γὰρ αὐτὸν δεῖν ἀξιόπιστον παρέχειν (from Androcydes, thus Corssen, *Rh. M.*, LXVII, 1912, p. 258).

[20] Cf. Hirzel, *op. cit.*, p. 112, who points out the difference between this attitude and that of the Jews and Christians.

[21] Diodorus, X, 9, 2: ὅτι Πυθαγόρας παρήγγελε τοῖς μανθάνουσι σπανίως μὲν ὀμνύναι, . . . ; cf. Hirzel, *op. cit.*, pp. 98 ff.; Burckhardt, *Griechische Kulturgeschichte*, III, p. 320. H. Diels, *Archiv f. Geschichte d. Philosophie*, III, 1890, p. 457, does not do justice to this divergence of the tradition. Diodorus' statement most probably goes back to Aristoxenus on whom he largely depends, cf. E.

late Pythagoreans, though they seem to have been stricter in this respect, did not renounce vows altogether. Just as the physician is supposed to take an oath when he settles down to practice, so those who intended to become members of the Pythagorean society took an oath of allegiance.[22]

At this point, I think, I can say without hesitation that the so-called Oath of Hippocrates is a document, uniformly conceived and thoroughly saturated with Pythagorean philosophy. In spirit and in letter, in form and content, it is a Pythagorean manifesto. The main features of the Oath are understandable only in connection with Pythagoreanism; all its details are in complete agreement with this system of thought. If only one or another characteristic had been uncovered, one might consider the coincidence fortuitous. Since the concord is complete, and since there is no counterinstance of any other influence, all indications point to the conclusion that the Oath is a Pythagorean document.

Schwartz, s.v. Diodorus, Pauly-Wissowa, V, p. 679, for it is in perfect agreement with Aristoxenus' compromising attitude, cf. above, p. 30, n. 92.

[22] For the Neo-Pythagoreans in general, cf. Zeller, op. cit., III, 2, p. 146 (I, 1, p. 462, n. 7), and again for the similarity of the Pythagorean attitude with that of the Essenians, ibid., III, 2, p. 284, n. 5; cf. also Hirzel, op. cit., pp. 99-100. Julian, VII, 236 D, probably in opposition to the Christians, says: . . . οὔτε τὸ ὅρκῳ χρῆσθαι προπετῶς τοῖς τῶν θεῶν ὀνόμασιν [sc. ἐπέτρεπεν]. Pétrequin, op. cit., p. 173, was the first to compare the Hippocratic Oath with Pythagorean fidelity to a vow.

IV

DATE AND PURPOSE OF THE OATH

The origin of the Hippocratic Oath having been established, it should now be possible to determine the time when the Oath was written and the purpose for which it was intended. What answers regarding these questions are to be deduced from the analysis of the document?

As for the date, it seems one must conclude that the Oath was not composed before the 4th century B. C. All the doctrines followed in the treatise are characteristic of Pythagoreanism as it was envisaged in the 4th century B. C.[1] It is most probable even that the Oath was outlined only in the second half or towards the end of the 4th century, for the greater part of the parallels adduced are taken from the works of pupils of Aristotle.

Yet is such an assumption not irreconcilable with certain external data? Aristophanes, it is said, in one of his comedies performed in 411 B. C. makes mention of the Hippocratic Oath.[2] Not even the ancient commentators dared to claim that the Hippocrates referred to here was the physician of Cos. Eager as they were to find allusions to great historical names wherever that was possible, and even where it was most unlikely, in the case in question they expressly stated that the Hippocrates whom Aristophanes names was an Athenian general.[3] Nor can one infer from linguistic considerations that the

---

[1] The only exceptions to this statement are the references to Sotion and to the *Carmen Aureum* (cf. above, p. 46, n. 25). I think it permissible to say that, the whole argument taken into consideration, these two instances do not invalidate the claim that the interpretation given rests on the testimony of 4th century authors.

[2] D. Triller in the 18th century seems to have been the originator of this claim. Littré first followed him, *op. cit.*, I, p. 31, but later rejected the theory, cf. *ibid.*, II, p. xlviii; IV, p. 610. Pétrequin, however, repeated Triller's argument, *op. cit.*, p. 172, n. 1, and it has again been brought forward by Jones, *op. cit.*, p. 40.

[3] Cf. Aristophanes, *Scholia in Thesmophoriazusas*, ϝ. 273; in *Nubes*, v. 1001; and Daremberg, *op. cit.*, p. 1, n. 1. I must confess that I fail to discover any reference to an Oath of Hippocrates in the lines in question. Euripides swears by Aether, the abode of Zeus (272). The interlocutor asks why he does so instead of swearing τὴν Ἱπποκράτους ξυνοικίαν. This, Jones, *op. cit.*, p. 40, takes to mean: "by the community of Hippocrates." But ξυνοικία is a tenement house in which many families live, and it is apparently the joke of the whole statement that the inter-

Oath was written in the 5th century. Granted for the sake of argument that the great Hippocrates was the author of the Oath; that he was in Athens in the year 421 B. C.; that the words "covenant" and "law" in Athens between March and October, 421, were used interchangeably to cover the same meaning, just as they are supposedly used in the Oath—all this would have no bearing on the date of this document, for it is written in the Ionic, not in the Attic dialect.[4] There is, then, no reason for rejecting the date that seems to follow from the internal evidence on the basis of external data.[5]

On the other hand, one may argue: it is true, the Oath agrees with reports of 4th century writers on Pythagoreanism; yet these accounts, though they stem from the 4th century, must not necessarily describe the Pythagorean system as it was evolved or understood at that time; the passages may in part at least reflect older conditions or reproduce more ancient traditions; the composition of the Hippocratic Oath, therefore, could well fall into an earlier period. However, such reasoning is not probable. I shall not dwell on the fact that the Pythagorean system of the 5th or even of the 6th century is practically unknown, that whatever is reported about the old Pythagorean teaching as a whole is, if not the invention, at least the interpretation of authors of the 4th century.[6] Two of the main pro-

locutor does not understand why the oath should be made by the house of Zeus rather than by the house of Hippocrates. That by ξυνοικία "Aristophanes probably had in mind the opening words of Oath, with their comprehensive ξυνοικία of divinities" (Jones, ibid.), I cannot believe, the less so, since ξυνοικία is never used in the sense required by Jones' interpretation. It should also be noted that Athenaeus, III, 96 e-f, says that "the sons of Hippocrates were ridiculed in comedy for swinishness," a statement which certainly refers to the Aristophanes passages under discussion.

[4] Cf. Nittis, *Bulletin of the History of Medicine*, 1940, p. 1020. I am far from admitting that Nittis' statements concerning the terms νόμος and ξυγγραφή are convincing, but for the reason given above I see no need to go into the details of his theory. In regard to the external evidence, I should mention at least that the Hippocratic *Oath* in reality is first mentioned by Erotianus and by Scribonius Largus in the first century A. D. Erotianus' list of Hippocratic writings probably goes back to Hellenistic sources, but even so the *Oath* would not be attested before the 3rd century B. C. (cf. Deichgräber, *op. cit.*, n. 1).

[5] That the fifth century origin of the *Oath* cannot be proved by reference to general sociological laws has been shown above, p. 41.

[6] Cf. above, pp. 18 f.; in general Ueberweg-Praechter, *op. cit.*, pp. 67 ff.; cf. also *ibid.*, p. 66: "Im allgemeinen gilt, abgesehen von jener Lehre (*sc.* that of metem-

visions of the Oath are connected with theories that are attributed either directly or indirectly to Philolaus, a contemporary of Plato. This makes the turn of the 5th to the 4th century the *terminus post quem* for the composition of the Oath.[7] Moreover, even if one or another ethical precept ascribed to the Pythagoreans by Aristoxenus and accepted in the Hippocratic Oath was held also by older Pythagoreans, the whole program of instruction envisaged in the Oath in conformity with the Pythagorean model is characteristic f 4th century Pythagoreanism; for it presupposes the destruction of the Pythagorean society in the last decades of the 5th century.[8] As Aristoxenus relates, it was after the uprising in Italy that Lysis went to Thebes where he taught Epaminondas and was revered by him as his adopted father. In a letter ascribed to him, Lysis protes's against those who after the dissolution of the society made the Pythagorean dogma available to everybody. Pythagoras himself, Lysis asserts, had charged his daughter never to give his writings to those " outside of the house."[9] Whether this letter is genuine or not, it must have been for some such reasons that Lysis bound Epaminondas to himself as his adopted son. This afforded the only solution which made it possible to initiate outsiders into the Pythagorean doctrine, and yet to keep it a secret, a " family secret," as is also the intention of the Oath.[10] But such a relationship between teacher and pupil could be

psychosis), jedenfalls der Satz, dass wir nur von einer Philosophie der Pythagoreer, nicht des Pythagoras sprechen können, wie dies in der Tat auch schon bei Aristoteles geschieht." And these Pythagoreans, as far as their names are known, are Philolaus and his contemporaries or successors, cf. *ibid.*, p. 61.

[7] For Philolaus and his relation to Plato, cf. *e. g.* Ueberweg-Praechter, *op. cit.*, p. 65 (44 A 5 [Diels-Kranz]) ; cf. above, p. 15 and p. 17.

[8] For the time of the dissolution of the Pythagorean society through which the members of the school were brought from Italy to Greece, cf. Zeller, *op. cit.*, I, 1, pp. 332 ff; Ueberweg-Praechter, *op. cit.*, p. 65; K. v. Fritz, Pythagorean Politics in Southern Italy, 1940, p. 92.

[9] Cf. p. 104, 1 ff. [Diels-Kranz], and Diogenes Laertius, VIII, 42; Hercher, *Epistolographi Graeci*, p. 603, 5. For the authenticity of the letter, cf. p. 421, 12 ff. [Diels-Kranz]. The situation is viewed in the same manner by Aristoxenus, cf. Diogenes Laertius, VIII, 15, and Timaeus, cf. *ibid.*, 54. Nicomachus also summarizes the situation by asserting that the Pythagoreans restricted their teaching to the members of their own families, cf. Iamblichus, *De Vita Pythagorica*, 253; 251; Porphyry, *Vita Pythagorae*, 58. Nicomachus uses the same words ἔξω τῆς οἰκίας which appear in the letter of Lysis.

[10] Cf. above, p. 45. The belief in a spiritual kinship between teacher and pupil (cf.

instituted only after the disappearance of the great fraternity that had existed before. Only at that moment did the transmission of the Pythagorean doctrine become the concern of the individual Pythagorean; in earlier times it had been promoted by the society itself. The Hippocratic Oath which calls the teacher the adopted father of the pupil can hardly have been composed, therefore, before the 4th century B. C.[11]

Nor is it likely that the document is of later origin. In the 4th century B. C. Pythagoreanism reached the peak of its importance. Its influence gradually began to wane from the beginning of the Hellenistic period. When in the 1st century B. C. the Pythagorean system was revived and again became a potent factor in philosophical speculation, it took on traits very different from those which are characteristic of the earlier dogma and the prescripts of the Oath.[12]

above, p. 41) may also have been influential in the founding of this system of education, for even in their ethical behavior the Pythagoreans were bidden to take toward each other the attitude of the good father toward his children, cf. p. 471, 24 [Diels-Kranz]; *ibid.*, 477, 15 (Aristoxenus), where again this fatherly love is compared with that of the benefactor; both must be free from envy. If men owe to nature their lives, but to education their knowledge of the right life (Diodorus, XII, 13, 3 [Charondas]; cf. Rohde, *op. cit.*, p. 168), the teacher can well be called the spiritual father of the pupil. But basically the insistence on an adoption of the pupil is determined by external factors, by the new situation in which the Pythagoreans found themselves in the 4th century B. C. In this connection it seems worth pointing out that in the Platonic *Phaedo* which is strongly influenced by Pythagorean concepts Socrates is once referred to as the father of his pupils (116 a), just as late Neo-Platonists for whom the Platonic and Pythagorean dogmas coincide, again speak of their teacher as their father and even of the teacher's teacher as their grandfather, cf. Marinus, *Vita Procli*, 29. For the importance of the father-son relation in later mystery cults, cf. R. Reitzenstein, *Die hellenistischen Mysterienreligionen*[3], 1927, p. 20 (cf. also first edition, 1910, p. 27).

[11] That the *Oath* cannot be traced to pre-Sophistic times for the reasons adduced by Hoffmann, has been shown above, p. 42. Meyer-Steineg–Schonack, *op. cit.*, p. 4, assume the date of the 6th century without even attempting to give a proof for their assertion; cf. also Deichgräber, *op. cit.*, n. 24.

[12] For the general development of Pythagoreanism, cf. Ueberweg-Prächter, *op. cit.*, p. 65; pp. 513 ff.; esp. p. 516. Even if the Pythagorean school was not entirely in eclipse in Hellenistic centuries, it certainly had lost its strong hold over the philosophical mind. Yet in the 4th century B. C. Pythagoreanism through Plato, Aristotle and their schools had become a subject of general interest for the educated. As the references in the Middle Comedy prove, the followers of Pythagoras were also figures familiar to everyone. The Neo-Pythagorean movement of the 1st century B. C. is influenced by mystic tendencies; the ascetic features are

Moreover, in Alexandria medical ethics was integrated into the teaching of the medical sects. Closely connected as these newly established schools were with philosophy, Pythagoreanism played no part in their teaching. A direct influence of Pythagorean philosophy on medicine, however, is not probable.[13]

Yet in the 4th century B. C. the Hippocratic Oath in every respect was a timely manifesto. In that period many individual attempts were made to improve medical conditions. Abuses, to be sure, had been criticized even before.[14] But it is in those Hippocratic treatises that were written in the second half of the 4th century or even later, that one finds the first outlines of a system of medical deontology. Moreover, these endeavors at reform were instigated by the reflection on ethical problems as it developed in the rising philosophical schools.[15] Thus a medical ethics devised in accordance with Pythagoreanism is well in agreement with the general trend of thought in that period. On the other hand, from the point of view of 4th century Pythagoreanism it was quite justifiable that those concepts which

overstressed; the practical interest in human affairs which the *Oath* presupposes, cf. below, p. 60, is almost entirely lacking. That is why I cannot believe that the *Oath* is in any way connected with this late teaching.

[13] It has sometimes been claimed that the Hippocratic *Oath* was written in Hellenistic times. The proof offered is the fact that medicine is here divided into dietetics, pharmacology and surgery, cf. Münzer, *Münchener medizinische Wochenschrift*, 1919, p. 309; cf. Körner, *op. cit.*, p. 7. That this division is not typical of Alexandrian medicine has been shown above, p. 20, n. 49. C. Singer, *From Magic to Science*, 1928, p. 18, goes so far as to say: "Despite the Ionic Greek dress in which this formula is known to us, there is evidence that it is of Imperial date, and of Roman rather than of Greek origin"; cf. the same, *A Short History of Medicine*, 1928, pp. 16 ff.: parts earlier than Hippocrates, the *Oath* as such very much later. Singer does not make explicit why he holds this belief.

[14] Cf. especially the surgical books of the *Corpus Hippocraticum* which are usually ascribed to the 5th century; cf. *e. g.* K. Deichgräber, Die Epidemien und das Corpus Hippocraticum, *Abh. Berl. Akad.*, 1933, nr. 3, p. 98. In general L. Edelstein, *Problemata*, IV, pp. 100 ff.

[15] I am referring to the books *Decorum, Physician* and *Precepts*. For their late date and for the Epicurean or Stoic influence on them, cf. Jones in his introduction to these treatises, Loeb vols. I and II; cf. also the chapter "Ancient medical etiquette," *ibid.*, II, pp. xxxiii ff. The Ps. Hippocratic *Law*, another book of this type, has been connected with the Democritean school by Wilamowitz, *Hermes*, LIV, 1919, pp. 46 ff.; cf. however, F. Müller, *Hermes*, LXXV, 1940, pp. 39 ff., who dates the treatise in the 5th century. I was unable to secure this article which is abstracted in *Classical Weekly*, XXXVI, 1942, p. 84.

underlay philosophical instruction were applied also to the teaching of the healing art, and that Pythagorean ethics was infused into the practice of medicine. The school ranked medicine together with music and mantic as the supreme sciences. Medical skill, to its members, was the greatest wisdom attainable by men.[16] The standards of medical education, therefore, could not be set too high. Moreover, the Pythagoreans thought that "love for what is truly noble" manifests itself in practical pursuits and in the sciences—for here the love for good habits and the devotion to them become apparent—and consequently they called the fair and dignified sciences "full of love for the noble." To imbue medicine with the spirit of Pythagorean holiness and purity was a task enjoined by the Pythagorean dogma itself.[17]

It stands to reason, then, that it was in the 4th century B. C. that Pythagorean philosophy led to the formulation of the Hippocratic Oath. Does this imply that the document must have been outlined by a philosopher rather than by a physician? Not at all. The Hippocratic Oath is a program of medical ethics, and there is no reason to question that it was composed by a doctor. But ancient physicians often belonged to philosophical schools or studied with philosophers. The Pythagorean teaching aroused considerable interest among the physicians of the 4th century.[18] It is quite possible that a physician,

[16] Cf. 58 D 1, p. 467, 3 [Diels-Kranz]: τῶν δ' ἐπιστημῶν οὐχ ἥκιστά φασιν τοὺς Πυθαγορείους τιμᾶν μουσικήν τε καὶ ἰατρικὴν καὶ μαντικήν (Aristoxenus); cf. ibid., p. 464, 9: τί σοφώτατον τῶν παρ' ἡμῖν; ἰατρική (old Ἄκουσμα).

[17] Cf. p. 478, 17 ff. [Diels-Kranz]: τὴν ἀληθῆ φιλοκαλίαν ἐν τοῖς ἐπιτηδεύμασι καὶ ἐν ταῖς ἐπιστήμαις ἔλεγεν εἶναι· . . . ὡσαύτως δὲ καὶ τῶν ἐπιστημῶν τε καὶ ἐμπειριῶν τὰς καλὰς καὶ εὐσχήμονας ἀληθῶς εἶναι φιλοκάλους . . . (Aristoxenus). What men gain in the usual pursuits of life only is λάφυρά που τῆς ἀληθινῆς . . . φιλοκαλίας. The term φιλοκαλία itself seems to be preeminently a Peripatetic concept, cf. N. E., 1125 b 12; 1179 b 9; cf. also E. E., 1250 b 34; 1251 b 36. It almost approaches the meaning of "love of honor," cf. Xenophon, Symposium, IV, 15. Zeller's interpretation of the fragment ("Die Wissenschaft . . . kann nur da gedeihen, wo sie mit Lust und Liebe betrieben wird," op. cit., I, 1, p. 462) does not do justice to the words.

[18] Thus Philolaus is mentioned in Meno's history of medicine, 44 A 27 [Diels-Kranz]. Androcydes, a physician, wrote on Pythagorean symbols, cf. C. Hölk; De acusmatis sive symbolis Pythagoricis, Diss. Kiel, 1894, pp. 40 ff.; Corssen, Rh. M., LXVII, 1912, pp. 240 ff. Another Pythagorean physician of that time (Phaon) is perhaps referred to in a fragment preserved from the Middle Comedy, p. 479, 26 [Diels-Kranz].

strongly impressed by what he had learned from the Pythagoreans either through personal contact or through books, conceived this medical code in conformity with Pythagorean ideals.[19]

One last question remains: what is the purpose of the Oath? Is this document an ideal program with no direct bearing on reality? Or was the Oath actually administered?[20] In my opinion one need not doubt that this vow was made by many an ancient physician, that it was sworn to and regarded by them as their "Golden Rule" of conduct. If it is true that Epaminondas considered his teacher his adopted father, a physician could honor his master in the same way. If it is true that Epaminondas, the great statesman, in his life strove to practice Pythagorean virtue, a physician could do so as well.[21]

To be sure, no special societies of Pythagorean physicians are attested, no guilds are known for which Pythagorean philosophy was the statute of organization. But the covenant is a private agreement between pupil and teacher.[22] The Oath as a whole is hardly an obligation enforced upon the physician by any authority but rather one which he accepted of his own free will. It is not a legal engagement; as the wording indicates, it is a solemn promise given and vouchsafed only by the conscience of him who swears.[23] This again is in keeping with Pythagorean ethics. For the school insisted that all instruction must be based on the willingness of teacher and pupil, on voluntary

[19] That the covenant is probably modelled according to a general pattern of Pythagorean training has been suggested above, p. 49, n. 1. Nevertheless the work as a whole could be that of a physician, and the rules concerning medical conduct could hardly have been drawn by anybody except a practitioner.

[20] Cf. Jones, op. cit., p. 57: "We must clearly understand, however, that the extant evidence does not prove conclusively that the Oath was ever actually administered. It is conceivable that it was a mere ideal, a counsel of perfection expressed in the form of an oath . . . ." Cf. also Deichgräber, op. cit., p. 32 (before he uses the Oath as the basis for his reconstruction of the early history of Greek crafts!): "Für die sichere Beantwortung dieser Fragen (sc. when and where the Oath was sworn) fehlt es an näheren Nachrichten und übertragbaren Analogien."

[21] For the exemplary character of Epaminondas' life, cf. e. g. Nepos, Epaminondas, ch. 3.

[22] Cf. above, p. 40.

[23] Hirzel, op. cit., p. 140, has shown that those oaths which in the end ask for reward or punishment (cf. above, p. 51) are indicative of a transition from the legal to the merely ethical sphere.

rule as well as on voluntary obedience.[24] And was not the whole reform which Pythagoras instituted a reform of the life of the individual, an appeal to man, not as a citizen, but as a private person, to lead a better, a purer, a holier existence? As Plato· saw it, the Pythagorean "way of life" meant not a political or a group movement; Pythagoras wanted to stir up the conscience of the individual.[25] Throughout antiquity many responded to this summons. Certainly, in its application to the task of the physician it also found its devotees.

[24] Cf. p. 470, 35 [Diels-Kranz] (Aristoxenus) : . . . καὶ τὰς μαθήσεις τὰς ὀρθῶς γινομένας ἑκουσίως δεῖν ἔφασαν γίνεσθαι, ἀμφοτέρων βουλομένων, τοῦ τε διδάσκοντος καὶ τοῦ μανθάνοντος· ἀντιτείνοντος γὰρ ὁποτέρου δήποτε τῶν εἰρημένων οὐκ ἂν ἐπιτελεσθῆναι κατὰ τρόπον τὸ προκείμενον ἔργον.

[25] Cf. Plato, *Republic*, X, 600 a ff.; Burckhardt, *Griechische Kulturgeschichte*, III, p. 320; *Vorträge*, pp. 199 ff. It is Burckhardt who has brought out this essential point, proving it from the fact that Plato contrasted Pythagoras and Orpheus with men like Charondas and Solon. In accepting Burckhardt's characterization of the intent of Pythagorean philosophy, I do not wish to pass judgment on the controversy whether the Pythagorean movement in Italy actually was a political movement or not, cf. v. Fritz, *op. cit., passim*. Within the limits of this investigation it is not the early Pythagorean school, but Pythagoreanism as represented in the 4th century B. C. that has to be considered, cf. above, p. 18, and for this form of the Pythagorean dogma Burckhardt's interpretation is undoubtedly correct and in agreement also with the reports of Aristoxenus. Cf. also J. Burnet, *Early Greek Philosophy*[4], 1930, p. 89 (cf. also E. Frank's review of v. Fritz' book, *American Journal of Philology*, LXIV, 1943, pp. 220 ff., which appeared when this study was already in print).

V

CONCLUSION

The so-called Hippocratic Oath has always been regarded as a message of timeless validity. From the interpretation given it follows that the document originated in a group representing a small segment of Greek opinion. That the Oath at first was not accepted by all ancient physicians is certain. Medical writings, from the time of Hippocrates down to that of Galen, give evidence of the violation of almost every one of its injunctions. This is true not only in regard to the general rules concerning helpfulness, continence and secrecy. Such deviations one would naturally expect. But for centuries ancient physicians, in opposition to the demands made in the Oath, put poison in the hands of those among their patients who intended to commit suicide; they administered abortive remedies; they practiced surgery.

At the end of antiquity a decided change took place. Medical practice began to conform to that state of affairs which the Oath had envisaged. Surgery was separated from general practice. Resistance against suicide, against abortion, became common. Now the Oath began to be popular. It circulated in various forms adapted to the varying circumstances and purposes of the centuries.[1] Generally considered the work of the great Hippocrates, its study became part of the medical curriculum. The commentators supposed that the master had written the Oath as the first of all his books and made it incumbent on the beginner to read this treatise first.[2]

Small wonder! A new religion arose that changed the very foundations of ancient civilization. Yet, Pythagoreanism seemed to bridge the gulf between heathendom and the new belief. Christianity found

[1] For the manuscript tradition in general, cf. Jones, *op. cit.*, pp. 2 ff.; 12 ff.; cf. also J. H. Oliver–P. Maas, *Bulletin of the History of Medicine*, VII, 1939, pp. 315 ff. (a medical Paean); and for the *Oath* in non-medical ancient literature, cf. E. Nachmanson, *Symbolae Philologicae, O. A. Danielsson dedicatae*, Upsala, 1932, pp. 185 ff.

[2] Cf. Ps. Oribasius, *Commentarius in Aphorismos Hippocratis*, Basileae, 1535, p. 7. I need not deal here with the historical process by which ancient medical works came to be ascribed to Hippocrates, cf. L. Edelstein, The Genuine Works of Hippocrates, *Bulletin of the History of Medicine*, VII, 1939, pp. 236 ff.; cf. the same, *Problemata*, IV, ch. IV.

itself in agreement with the principles of Pythagorean ethics, its concepts of holiness and purity, justice and forbearance.[3] The Pythagorean god who forbade suicide to men, his creatures, was also the God of the Jews and the Christians. As early as in the " Teaching of the Twelve Apostles " the command was given : " Thou shalt not use philtres; thou shalt not procure abortion; nor commit infanticide." Even the Church Fathers abounded in praise of the high-mindedness of Hippocrates and his regulations for the practice of medicine.[4]

As time went on, the Hippocratic Oath became the nucleus of all medical ethics. In all countries, in all epochs in which monotheism, in its purely religious or in its more secularized form, was the accepted creed, the Hippocratic Oath was applauded as the embodiment of truth. Not only Jews and Christians, but the Arabs, the mediaeval doctors, men of the Renaissance, scientists of the Enlightenment, and scholars of the 19th century embraced the ideals of the Oath.[5] I am not qualified to outline the successive stages of this historical process. But I venture to suggest that he who undertakes to study this development will find it better understandable if he realizes that the Hippocratic Oath is a Pythagorean manifesto and not the expression of an absolute standard of medical conduct.

[3] Cf. above, p. 17, n. 40; p. 54, n. 22, where the coincidence of certain Pythagorean doctrines with Jewish (Essenian) and Christian teachings was noted. Cf. also the material collected by Meibom, op. cit., pp. 131 ff., who speaks of " Hippocratis religiositas."

[4] Cf. the so-called Διαδοχὴ τῶν δώδεκα 'Αποστόλων, The Apostolic Fathers, with an English translation by Kirsopp Lake, I, 1925, pp. 310-312 [Loeb] ; cf. also Gregory of Nazianzus, XXXV, col. 767 A [Migne] ; Hieronymus, Epist., 52, 15 (XXII, col. 539 [Migne]).

[5] It would be difficult here to substantiate this general statement; a few references to the pertinent literature must suffice. For the Jews and Arabs, cf. H. Friedenwald-G. Sarton, with reference to M. Meyerhof, Isis, XXII, 1934, pp. 222-23; cf. also Jones, op. cit., pp. 29 ff.; Deichgräber, op. cit., pp. 38 f. Some mediaeval references are collected ibid., pp. 39-40, cf. also E. Hirschfeld, Deontologische Texte des frühen Mittelalters, Archiv f. Geschichte d. Medizin, XX, 1928, p. 369. For the Renaissance and later centuries the commentaries on the Oath quoted above, p. 25, n. 72, furnish some evidence of the importance of the document; cf. besides S. V. Larkey, The Hippocratic Oath in Elizabethan England, Bulletin of the History of Medicine, IV, 1936, pp. 201 ff. Cf. also Erasmus, Methodus ad Veram Theologiam, ed. H. Holborn, 1933, p. 151; p. 180. For the 18th century, cf. e. g. J. P. Frank, The People's Misery : Mother of Diseases, H. E. Sigerist, Bulletin of the History of Medicine, IX, 1941, p. 100. Goethe, too, took over the principles of the Oath in his Wilhelm Meister, cf. Hoffmann, op. cit., pp. 18 ff.

THE PROFESSIONAL ETHICS OF THE GREEK PHYSICIAN [1]

LUDWIG EDELSTEIN

William Osler, for whom this lecture in the history of medicine is named, has many claims to fame. No one is greater, I venture to think, than that, in the midst of a busy life devoted to the bodily welfare of man, he never for one moment forgot about man's intellectual and moral aspirations. An unexamined life, to use a phrase of Plato, he found not worth living. The physician and scientist turned historian, even philosopher, because he wanted to understand the meaning of human existence. And once he had made his own decision, he also felt impelled to speak out in advocacy of the " Way of Life " he thought he had discovered.

To his truly humanistic teaching—namely that the task and the dignity of the human being consist in the individual's willingness to live up to an ideal and to be of help to others—Osler finally gave expression in categories of William James' pragmatism, the philosophy that gained ascendancy in his later years. On the other hand, he was quite aware of the fact that his creed was not of today or yesterday, but took its origin and was put into practice long ago. When formulating his basic tenets for the last time, he characterized as the heritage of Plato and as " the

[1] The William Osler Lecture in the History of Medicine, Faculty of Medicine, McGill University. This lecture was given in the Amphitheatre of the Montreal General Hospital on December 9, 1955. It is here printed in a somewhat extended form, though substantially unchanged. I have added some footnotes referring to the pertinent literature and giving fuller documentation concerning certain points than was possible in the lecture.

Greek message to modern democracy" that "need for individual reconstruction" with which "is blended the note of individual service to the
community." At the same time, he pointed out that such an idealism once
existed in Greece even in the daily pursuits of men of action. For to the
ancient physician "the love of humanity [was] associated with the love
of his craft—*philanthropia* and *philotechnia*—the joy of working joined in
each one to a true love of his brother." [2]

It is this appreciation of the humanism of the Greek doctor on the
part of the humanist Osler that determined me to choose as my topic the
professional ethics of the Greek physician. No other subject within my
reach seemed more appropriate for a lecture in his memory. I wish to
outline the various ethical positions taken by ancient physicians. In
particular, it will be my aim to find out when and where the idea originated that medicine itself imposes certain obligations upon the physician,
obligations summed up in the magic phrase "love of humanity." For, in
my opinion, this lofty ideal was not the only one in antiquity that
motivated the help proffered by medical men to those who suffer and are
in distress. Over a long period of time other concepts of medicine and
therefore other obligations and duties were held in high esteem. Rome
was not built in one day.

Now at first glance it may seem as if such a contention were in fact
quite unwarranted. For is it not in one of the Hippocratic writings, the
essay called *Precepts,* that the statement occurs which Osler quoted:
"Where there is love of man, there is also love of the art" (ch. 6)? Is
it not said in another Hippocratic book, the treatise *On the Physician,*
that the doctor must be a "lover of man" (ch. 1)? And does not Galen,
no mean judge in these matters, expressly assert that Hippocrates,
Empedocles, Diocles, and not a few of the other early physicians healed
the sick because of their love of mankind (*De Placitis Hippocratis et
Platonis,* ed. I. Müller, p. 765)? In the classical age of Greek civilization, then, the ethic of philanthropy seems already to have been
securely established.

But if one scrutinizes carefully the context in which the word "philanthropy" appears in the so-called Hippocratic writings just mentioned,
he realizes that it means no more than a certain friendliness of disposition, a kindliness, as opposed to any misanthropic attitude. A "philanthropic" doctor in the sense in which the term is used in the treatise

---

[2] *The Old Humanities and the New Science,* 1920, p. 62 f. For Osler's humanism and
his adherence to James' pragmatism, cf. L. Edelstein, "William Osler's Philosophy,"
Bull. Hist. Med. 20, 1946, pp. 280 ff.

On the Physician (ch. 1) will comport himself in a dignified manner; for aggressiveness and obtrusiveness are despicable; sour looks, harshness, arrogance, vulgarity, are disagreeable.[3] Likewise, the Hippocratic *Precepts* (ch. 6) understands by the doctor's "philanthropy" his kindheartedness and his willingness to accommodate his fees to the patient's cirmumstances. He should also treat strangers and paupers, even if they are unable to pay him. That is, he should be charitable, recalling some of the benefits which he may have received himself in the past, or thinking of the good name that his charitableness is likely to make for him in the future. If he acts thus, if such "philanthropy" is present on his part, then also "love of the (medical) art" will be kindled in his patients, a state of mind that greatly contributes to their speedy recovery, especially when they are dangerously sick. No more—and no less—is implied by the famous aphorism: "Where there is love of man, there is also love of the art."[4]

[3] U. Fleischer, *Untersuchungen zu den pseudohippokratischen Schriften* Παραγγελίαι, Περὶ ἰητροῦ *und* Περὶ εὐσχημοσύνης (Neue Deutsche Forschungen, Abt. Klass. Philologie), 1939, pp. 1; 54, seems to take φιλάνθρωπος to refer to "love of mankind." Yet Jones is surely right in translating the word as "kind to all," and μισάνθρωπος, the term contrasted with it immediately afterwards, as "unkind" (*Hippocrates*, II, pp. 311; 313 [Loeb Classical Library]; cf. also E. Littré, *Oeuvres complètes d'Hippocrate*, vol. 9, 1861, pp. 205-7: *humain—dur*).

[4] The usual interpretation, "where there is love of man (on the part of the physician), there is also love of the art (on his part)," is refuted by the immediately following words: "For some patients, though conscious that their condition is perilous, recover their health simply through their contentment with the goodness of the physician." The previous sentence then must contain an assertion as to the patients' attitude, and it can only be "love of the art" felt by them in consequence of the doctor's philanthropy, contentment with the goodness of the physician, of which the author is speaking. In his opinion the question of fees discussed in ch. 6 has psychologically important consequences for the recovery of the sick. If the doctor is reasonable in his charges, or even willing to undertake the treatment without compensation, he creates an atmosphere of confidence that is helpful for the restoration of health. In the same spirit the writer, in an earlier chapter (4), has warned against discussing fees at the beginning of the cure because worry regarding fees is "harmful to a troubled patient, particularly if the disease is acute." Fleischer, *op. cit.*, p. 38, has clearly seen that the sequence of the statements made in chapter 6 points to the meaning: "wenn der Arzt Menschenfreund ist, sind die Menschen Freunde seiner Kunst." Nevertheless he tries to save the common interpretation, believing that the term "love of the art" is more often predicated of the representative of the art and that the latter's "wish for knowledge" forms the starting point of the discussion. But the context is quite a different one, as I have tried to show in the text. Nor is it "love of mankind" that is here made "the motive of medical practice." In *Precepts* too the author speaks of "love of man," having warned at the beginning of the chapter against "disdain of man" (ἀπανθρωπίη, "not to be unkind," Jones, *op. cit.*, I, p. 319; âpreté, Littré, *op. cit.*, vol. 9, p. 259). "Philanthropy" then appears here in exactly the same contrast as in the treatise *On the Physician*.

"Philanthropy," then, in the two Hippocratic treatises designates a proper behavior toward those with whom the physician comes in contact during treatment; it is viewed as a minor social virtue, so to say. And it was indeed in this way that the word, which later came to have such an exalted connotation, was commonly understood in the classical age and far down into the Hellenistic era.[5] Moreover, according to recent investigations, the book *On the Physician* was composed at the earliest between 350 and 300 B. C. *Precepts* cannot have been written before the first century B. C. or A. D. Neither the one nor the other treatise provides evidence for the ethics of the early Greek physician.[6] I trust that Osler, the scholar, would forgive me for dissenting from him in a question of interpretation and of chronology in which he followed the opinion of his time. I am sure he would not have wished me to put acceptance of authority before acceptance of the results of continued research.

As for Galen and his verdict, far be it from me to deny that even in the classical period there may have been men who dedicated themselves to medicine out of an instinctive compassion for the sufferings of their fellow men. But to assume that such a feeling, made conscious and, under whatever name, elevated to an ideal, could have extended to all mankind, would be the unhistorical projection of later concepts into an age entirely ignorant of them. To be sure, some of the Sophists taught that by nature all human beings—free, slave, and barbarian—are equal. The adherents of the rising enlightenment questioned existing conditions and extolled a natural or divine law of morality over the changing demands of the day. However, the time had not yet come to think in terms of obligations toward humanity.[7]

[5] The word φιλάνθρωπος originally was used only of gods and kings to denote their benevolent attitude toward men, *i. e.* toward their inferiors (or of animals who are friendly toward men). From the second half of the fourth century B. C. it began to be applied more generally and to be interpreted as kindliness and friendliness of individuals in their social contacts (cf. S. Lorenz, *De progressu notionis φιλανθρωπίας*, Diss. Leipzig, 1914, pp. 8 ff.; 14 ff.; 19 ff.; also J. Heinemann, *s. v.* "Humanismus," *Realencyclopädie der classischen Altertumswissenschaft*, Supplementband 5, 1931, col. 298). The contrast φιλάνθρωπος—μισάνθρωπος is usual in the fourth century (Lorenz, p. 25 f.); for the Peripatetic and Stoic interpretations of the term φιλανθρωπία as kindness, which is reflected in the Hippocratic respective treatises, cf. below, notes 19 and 20.

[6] For the late date of *On the Physician* and *Precepts* in general, cf. now Fleischer, *passim*, and below, notes 19, 20.

[7] W. W. Tarn, "Alexander, Cynics and Stoics," *Amer. Journ. Philol.*, 60, 1939, p. 44, rightly says that even the cosmopolitanism of the fourth-century Cynics has nothing to do "with any belief in the unity of mankind or a human brotherhood." It is a negative rather than a positive creed (cf. also Heinemann, *loc. cit.*, col. 291). And the same holds true of the advocacy of the equality and kinship of men by Hippias and others (cf. Heine-

Most important, those treatises of the *Corpus Hippocraticum* which were written during the fifth and fourth centuries B. C. and reflect the situation then prevailing, show clearly, I suggest, that even the best among the physicians were not concerned at all with such considerations as Galen imputes to them. Their ethics was not one of the heart or of inner intention. It was shaped by rather different values.

For the early Hippocratic books are concerned exclusively with a body of rules prescribing a certain behavior during the physician's working hours, with medical etiquette, one might say. It is explained how the doctor's office—his *iatreion*—should be set up, how it should or should not be equipped. Bedside manners are discussed, the right way to enter a sick room, to converse with the patient; whether or not to give a prognosis of the outcome of the disease if there is danger of a fatal issue. The surgeon is admonished not to make a show of the application of bandages or of operations, since to do what is proper is preferable to indulging in the mere display of one's dexterity. It is urged that a treatment once started should be completed, and that the physician should not withdraw his help from the sick so as to avoid blame or other unwelcome consequences.[8]

Such injunctions, and many more that could be cited, are dictated by the wish to uphold a certain standard of performance and serve to distinguish the expert from the charlatan. From Homeric times the physician had been an itinerant craftsman; even in the classical age, few physicians stayed in the cities of their birth or took up permanent residence elsewhere. Living here today, there tomorrow, they were not subject to the ordinary social strictures and pressures which result from the integration of the crafts into a community, and which tend to insure the reliability of the workmen. Besides, no medical schools existed; training was not required, everybody was free to practice medicine, the state did not issue

mann, *ibid.*, col. 287), or the "cosmopolitanism" to be found in Democritus and Euripides (cf. W. Nestle, *Vom Mythos zum Logos*, 1942², p. 380 f.). Lorenz' attempt to show that at least in the philosophical language of the fourth century philanthropy had the wider sense which it had later on (*op. cit.*, pp. 35 ff.), is refuted by the testimonies themselves. Still in Aristotle φιλανθρωπία · is but an emotion, an instinctive feeling of friendliness and kinship that exists between men as members of the same species, just as animals of the same race feel akin to one another (cf. J. Burnet, *The Ethics of Aristotle*, 1900, *ad* 1155 a 16 ff.; also H. v. Arnim, *Arius Didymus' Abriss der peripatetischen Ethik*, Sitzb. Wien, philos. hist. Kl., 204, No. 3, 1926, p. 107).

[8] For a more detailed picture of the rules of behavior, cf. L. Edelstein, Περὶ ἀέρων *und die Sammlung der Hippokratischen Schiften* (Problemata, 4), 1931, pp. 93 ff. (this will be quoted as *Problemata*). Cf. also W. H. S. Jones, *Hippocrates*, II, Introductory Essay V.

any license. Under these circumstances abuses abounded and went unpunished. They could be prevented only by the individual's decision to make himself responsible before the bar of his own conscience, the conscience of a good craftsman, and this responsibility he assumed by the adoption of a strict etiquette. A great achievement indeed! For not only did the physician thus voluntarily establish a set of values governing sound treatment, he also gave, so to say, a personal pledge of safety to his patients, badly needed in a world that knew of no other protection for them.[9]

Yet at no point does the Hippocratic physician aim farther. Medicine to him is but the proper application of his knowledge to the treatment of diseases. "The medical art," it is maintained in one of the rare expositions of the character of medicine to be found in the *Corpus Hippocraticum,* "has to consider three factors, the disease, the patient, the physician. The physician is the servant of his art, and the patient must cooperate with the doctor in combatting the disease" (*Epidemics,* I, 11). In other words, it is the sole purpose of the good physician to achieve the objective of his art, to save his patient from the threat of death, if possible; to help him, or at least not to harm him, as the famous saying has it (*ibid.*). His ethic consists in doing his task well, in perfecting his skill; it is an ethic of outward achievement rather than of inner intention.[10]

As for the physician's motives in practicing medicine, he was engaged in it in order to make a living. Nor was there any conflict between his pecuniary interests and the exigencies of craftsmanship, as long as he remembered that love of money, of easy success, should not induce him to act without regard for the benefit of the patient, or, to speak with Ruskin, that the good workman rarely thinks first of his pay, and that the knack of getting well paid does not always go with the ability to do the work well. If he learned to forget personal advantage for the sake of doing the right thing, he had, in his opinion, done all that was necessary.[11]

[9] The term used by the true physician in setting himself apart from the charlatan is that of "expertness," which is at the same time "goodness" (ἀνδραγαθικώτερον καὶ τεχνικώτερον); cf. *e. g.* Hippocratis Opera, ed. H. Kuehlewein, II, 1902, pp. 236, 18–237, 1; and in general, *Problemata,* pp. 95-98. For the lack of supervision of the medical art on the part of civil authorities, cf. *ibid.,* p. 89 f.

[10] Here I am concerned only with the ideal of medical practice, as it emerges from the Hippocratic writings. How far reality could fall behind this ideal, how far the ancient physician could deviate from strictly medical considerations in order to attract patients, I have tried to show in *Problemata,* chs. 2 and 3.

[11] That the competent Hippocratic physician was willing to forego momentary success and easy gain, follows *e. g.* from the surgical writings (cf. *Hippocratis Opera,* ed. Kuehlewein, II, pp. 168, 3 ff.; 175, 8 ff.; *Problemata,* pp. 97-99, where I should not have quoted

And **society fully** approved of such an attitude, as follows with certainty from a memorable passage in the first book of Plato's *Republic* (340 C ff.). The question there debated is whether self-interest is at the root of all human endeavor and therefore also of political activity. Parallels from the various arts, and especially the comparison with medicine, are used in order to decide the issue. The physician in the precise sense of the term is not a money maker or an earner of fees, Socrates holds, but a healer of the sick (341 C), just as it may be said of all the other arts that they were invented not for the sake of personal advantage, but rather for the purpose of performing a service, and most effectively at that. Medicine itself therefore has no concern for the advantage of medicine or of the physician, but only for that of the patient and his bodily welfare (342 C). Like every art, *qua* art, it looks out for the good of that which is its object. And when Socrates is asked rather mockingly: " Is this true of the shepherd also? Does he too have the good of his flock in mind? " (343 A ff.), he answers emphatically: " *qua* shepherd, yes." The fact that he sells the wool and makes money by so doing is not an intrinsic property of the art of shepherding; it belongs to another art, that of money making. For " if we are to consider it ' precisely ' medicine produces health but the fee-earning art the pay, and architecture a house but the fee-earning art accompanying it the fee, and so with all the others, each performs its own task and benefits that over which it is set " (346 D). Yet the subsidiary art of fee earning cannot be entirely separated from the art producing health. " Unless pay is added to it," there would be no benefit for the craftsman, and consequently he would be unwilling to go to the trouble of taking care of the troubles of others. This is why everybody expects to make money with his craft, and why pay must be provided by those who benefit from the craft. Otherwise the self-interest of the craftsman would not be satisfied (346 E-347 A).

All the interlocutors in the dialogue agree on this conclusion—and I think none of their contemporaries would have gainsaid their admission: the artisan has fulfilled his duty if he is intent primarily upon the aim of his art—that is, in the case of medicine, upon restoring health to the body—and thinks of his income afterwards. No other obligations are incumbent upon him, no other personal qualities are demanded of him.[12]

however a passage from the later *Precepts*.) The Ruskin quotation I have borrowed from P. Shorey (*Plato, The Republic*, I, [Loeb], *ad* 346 A).

[12] In the Platonic passage referred to Socrates argues according to the beliefs generally held; the passage therefore is especially illuminating for the common attitude towards the crafts. Aristotle too maintains that the function of medicine is that of causing health, not of producing wealth (*Politics*, 1258 a 10 ff.), though by some it is wrongly turned

It is also clear that in the society of the fifth and fourth centuries, medicine is a craft like all the others and in no way differentiated from them. Completely free of any idealization of work as such, and considering it a dire necessity rather than an ennobling activity, the classical age judged all manual labor only by the standard of expertness and performance. What can, properly speaking, be called morality, it found realized in man's private life, and preeminently in his life as a citizen. Even medicine, therefore, remained impervious to moral considerations.[13]

But at this point your patience with my argument should be exhausted, and I must face the objection which no doubt will have been on your minds for some time: how does all this square with the content of the Hippocratic *Oath*? Certainly, the *Oath* prescribes a most refined personal ethics for the physician. It enjoins upon him a life pleasing to gods and men, a life almost saintly and bound by the strictest rules of purity and holiness. It makes him renounce all intentional injustice or mischief. Here a morality of the highest order is infused into medical practice. Have not centuries upon centuries seen in the Hippocratic *Oath* the prototype of all medical ethics?

I trust that I am second to none in my appreciation of this document. Yet its picture of the true physician is evidence not of the thought of the classical era which I have so far considered, but of a movement which started in the latter part of the fourth century B. C.—the time when the *Oath* was composed—and extended through the Hellenistic period down to the time of Galen. Through it, the ethics of the medical craftsman was reshaped in accordance with the various systems of philosophy. The new standards characteristic of the second stage in the development of ancient medical ethics originated in a revaluation of the arts and crafts and in the transformation of the medical craft into a scientific pursuit.

into mere money making, as if this were the aim of medicine (*ibid.*). From the point of view of economic theory, medicine belongs to that "art of acquisition" which deals with exchange, and is "labor for hire" ($\mu\iota\sigma\theta\alpha\rho\nu\iota\alpha$ 1258 b 25).

[13] That the classical age did not know of the concept of "professions" but ranged the artist, the physician, and others with the common workmen or craftsmen ($\tau\epsilon\chi\nu\hat{\iota}\tau\alpha\iota$) has been emphasized especially by A. E. Zimmern, *The Greek Commonwealth*, 1915[2], pp. 257 ff. For the contrast between the classical attitude toward work and the modern concept of the "nobility of toil," cf. H. Michell, *The Economics of Ancient Greece*, 1940, p. 14. It is because of the facts referred to that I cannot agree with W. Müri's statement that the Hippocratic physician is the "Vertreter des Standes" and as such "in seinem Auftreten nicht mehr ganz frei" (*Arzt und Patient bei Hippokrates*, Beilage z. Jahresber. über d. städt. Gymnasium in Bern, 1936, p. 35). W. A. Heidel's chapter on the medical profession (*Hippocratic Medicine*, 1941, pp. 26-39) also is vitiated by his failure to consider the particular social and moral values prevailing in the world in which the Hippocratic "doctor" practiced.

To speak first of the change in attitude toward the crafts, Aristotle already raised the problem " whether artisans too ought not to have goodness, seeing that they often fall short of their duties through intemperance." But he decided that unlike the slave who is subject to " unlimited servitude," the artisan is subject only to " limited servitude," namely the performance of his particular job, and therefore is obligated only to do his task; his moral goodness is his own affair (*Politics*, 1260 a 36-b2; cf. *Nic. Eth.*, 1105 a 26 ff.). The so-called Pythagoreans of Aristotle's time, however, insisted on the moral implications of workmanship and considered it, if not a " noble toil " in the modern sense of the term, at least a matter of moral concern. They even claimed that " the good " could be achieved especially well through the crafts.[14] In Hellenistic philosophy such a belief became more widespread. Aristotle's successors distinguished the " happy life " and the " good life "—the one presupposing independent means, the other to be led by him who has to have an occupation. In both, man is asked to fulfill the moral law. Finally, the Stoa recognized the acquisition of money through any kind of work as compatible with the moral order and taught that in whatever station in life one may find oneself, one can and must live up to the rules of ethics.[15]

[14] The attitude of the Pythagoreans of the late fourth century toward the crafts I have discussed in *The Hippocratic Oath*, 1943, p. 60. Their views are the more significant since, generally speaking, the fifth and fourth centuries considered the workman not only déclassé, but evinced a definite prejudice against him, contrary to the pre-classical generations, a prejudice to be found in aristocratic and democratic societies alike (cf. Michell, *op. cit.*, pp. 11 ff.; also M. Pohlenz, " Die Lebensformen, Arbeit und Erwerb " in *Der Hellenische Mensch*, ch. XIII, pp. 357 ff. That an exception was made in regard to the physician [*ibid.*, p. 359] is not attested). Among the few who at least maintained that for the poor it is shameful to remain idle rather than to work was the " historical " Socrates (cf. Pohlenz, *ibid.*, p. 358), whose teaching seems to have been important also for the development of a concept of professional ethics. Cf. below, note 39.

[15] The Stoic philosophy of work, as it was formulated by Chrysippus, has been most adequately interpreted by A. Bonhöffer, *Die Ethik des Stoikers Epictet*, 1894, " Exkurs " IV, pp. 233 ff. For the importance of Stoic theories of the second and first centuries A. D. with regard to medical ethics, cf. below, pp. 411 ff. The Peripatetic doctrine concerning the life of the ordinary citizen and the art of acquisition is attested by Stobaeus (*Eclogae*, II, pp. 143, 24 ff.; 149, 21-23, ed. Wachsmuth, and Arnim, *op. cit.*, p. 90). I need not enter here into a discussion of the question whether the system outlined in Stobaeus can be traced altogether to Theophrastus (cf. Arnim, *op. cit.*, pp. 83 ff.), or whether it is influenced at least in part by Stoicism (R. Walzer, *Magna Moralia und Aristotelische Ethik* [Neue Philol. Unters., VII], 1929, p. 191 f.; also O. Regenbogen, *s. v.* " Theophrastos," *Realencycl.*, Suppl. VII, cols. 1492-94). However, it is important to note that the verdict of Aristotle's *Politics* according to which workmanship may be noble or ignoble depending on how much or how little virtue it requires as an accessory (1258 b 38 f.), must be considered an interpolation along the lines of later Peripatetic ethics. For it is in contradiction to Aristotle's general position. That the sentence in question

Such an entirely new appraisal of the crafts surely was facilitated by the fact that virtue or morality was increasingly identified not with the objective content of human actions, but rather with the inner attitude of the human agent. The principal criterion of right or wrong came to be found almost exclusively in the proper use of things, good, bad, or indifferent, rather than in the things themselves.[16]

Now, once it was realized that the craftsman can partake in virtue, the narrow limitations of the old ethics of good craftsmanship were swept aside. The moral issues latent in the pursuit of medicine, which the classical age had either failed to see, or failed to emphasize, were brought out into the open. The so-called deontological writings of the *Corpus Hippocraticum,* the *Oath,* the treatise *On the Physician, Precepts,* and *On Decorum*—the three latter composed in Hellenistic times, if not at the beginning of the Christian era—take up the various questions concerning medical ethics and try to give an answer to them from different philosophical points of view.[17]

Does not the practice of medicine involve the physician in the most intimate contact with other human beings? Is he not sometimes called upon to make decisions that reach far beyond the mere application of technical knowledge and skill? In the Hippocratic *Oath* that responsibility which is peculiarly the doctor's is defined in agreement with the way of life instituted by Pythagoras.[18] And what about the patient who is putting himself and " his all " into the hands of the physician? How can he be sure that he may have trust in the doctor, not only in his knowledge,

is an addition has been suspected for other reasons by W. L. Newman, *The Politics of Aristotle,* II, 1887, p. 203; the whole chapter in which the statement occurs differs in many respects from the rest of the text, cf. E. Barker, *The Politics of Aristotle,* 1946, p. 29, note 3.

[16] I should mention at least that at the turn of the fourth to the third century economic theory also began to consider the crafts in a new light. The Ps. Platonic dialogue *Eryxias* discussing the relation between wealth and virtue (393 A) entertains the notion that the crafts are not barter or " limited service," as Aristotle held (cf. above, note 12), but rather are to be classified under possession of wealth, and are thus more noble. The " expert pilot " and the " skilled physician " are the examples adduced (394 E) ; cf. M. L. W. Laistner, *Greek Economics,* 1923, p. xxviii f. The right, that is, the moral use of such " wealth " of practical skill forms the subject of a considerable part of the conversation reported in this dialogue, the only extant Greek treatise which deals exclusively with economic problems.

[17] The following analysis of the deontological writings which go into minute details of medical practice, is not intended to be exhaustive. I shall simply consider a number of salient features that within the context of my discussion seem to characterize the teaching of these essays.

[18] For the Pythagorean origin of the *Oath* and its date, cf. Edelstein, *The Hippocratic Oath,* especially p. 59 f.

but also in the man himself? Such confidence, according to the book *On the Physician,* can be aroused only if the physician asks himself what he should be like " in regard to his soul." Consequently the author of this treatise—perhaps the oldest known " introduction to medicine " which is posterior to the *Oath* by approximately two or three generations—prescribes for " the soul " of the physician self-control, regularity of habits, justness and fairness, a proper and good behavior, in short, all the virtues of the " gentleman ". It is the doctrine of the Aristotelian school, I think, which is here adapted to medicine.[19]

Again, in the *Precepts* and in the book *On Decorum* it is the Stoic outlook which predominates. In the former treatise, gentleness and kind-heartedness are commended. The physician ought to be charitable, especially toward him who is a stranger and in financial straits (ch. 6). In keeping with such a kindly and tolerant attitude the good physician—the " fellow workman," as he is called (ch. 7)—must also be ready at all times to call in another physician as a consultant, and he must not quarrel with his confrères either. Thus, aspects of medical practice neglected in the *Oath* and in the essay *On the Physician,* are elucidated in

[19] Fleischer's dating of the treatise *On the Physician* in the third century (*op. cit.,* p. 56 f.) seems convincing to me. (H. Diller, *Gnomon,* 17, 1941, p. 30, thinks it unlikely that the book was written after 300 B. C.). The short summary of ethics given by the " Hippocratic " author is usually related to the protreptic-paraenetic literature of the time (cf. J. F. Bensel, " De medico libellus ad codicum fidem recensitus," *Philologus,* 78, 1922, pp. 102-4; also Müri, *op. cit.,* p. 37), or is linked in addition with the content of introductory manuals on the crafts which became common in the Hellenistic era (Fleischer, *op. cit.,* p. 54 f.). Yet, the right behavior of the physician is defined at least once in the typically Aristotelian manner as " a mean between extremes." (" In appearance let him be of a serious, but not harsh countenance, for surliness is taken for arrogance and unkindness, while a man of uncontrolled laughter and excessive gaiety is considered vulgar "). Details of the precept also fall in line with Peripatetic terminology and doctrine. The concept of surliness (αὐθάδεια) is used here in the restricted and derogatory sense which it came to have in the Peripatetic school (*Magna Moralia,* 1192 b 31; Stobaeus, p. 146, 8, and Walzer, *op. cit.,* p. 161, n. 1). As Bensel already noted (p. 105), the word " vulgar " (φορτικός) is applied to him who indulges in excessive laughter, just as it is in *Nic. Eth.,* 1128 a 3 ff. Self-control (ἐγκράτεια) commended in the Hippocratic essay is treated as one of the main virtues in *Magna Moralia,* in contrast to the genuine Aristotelian ethics (Walzer, *op. cit.,* pp. 98; 106). The use of the term friendliness (φιλάνθρωπος, cf. above, note 3) agrees with that to be found in the Ps. Aristotelian treatise *On Virtues and Vices* (1251 b 35; cf. 1251 b 16; 1250 b 33; also Theophrastus *apud* Stobaeus, *Florilegium,* 3, 50). Finally, the ideal of the " gentleman " (τὸ δὲ ἦθος εἶναι καλὸν καὶ ἀγαθόν) remains valid throughout the history of Peripatetic ethics (Stobaeus, p. 147, 23). It is true, the ethics propounded in the book *On the Physician* is that of common morality, but as one has rightly said, the later Peripatos restored " bourgeois morality " (Walzer, *op. cit.,* p. 188). For the Peripatetic concern with the life of the ordinary citizen, cf. above, note 15. I should add that the Peripatetic flavor of the " Hippocratic " essay speaks for its being dated after 300 B. C.

the light of general moral considerations.[20] The essay *On Decorum*, on the other hand, though abounding in detailed advice on moral situations as they may arise in the course of a treatment, mainly discusses the "wisdom" of the physician. For "between wisdom and medicine there is no gulf; in fact, medicine possesses all the qualities that make for wisdom" (ch. 5), that is, wisdom "applied to life," "directed toward seemliness and good repute" (ch. 1), which should be carefully distinguished from its opposite, from false or sham philosophy. A physician who has the right kind of philosophy is indeed "the equal of a god"; his are all the virtues one can think of (ch. 5). To put it in the technical language of the Stoic school, to which the author of the treatise owes allegiance, the true physician is the peer of the sage.[21]

Perhaps you are astonished at the fact that all these treatises which I have characterized briefly are so strongly imbued with philosophy. And thinking again of the Hippocratic *Oath* you may wonder why the ancient physician could not rest satisfied with the stipulation of his oath which seems to tell him all he has to know about his duties. But the Hippocratic *Oath* originally was a literary manifesto, a programme laid down by one who wished to set matters right in accordance with his own convictions. It was not an oath taken by all physicians, if indeed it was ever taken at all by any one before the end of antiquity.[22] Throughout

[20] *Precepts* is usually held to be Epicurean in origin, cf. now Fleischer, *op. cit.*, pp. 10 ff. However Bensel, *op. cit.*, pp. 96; 98, rightly doubted an influence of Epicurus on any of the deontological writings because Epicurus (Fr. 196 ed. Usener) considers all forms of life which are not directed toward the happy life merely vulgar activities. Epicurean philosophy seems the only Hellenistic system that does not share in the rehabilitation of the crafts (cf. Philodemus, *On Oeconomics*, XXIII, 18 ff.). And indeed, the moral teaching of *Precepts* is Stoic rather than Epicurean. The term φιλανθρωπία, as it is used here (cf. above, note 4), corresponds to the meaning which the word has for the Chrysippean Stoa (φιλικὴ χρῆσις ἀνθρώπων [*Stoicorum Veterum Fragmenta*, III, 292 ed. Arnim]), and in its emphatically moral connotation differs significantly from the more utilitarian recommendation of φιλανθρωπία by the Epicureans (Philodemus, *op. cit.*, XXIV, 29). The injunction on fees laid down in *Precepts* is paralleled by Chrysippus' statements on fees for teaching (*St. V. Fr.*, III, 701). The definition of medicine as "habit" (ἕξις, ch. 2) is that of the Stoa (cf. *e. g.*, *St. V. Fr.*, II, 393; III, 111). That the epistemological theories, too, are Stoic rather than Epicurean, I hope to show elsewhere. The date of *Precepts* has been fixed by Fleischer (*op. cit.*, p. 24) in the first or second century A. D. At any rate, the book must be late Hellenistic.

[21] The Stoic influence on the treatise *On Decorum* is generally recognized (*e. g.* Jones, *Hippocrates*, II, p. 270 f.) and has been traced in detail by Fleischer (*op. cit.*, especially pp. 78; 90: 101 ff.). The latter also dates the essay in the first-second century A. D. A reexamination of the background of the Stoic theories here adopted may perhaps lead to the assumption of a slightly earlier date. But this too I must leave for another investigation.

[22] Scribonius Largus, perhaps the first to mention the *Oath*, maintains that Hippocrates

Hellenistic times and in the first centuries of the Christian era no common agreement existed concerning an ethical code binding for the medical practitioner. As was the case with the medical etiquette of old, so moral stipulations were accepted voluntarily. The writers of whom I have spoken were individuals trying to find out for themselves how to conduct their business in the right way. Just like Osler, they believed they could see their own work in truer perspective by taking " the larger view." And in this endeavor where could they turn for instruction except to philosophy? Ancient religion had no moral or metaphysical message. In the vacuum that resulted from the disappearance of the city state, from the breakdown of the old ideal of civic virtue, philosophy alone could still provide guidance. It was, and it intended to be, not merely the domain of academics, but rather the inspiration of everybody who refused to get lost in doing his daily chores and was in search of standards on which to orientate himself. To be sure, adherence to whatever dogma seemed to the individual nearest to the truth did not yet make him a " philosopher-in-precept," and this holds also for the authors of the deontological writings. Philosophy gave them a *Weltanschauung* which enabled them to solve the task they had set for themselves.[23]

Yet I must turn now to a consideration of the other factor which, as I suggested before, was responsible for the acceptance of a philosophical ethic on the part of the physician: I mean the change of the medical art into medical science. Ever since the fifth and fourth centuries some physicians had interested themselves in the physiological and biological

began medical instruction by administering this vow (*Compositiones*, p. 2, 27 f. ed. Helmreich). This of course is mere conjecture. Such books as Ps. Soranus, *Introductio ad medicinam* (V. Rose, *Anecdota Graeca et Graeco-Latina*, II, 1870) speak of a medical oath and of the oath of Hippocrates (pp. 244, 27; 245, 16 f.). In the fourth century A. D. Libanius (Κατὰ ἰατροῦ φαρμακέως, 9) refers to "the oath taken by physicians when entering upon the practice of their profession" (cf. R. Pack, "Note on a ' Progymnasma' of Libanius," *Amer. Jour. Philol.*, 69, 1948, p. 300), and many such oaths were in fact current (Pack, *ibid.*). That any of them were obligatory, cannot be proved. According to Ps. Oribasius, *Comment. in Aphorismos Hippocratis*, ed. Basileae, 1535, p. 7, the *Oath* was the first book to be read by the beginner, cf. K. Deichgräber, "Die ärztliche Standesethik des hippokratischen Eides," *Quellen u. Stud. z. Gesch. d. Naturwiss. u. d. Medizin*, III, 2, 1932, p. 93, n. 1, and the material there given on other oaths, p. 95, n. 33; p. 97, n. 42.

[23] It is usual to designate the ethics of the *Oath* as "*Berufsethos*" (cf. *e. g.* Pohlenz, *op. cit.*, p. 334); Müri uses this term in his analysis of the picture of the ideal physician, as it is given in the deontological writings (*op. cit.*, p. 39). In a loose sense, such a characterization is surely not unjustified. But it is important to note that none of the " Hippocratic " treatises here discussed considers the obligations of the physician as inherent in his medical task. They rather adapt philosophical ethics to medicine, cf. below, p. 408.

theories of the philosophers and had made use of them in their own work. Thereby they created scientific medicine, if I may use this term to designate the type of medicine that went beyond the practical application of traditional knowledge and demanded research into the nature of the body and of all the factors that may have a bearing upon it.[24] While throughout antiquity merely technical skill and empirical proficiency constituted the equipment of the average physician who as a craftsman was trained through apprenticeship with another physician-craftsman, the medical " scientists " studied philosophy. In the Hellenistic era they belonged to the various medical sects for which the unity of philosophy and medicine was axiomatic. And the new spirit in which medicine was thus approached soon made itself felt also in medical practice. The ethics of these physicians became identical with that of the philosophical school to which they professed allegiance as scientists.

The first testimony to this effect is perhaps the Hippocratic *Law* written at approximately the same time as the *Oath*. Many physicians, the author of the short and almost enigmatic treatise holds, are physicians " by repute "; very few are physicians " in reality." Rather have the majority, " like the supernumeraries in tragedies," merely " the appearance, dress, and mask of an actor without being actors " (ch. 1). He who wishes to win the reputation of being a physician " not only in name, but in deed," must go through a proper training, that is, a philosophical training. Its result will also be " cheerfulness " and " joyousness," instead of " cowardice " and " rashness," which betray " helplessness " and " want of knowledge " (ch. 4). This is the Democritean ideal of theoretical speculation, according to which the man of true insight is at the same time necessarily the man of truly good character.[25]

[24] For a more detailed interpretation of " scientific " medicine, cf. L. Edelstein, " The Relation of Ancient Philosophy to Medicine," *Bull. Hist. Med.*, 26, 1952, pp. 301 ff.

[25] In the interpretation of the *Law* I follow Wilamowitz, *Hermes*, 54, 1919, pp. 46 ff. F. Müller's attempt (*Hermes*, 75, 1940, pp. 39 ff.) to date the *Law* in the fifth century B. C. to me is unconvincing. As Fleischer says (*op. cit.*, p. 46), it is perhaps impossible to date the essay exactly, because many of its concepts became common stock in the discussion of moral problems. Yet the book cannot be earlier than Democritus, some of whose central ethical concepts are here presupposed, as Wilamowitz has shown. Nor will it be much later than the end of the fourth century, since unalloyed Democritean teaching did not long survive. Jones (*Hippocrates*, II, p. 275) connects the *Law* with the doctrine of secret medical societies, which he thinks might have existed in Greece, since at the end of the *Law* it is proclaimed: " Holy things are shown to holy men; to the profane it is not lawful to show them until these have been initiated into the rites of knowledge." But the description of " knowledge " through the metaphor of the mysteries is not uncommon with Greek philosophers (cf. E. Frank, *Knowledge, Will and Belief*, 1955, pp. 63 f.; 67). Wilamowitz, *op. cit.*, p. 49, already compared ἱερὰ πρήγματα

While here the ethics of the scientific physician still remains vague and shadowy, it manifests itself in its fully developed form in the doctrine of the Hellenistic Empiricists whose sect was of the sceptic persuasion. The empirical physician therefore, like all sceptic philosophers, accepts the established rules of life which, though by no means representing absolute truth, have the sanction of probability. In accordance with the common aim of men, he practices medicine for the sake of reputation or of money, of neither of which he desires to have too much or too little, but just as much as is adequate and guarantees peace of mind. In his character and behavior he evinces tranquillity and gentleness. In his work he is not given to unnecessary talk, but prefers action; talking much or talking big is the habit of those who, unlike the empiricist and sceptic, believe in speculative theories. In his writings and in his research he is truthful, not intent on winning an argument *à tout prix,* or on displaying his conceit. On the whole, then, he follows in the wake of the day, relying on indubitable data of sense perception and experience; living thus, he lives like Hippocrates himself who, in the opinion of the sceptics, had of course been a sceptic, and as a sceptic had equalled the fame of Asclepius.[26]

Evidence on the ethical teaching of the early dogmatic sects is almost entirely lacking. A happy chance has preserved at least one testimony which bears witness to the preoccupation of Erasistratus with medical ethics. "Most fortunate indeed," he says, "wherever it happens that the physician is both, perfect in his art and most excellent in his moral conduct. But if one of the two should have to be missing, then it is better to be a good man devoid of learning than to be a perfect practitioner of bad moral conduct, and an untrustworthy man—if indeed it is true that good morals compensate for what is missing in art, while bad morals can corrupt and confound even perfect art."[27] Further details of the de-

---

in the *Law* with the ἱερὸν πνεῦμα that, according to Democritus, inspires the poet. Jones' translation of ἠδελφισμένος (*Precepts*, ch. 5) as "one made a brother" (of a secret society) involves an unnecessary change of the best manuscript tradition ἠδελφισμένως, for the meaning of which cf. Fleischer, *op. cit.*, p. 36.

[26] Cf. K. Deichgräber, *Die griechische Empirikerschule*, 1930, p. 322 f. Especially important is the statement, p. 82, 29 ff.: οἷός δ' ἐστι καθ' ὅλον τὸν βίον ὁ σκεπτικός, τοιοῦτός ἐστι περὶ τὴν ἰατρικὴν ὁ ἐμπειρικός. Ch. 11 of Galen's *Subfiguratio Empirica* treats "De moribus et dictis que debent esse in empericis." For the sceptics' conformance with the established laws, cf. *e. g.* M. M. Patrick, *The Greek Sceptics*, 1929, p. 51.

[27] Cf. Ps. Soranus, *Introductio ad medicinam* (Rose, *Anecdota Graeca et Graeco-Latina,* II, p. 244, 16-23): "Disciplinarum autem ceterarum minime sit expers [sc. medicus], sed et circa mores habeat diligentiam. iuxta enim Erasistratum felicissimum quidem est ubi utraeque res fuerint, uti et in arte sit perfectus et moribus sit optimus. si autem unum de duobus defuerit, melius est virum esse bonum absque doctrina quam artificem perfectum mores habentem malos et improbum esse. modesti si quidem mores quod in

ontology of the Herophilean and Erasistratean sects may be contained in the writings of Galen, the great systematizer of medicine. At any rate, his little essay *That the Best Physician also is a Philosopher* gives an exhaustive account of later dogmatic ethics. It can be summed up in the demand that the physician should be contemptuous of money, interested in his work, self-controlled and just. Once he is in possession of these basic virtues, he will have all the others at his command as well (ch. 3). And how is such moral eminence to be achieved? Like Galen, the true physician must become a philosopher himself, an adherent of Plato, or rather of the Platonism of Galen's time, which was fused with Aristotelianism and Stoicism.[28]

With this short description of Galen's views I have come to the end of my analysis of the various attitudes taken by the scientist-physicians and by the craftsmen-physicians during the second stage in the development of medical ethics. The important consequence of the movement which I have described hardly needs reemphasis. The morality of outward performance characteristic of the classical era was now supplemented by a morality of inner intention. The physician—whether as an amateur philosopher or as a philosopher in his own right—had learned to regard his patient not only as the object of his art, but also as a fellowman to whom he owed more than knowledge alone, however great, can provide. He had learned to face him not only as a master of techniques, but also as a virtuoso in moral conduct.

Can one then go one step further and claim that between the end of the fourth century B. C. and the second century A. D. medicine had been elevated to the rank of the most philanthropic art? Have I answered also the specific question raised at the very beginning of my discussion? Have I uncovered the origin of the humanism which Osler admired in Greek medicine? It may almost seem so. For surely, in Galen's opinion,

arte deest honestate repensare videntur, culpa autem morum artem perfectam corrumpere atque improbare potest." The *Introductio* which forms part of a collection of *Quaestiones Medicinales* (cf. Rose, *op. cit.*, p. 169), though hardly by Soranus, is based on good ancient sources. There is no reason to doubt the authenticity of the quotation from Erasistratus.

[28] E. Wenkebach, "Der hippokratische Arzt als das Ideal Galens," *Quell. u. Stud. z. Gesch. d. Nat. u. d. Med.*, III, 1932-33, p. 372 f., stresses the influence of Hippocratic medicine on Galen's ideal as outlined in the treatise referred to. But although Galen identifies his philosophy with that of Hippocrates, one must remember that for him, Hippocrates and Plato agree in almost all points. Besides, he says expressly (ch. 3) that philosophy is indispensable for medical practice, just as it is for medical theory; in addition to logic and physics, the physician must take up the third part of philosophy, namely ethics.

the physician who accepts his philosophy will be led to practice medicine
out of love of humanity, the motive which Galen is willing to attribute
even to Hippocrates, as I mentioned before. And since nowhere else,
neither in the deontological writings of the *Corpus Hippocraticum,* nor
in the teaching of any of the other medical sects, philanthropy is mentioned
as the inspiration of the doctor, one should conclude that it was dogmatic
medicine, as formulated by Galen or maybe by one of his predecessors,
which gave rise to medical humanism.[29]

But Galen's own appraisal of the possible motivations of medical
practice, I am afraid, makes it impossible to rest satisfied as yet. For as
he says (*De Placitis,* p. 763 f. ed. Müller) on the authority of the same
passage in Plato's *Republic* to which I referred in my analysis of classical
medicine, the physician's particular job is to take care of the health of
the body, although it may be for a variety of reasons that he practices
medicine. Some physicians engage in it for the sake of money, some for
the sake of exemption from public duties—physicians in Galen's time
were sometimes granted such privileges [30]—some few for love of mankind, just as still others for glory or honor. In so far as they are able
to bring health to their patients, all of them are named physicians; in so
far as they do what they do for different reasons, the one is called a
" philanthropist," the other a lover of honor, the third a lover of glory,
the fourth a lover of money. Therefore, Galen continues (p. 764 f.), the
aim of the physician as physician is not glory or money, as the Empiricist
Menodotus claimed; this may have been true of himself, but others in

[29] On the evidence of Galen's claim that " Diocles practiced medicine out of love of
mankind " (cf. above, p. 392), K. Deichgräber, *Professio medici, Zum Vorwort des
Scribonius Largus,* Abh. Akad. Mainz, Geistes- u. Sozialwiss. Klasse, 1950, No. 9),
tentatively suggests that the association between medicine and philanthropy may be due
to the influence of the Peripatos (p. 866, n. 1). Yet, for Aristotle, and even for Theophrastus, φιλανθρωπία is not " love of humanity " (cf. above, notes 7 and 19). As late
as in Stobaeus' report on Peripatetic ethics the κοινὴ φιλανθρωπία, as it is called in con-
tradistinction to the φιλία among friends (II, 121, 22; 120, 20), is not represented as
one of the main virtues (cf. Heinemann, *op. cit.,* col. 298) ; it rather is a natural sympathy
that prompts men to help other men in dire need and not think of themselves only (p. 120,
20–121, 22). Much as the Peripatos contributed to the Hellenistic concept of the unity of
men, it was the Stoa that stressed the rational duties inherent in the idea of humanity
(M. Pohlenz, *Die Stoa,* I, 1948, pp. 136-39). And even in the Stoic school justice was
at first the obligation stressed in connection with cosmopolitanism; love of mankind came
to be fully recognized only in the first century A. D. (Pohlenz, *ibid.,* p. 315; Bonhöffer,
op. cit., p. 106). I should be inclined, therefore, to believe that philanthropy became
integrated into the ethical teaching of the dogmatic physicians not long before Galen's
time, if indeed it was not Galen himself who accepted the ideal of philanthropy in
accordance with his Stoic leanings.

[30] Cf. below, p. 416.

the past surely had different aims in mind. The motive of glory or money or of philanthropy is a matter of personal choice; it has no intrinsic connection with the pursuit of medicine.[31] For in regard to every craft it is necessary to distinguish between its common characteristics and those which belong to the individual practicing it. Failure to make this distinction is bad logic, irreconcilable with the tenets of Plato and Hippocrates alike (p. 765 f.).

This argumentation of Galen, so utterly devoid of ethical overtones or of any feeling of moral indignation, shows clearly that in his opinion philanthropy is not indissolubly joined with the practice of medicine. It is, so to say, a superfluity of riches on the part of the physician. What is expected of him is only that he should be an expert in medicine. However, no rules of behavior can be stated absolutely. For Galen as well as for all the other moralizing physicians medical ethics remains relative to the respective philosophies to which they adhere at their own discretion. Whoever differs from their views is a bad philosopher, to be sure, but he is not necessarily a bad physician or a bad man. Various motivations of medical practice, therefore, are quite legitimate; no one single or definite virtue is enjoined upon the doctor by his task. From the point of view of medicine, his specific morality is incidental rather than essential.

Does this amount to the admission that the ancients never identified medicine with love of humanity? That they did not know of any strictly professional medical ethics dictated by the aim of medicine itself? By no means. Almost a hundred years before Galen there must have been a clear realization of a medical humanism inherent in the task of the physician. Scribonius Largus, a writer of the early first century A. D., speaks of it as something quite self-evident to himself and his readers. It still remains for me to elicit the full meaning of the doctrine in question from the few sentences in which Scribonius alludes to it, to determine its historical antecedents, and to sketch its later fate.[32]

Scribonius has embodied his views on the moral conduct of the physician in the preface to his book *On Remedies* in which he wishes to demonstrate the importance of treatment by drugs. Why is it, he asks

---

[31] In *That the Best Physician also is a Philosopher* Galen once speaks of medicine as a τέχνη οὕτω φιλάνθρωπος (ch. 2). The detailed refutation of Menodotus shows that by the term in question Galen can only mean that medicine is "philanthropic" because it removes the sufferings of men.

[32] The fact that Scribonius upholds a humanistic ethics has often been noticed, of course; cf. *e. g.* J. Hirschberg, *Vorlesungen über hippokratische Heilkunde*, 1922, p. 35. A detailed analysis of Scribonius' views has recently been given by K. Deichgräber, *op. cit.* (cf. above, note 29).

(p. 2, 8 ed. Helmreich), that his colleagues refrain from the application of drugs? Are they unfamiliar with them? This would be just reason for accusing them of negligence. Or are they aware of the usefulness of drugs, yet deny their use to others? If so, they are even more culpable, " because they burn with envy, an evil that must be despised by all men, and especially by the physician who is himself despised by gods and men if his heart is not full of sympathy (*misericordiae*) and humaneness (*humanitatis*) in accordance with the will (*voluntatem*) of medicine itself " (p. 2, 15-19).

But the sympathy and humaneness " willed " by medicine imply more than that the physician should not withhold his knowledge from his patients. The true physician, Scribonius continues, " is not allowed to harm anybody, not even the enemies of the state (*hostibus*). He may fight against them with every means as a soldier (*miles*) or as a good citizen (*vir bonus*), should this be demanded of him. [As a physician, he cannot and must not fight or harm them], since medicine does not judge men by their circumstances in life (*fortuna*), nor by their character (*personis*). Rather does medicine promise (*pollicetur*) her succor in equal measure to all who implore her help, and she professes (*profitetur*) never to be injurious to anyone " (p. 2, 19-26). For, as Scribonius reiterates in conclusion, " medicine is the knowledge of healing, not of hurting. If she does not try in every way to help the sick with all means at her disposal, she fails to offer to men the sympathy she promises " (*hominibus quam pollicetur misericordiam*, p. 3, 5-8).

Obviously, according to Scribonius, the sympathy and humaneness required of the physician are due to everybody in equal measure. Humaneness (*humanitas*) for him is not merely a friendliness of behavior, it is a " proficiency and benevolence toward all men without distinction," it truly is " love of mankind," as *humanitas* was defined at that time in correspondence with the then prevailing meaning of the Greek word φιλανθρωπία.[33] Besides, sympathy and love of humanity constitute positive rules, and obedience to them supersedes all other allegiances that the doctor may have as a good citizen or as a soldier. They are the special obligation of the physician which he cannot violate under any circumstances. Most important, the one and only right standard of conduct is enforced upon him by medicine itself, just as is the standard of adequate

---

[33] I am quoting the definition of *humanitas* which Gellius gives (*Noctes Atticae*, XIII, 17) as the one commonly accepted. Heinemann, *Realencycl.*, col. 306, has shown that in the literature of the first century A. D. the words *humanitas* and *humanus* and their Greek equivalents are used in the sense attested by Gellius.

knowledge. Unless he knows all that he ought to know and makes use of it for the benefit of the sick, he fails in his duty. He is as remiss, or even more so, if he does not fulfill his specific moral responsibility. Here, the ethics of inner intention and that of outward performance have become an inseparable unity; both are derived from the task to be achieved, from the " will " and " promise " of medicine itself, both are equally essential for medicine and the physician.

It is hardly by chance therefore that Scribonius calls medicine not merely an " art " or a " science," but a " profession " (*professio,* p. 2, 18; 27). This word, in the language of his time, was applied to workmanship in preference to the older and morally indefinite terms, in order to emphasize the ethical connotations of work, the idea of an obligation or a duty on the part of those engaged in the arts and crafts. It approximates most closely the Christian concept of " vocation " or " calling," except of course that for him who has been " called " to do a job his obligations are ordained by God, while for the member of an ancient profession his duties result from his own understanding of the nature of his profession.[34] But this difference of the ancient ethos of work from that of later ages does not lessen the strict validity of the rules to be observed. The true physician, Scribonius says, like a soldier, is " bound in lawful obedience to medicine by his military oath " (p. 2, 20-21). On the other hand, he who acts in a way unbecoming to a physician is a deserter, as it were; he is " deservedly despised by gods and men " (*diis hominibusque invisus merito,* ch. 199; cf. p. 2, 19: *diis et hominibus invisi esse debent*) ; he has " against the law transgressed the proper boundaries of the profession " (ch. 199).[35] He is, one might say, disqualified as a physician, for it is no longer up to him how he should conduct himself.

That such an ideal of medical humanism is foreign to the spirit of Hippocratic ethics, Scribonius admits himself. Even in the *Oath* which in his opinion is the work of Hippocrates, the " founder of our profession "

---

[34] M. Weber, " Die protestantische Ethik und der Geist des Kapitalismus," *Ges. Aufsätze z. Religionssoziologie,* I, 1920, analyzing the meaning of the term *Beruf* or " calling " has pointed up its difference from the classical concept of work (p. 63). He has also noted, however, that in Latin, such words as *officium* (cf. also below, n. 42), *munus,* and *professio* (originally denoting, it seems, the duty of making a tax declaration) came to assume " eine unserem Wort ' Beruf' in jeder Hinsicht ziemlich ähnliche Gesamtbedeutung . . . natürlich durchaus diesseitig, ohne jede religiöse Färbung " (p. 63, n. 1).

[35] The simile of fighting and military service used by Scribonius is quite common in Latin philosophy (cf. *e. g.* Pohlenz, *Die Stoa,* I, 1948, p. 314) ; it also occurs in the language of the mysteries so often applied to knowledge in general, cf. above, note 25, and *Amer. Journ. Philol.,* 72, 1951, p. 430, n. 6.

(p. 2, 27), he can find his views at best by implication. For, as he puts it, Hippocrates forbids the physician to give an abortive remedy to a woman, " and thereby has gone a long way toward preparing the mind of the learners for the love of humanity. For he who thinks it to be a crime to injure future life still in doubt, how much more criminal must he judge it to hurt a full grown human being " (p. 2, 30-3, 2)? [36] But if Scribonius' concept of medical ethics goes in fact beyond the demands of the classical period, if it is distinct from the teaching of all the deontological treatises and all the medical sects I have discussed, where and when did it originate?

That Scribonius himself formulated the code of behavior which he upholds, I cannot believe; for he does not argue about it, nor defend it, he simply presupposes it and takes it for granted, as I pointed out before. In addition, reading his account one cannot fail to be reminded of the doctrine concerning human life and human obligations which characterize the Stoic philosophy of humanism evolved in the second century B. C. by Panaetius and embedded in Cicero's book *On Duties,* the manual of all later humanism, ancient and Christian, secular and religious alike. Here if anywhere in antiquity, a programme of a professional ethics was firmly established.[37]

For first of all, Panaetius, as Cicero represents him, accepted and even enhanced the more positive evaluation of the arts and crafts which earlier philosophers had made of them, granting that virtue has its place even among craftsmen. Medicine, next to architecture and education, is expressly mentioned and singled out by Cicero as socially acceptable, because it demands a high degree of insight and contributes something useful to life; it is therefore, he says, a " proper " (*honestae*) occupation for those for whose station in life it is fitting (*On Duties,* I, 42, 151).[38]

[36] Scribonius concludes that Hippocrates apparently " thought it of great value for everyone to preserve the name and honor of medicine in purity and holiness, conducting himself after her design " (p. 3, 2-5). Thereby he translates into the language of his professional ethics the Pythagorean concepts of purity and holiness used in the *Oath* with reference to the art which the physician practices and to the life which he leads (ἁγνῶς δὲ καὶ ὁσίως διατηρήσω βίον ἐμὸν καὶ τέχνην ἐμήν). It is unwarranted, I think, to infer from this adaptation of the famous sentence in the *Oath* that Scribonius has a " religiös getönte Humanität " (Deichgräber, *op. cit.* [cf. above, note 29], p. 861).

[37] R. Reitzenstein, *Werden und Wesen der Humanität im Altertum,* 1907, p. 15, already suggested that the philosophy of Panaetius gave rise to a " *Standesethik* "; cf. also Heinemann, *op. cit.,* col. 294.

[38] In accordance with their own aristocratic prejudice and with the prejudice of the society in which they live, Panaetius and Cicero consider political and public activities the only ones proper for a gentleman (cf. M. Pohlenz, " Antikes Führertum," *Neue Wege*

But Panaetius' positive appreciation of the various occupations implies much more than a general approval of the activities indispensable for man's welfare and for civilization. Although philosophically speaking virtue is one and the same, and it is impossible to have any one virtue without having all of them (II, 10, 35 [Panaetius]), different aspects of this one and indivisible virtue in which all men share come to the fore in the various pursuits of human life and have to be practiced without fail. To give an example, the judge must always adhere to the truth, while the lawyer may sometimes defend the probable, even if this may not quite coincide with the truth (II, 14, 51 [Panaetius]). Obviously, here man's particular task imposes upon him certain obligations; each one has its own morality, from which there is no exception. For the judge is not permitted to indulge in any bias or favoritism out of friendship; while sitting as a judge, he is not supposed to act as a friend (III, 10, 43).[39]

If one asks why this should be so, the answer is that the individual who practices any occupation is playing a certain role. It may be one derived from chance circumstances, the place in society to which he is born and by which his inclination toward a particular career and also his opportunities for it are conditioned; it may be one which he assumes through his own free decision, through a deliberate choice of an occupation (I, 32, 115 ff.). But whether the role be inherited or chosen, one must act one's part as the role demands it, just as in the two roles which nature, in addition, has assigned to everyone—as a human being who has the same duties as all other human beings, and as an individual endowed with specific intellectual and emotional gifts (I, 30, 107 ff.)—one must live up to " the lines one has to speak." It is therefore that the judge must always utter the truth, that he is not permitted to listen to the voice of

z. *Antike*, 2. Reihe, H. 3, 1934, p. 83 f.). The views of the older Stoics in this respect had been more liberal; cf. above, note 15.

[39] Panaetius surely was not the first to discuss the particular virtues pertaining to an occupation. His teacher, Antipater (*St. V. Fr.*, III, 61 f.), had engaged in a famous dispute about " business ethics " with his predecessor, Diogenes (*St. V. Fr.*, III, 49). The casuistry of the old Stoa insists on the fact that for the physician it is permissible to lie (III, 513), that neither he, nor the judge is allowed to indulge in commiseration " with the suffering of his neighbors " (III, 451). The beginnings of such a " differenzierende Ethik " may be traced even to the Sophists, and especially to the Xenophontian Socrates (cf. E. Norden, in *Hermes*, *40*, 1905, pp. 521 ff.; F. Wehrli, " Ethik und Medizin," *Mus. Helveticum*, *8*, 1951, p. 45 f.). However, the recognition that virtuous action may differ with different people and different positions in life is still a far cry from the acknowledgement of professional virtues. At any rate, they seem not to have been appraised systematically before Panaetius.

friendship, "for he lays down the role (or mask) of the friend when putting on that of the judge" (III, 10, 43). What is fitting for the one, is not so for the other.[40]

Now is this not fundamentally the way in which Scribonius views medicine and the obligations imposed by it? The role which the physician plays in the tragedy, or comedy, of life demands of him the virtue of humaneness, sympathy, or commiseration. His lines are to be spoken in this spirit. Consequently as little as Cicero's judge in his professional activity can ever be in a situation justifying his failure to cling to the truth—though there are other professions in which this virtue may sometimes come second—so Scribonius' physician must never neglect love of humanity and all the duties it entails. Certainly, commiseration and humaneness are not demanded of him alone; but they are his professional virtues, just as truthfulness is the distinctive virtue of him who sits in court notwithstanding the fact that it is required of everybody. Only when he steps out of his role, so to say, is the member of a profession free to follow another code of morals. The physician may take on the role of a citizen or of a soldier, and in that case he may fight and kill the enemy. Yet as long as he acts his professional part, he has to stick to his cue. Otherwise, he would cease to be a physician, in the same manner in which the judge who indulges in favoritism ceases to be the representative of justice.

The similarity between Scribonius' concept of a profession and that of Cicero, in my opinion, is so striking that the former can hardly be thought to be independent of the latter.[41] Perhaps Scribonius consulted the same sources of which Cicero made use and found his inspiration there. Perhaps he drew from a lost treatise on medicine and its professional obligations influenced by Panaetius' Stoicism; treatises on other professions and their duties are known to have been written at the turn of the first century B. C. to the first century A. D. In whichever way Scribonius learned of the views of his predecessors, the principal tenets

[40] The discussion summarized in the text makes it clear that, in Cicero's view, each "profession" or career has its own ethos. The example of the judge is obviously used as particularly appropriate to Roman conditions; cf. also above, note 38.

[41] Deichgräber (op. cit., pp. 865 ff.) assumes that the ethics outlined by Scribonius is original with him, though with reference to ch. 199 he admits that "die Frage der professio der Medizin hat [for Scribonius] allgemeineren Charakter" (p. 859). This in itself is an indication, it seems, that he is merely applying to medicine a general theory of professional behavior. The physician to the emperor Claudius must surely have been familiar with Stoicism. He was the freer to accept Panaetius' teaching which did not influence the established medical sects, because he himself apparently did not belong to any of the schools of his age (Deichgräber, p. 865 f.).

of the creed which his book attests for the first time must have their roots in the Stoic humanism transmitted through Cicero.[42]

As for the later history of this strictly professional kind of ethics, few testimonies are extant. The novelist Apuleius refers to certain physicians who hold it unfitting for " the medical sect " to be guilty of anyone's death, because they have learned that " medicine is sought out not for the purpose of destroying men but rather for that of saving them " (*Metamorphoses*, X, 11). His contemporary, Soranus, the great rival of Galen, mentions some colleagues of his who regard it as their duty to banish abortives not only because Hippocrates said one should do so, but also " because it is the specific task of medicine to guard and preserve what has been engendered by nature " (*Gynaecology*, I, 60).[43] While these

[42] E. Norden has drawn attention to the specific literature " De officiis judicis " which starts to appear around the middle of the first century A. D. (*Hermes, 40*, 1905, p. 512 f.). It differs from the usual type of " Introductions " to any given art in that here only the moral obligations of the judge are considered. With Cicero and his contemporaries the word *officium* comes to mean not only the objective task of an art, but also, if not preeminently, the duties incumbent upon the artist (cf. E. Bernert, *De vi atque usu vocabuli officii*, Diss. Breslau, 1930, pp. 25 ff.; 29 ff.; and above, note 34). Gellius mentions books on the juridical " office " in both Latin and Greek (*Noctes Atticae*, XIV, 2, 1). Panaetius and his pupils, Posidonius and Hecaton, wrote Περὶ τοῦ καθήκοντος; other Stoic books " On Duties " are known from Seneca (cf. H. Gomoll, *Der stoische Philosoph Hekaton*, 1933, pp. 27 ff.); the work of the artisan is considered as an *officium*, as a moral obligation, by Cicero (*De officiis*, I, 7, 22) as well as by Seneca (*De beneficiis*, III, 18, 1; cf. Gomoll, p. 77 f.). In the Stoic treatises just referred to the obligations toward one's country and toward other groups to which the individual may belong were set forth, or they were defined according to certain virtues. For the importance of philanthropy in late Stoic ethics, cf. above, note 29; below, note 45. The details of the general theory of professions as it was developed in the Middle Stoa I hope to discuss in an investigation of Stoic ethics. That the works on duties began to pay attention also to medicine is the more likely since physicians by this time were granted citizenship, and medicine was practiced even by free-born Romans (cf. K. H. Below, *Der Arzt im römischen Recht*, Münch. Beitr. z. Papyrusforschung u. antiken Rechtsgeschichte, 37, 1953, p. 20 f.).

[43] I should mention that Galen's refutation of Menodotus (cf. above, p. 407 f.) may be an indirect reflection of the fight about the new professional ethics. Menodotus was a pupil of the Sceptic Antiochus (cf. Deichgräber, *Empirikerschule*, p. 212), who leaned toward Stoicism and deviated in many respects from his school. Possibly his assertion that the physician's aim is money or honor was intended as the antithesis of the ethos of philanthropy. Also, Seneca's contention that men owe more to the physician than financial remuneration (*De beneficiis*, VI, 16, 1) may be a reference to physicians of the type Scribonius depicts, although elsewhere he acknowledges the fact that medical knowledge and moral goodness do not always go together (*Ep.* 87, 17). Finally, could not Pliny's notorious diatribe against the physicians best be understood if his judgment was determined by the humanistic ideal? For Pliny is careful in mentioning that all the crimes committed by physicians should be attributed to the individuals and not to the medical art (XXIX, 21 f.).

passing remarks do hardly more than rephrase Scribonius' formulations, a poem composed by an otherwise unknown Stoic pholosopher, Sarapion —he too lived in the second century A. D.—shows, I think, a certain evolution of the original theory. For in this poem, entitled *On the Eternal Duties of the Physician,* and inscribed on stone in the Athenian temple of Asclepius, the god of medicine and of the physicians, the god who prided himself most of all on his virtue of philanthropy, the " eternal duties " of the doctor are said to be: " First to heal his mind and to give assistance to himself before giving it to anyone [else] " and to " cure with moral courage and with the proper moral attitude." [44] Then " he would be like god savior equally of slaves, of paupers, of rich men, of princes, and to all a brother, such help he would give. For we are all brothers. Therefore he would not hate anyone, nor would he harbor envy in his mind." Here, the thought of Scribonius, the philosophy advocated by Cicero, is restated in the language of late Stoicism, in its new terms of human brotherhood, which indeed foreshadow the categories of Christian medical ethics.[45]

Finally the quintessence of pagan medical humanism was expressed by Libanius in a moving speech which medicine addresses to the young

[44] Cf. P. L. Maas and James H. Oliver, " An Ancient Poem on the Duties of a Physician," *Bull. Hist. Med.,* 7, 1939, pp. 315 ff. The translation is Oliver's, whose emendation [αἰ]ώνια I also accept against Maas' [Παι]ώνια (cf. p. 320, n. 6).

[45] Maas in his commentary (*loc. cit.,* p. 323) says, *ad vv.* 12 ff.: " color Epicteteus, ne dicam Christianus." It seems to me that the poem can be adequately understood within the confines of late Stoicism that so often approximates Christian ethics. For the brotherhood of men cf. *e. g.* Epictetus, I, 13, 3 f.; Seneca, *Ep.,* 95, 52: "natura nos cognatos edidit . . . haec nobis amorem indidit mutuum." Sarapion enumerating man's various stations in life spells out Scribonius' claim that medicine does not judge men by their circumstances in life or by their personality. Both proscribe envy (Sarapion: [ζᾶλος]; Scribonius: *invidentia*). While Sarapion derives from the brotherhood of men the duty not to hate anyone, Scribonius expresses the same thought positively through his concept of *humanitas.* (In the lines of the poem which I have omitted there are certain parallels with the deontological writings of the *Corpus Hippocraticum* noted by Oliver, p. 318, notes 2, 3; p. 320, note 4). Later Christian passages closely resembling the main drift of Sarapion's poem are to be found *e. g.* in L. C. MacKinney, " Medical Ethics and Etiquette in the Early Middle Ages," *Bull. Hist. Med.,* 26, 1952, pp. 6; 11 f.; 27. Only one feature sharply distinguishes pagan humanism from the Christian attitude and that of the nineteenth-century humanist reformers (for whom cf. I. Galdston, " Humanism and Public Health," *Bull. Hist. Med.,* 8, 1940, pp. 1032 ff.) : pagan ethics lacks any recognition of social responsibilities on the part of the physician. Although sickness was understood in rational terms, and some diseases were traced to social conditions, even the gospel of brotherly love took account only of the relationship between the individual doctor and the individual patient. Immediate help rather than long-range improvement remained the watchword. In general, cf. O. Temkin in *Social Medicine: Its Derivations and Objectives,* ed. I. Galdston, 1949, pp. 3 ff.

physician starting out on his career: " You desired to be one of the healers (of sickness), you had the benefit of having (good) teachers. Now, practice your art faithfully. Be reliable; cultivate love of man; if you are called to your patient, hasten to go; when you enter the sickroom, apply all your mental ability to the case at hand; share in the pain of those who suffer; rejoice with those who have found relief; consider yourself a partner in the disease; muster all you know for the fight to be fought; consider yourself to be of your contemporaries the brother, of those who are your elders the son, of those who are younger the father. And if anyone of them neglects his own affairs, remember that this is not permissible for yourself, and that it is your duty to be to the sick what the Dioscuri are to the sailor (in distress)." [46]

Is it by chance that the evidence concerning the survival of the humanistic ideal does not seem to go beyond the second half of the fourth century A. D.? Since on the whole the material for the history of medical ethics is so fragmentary, one hesitates to hazard judgment. Yet one may say with assurance that from the third century, Stoic philosophy—of which the doctrine of professional ethos formed part and parcel—ceased to have influence. The Neo-Platonists established Galen as the unchallenged authority in medicine. Through him, the philosophical ethics of the scientist-physician, which had never quite lost its appeal, came to predominate among the learned. Among the general practitioners of late antiquity, the teaching of the deontological writings of the *Corpus Hippocraticum* seems to have prevailed.[47] As for the rising caste of especially privileged physicians—those who as city officials were granted immunity from public duties, and those who became court physicians—it is hard to believe that they should have been keen on following the precepts of brotherly love. As I mentioned before, Galen already noted that the city physicians accepted their position in order to be relieved from the staggering burden of " indirect taxation." The " courtly " ethics discernable even in his writings, according to which the physician will treat the emperor and his family, and all wealthy people for that matter, differently from what he proposes to do in the case of the poor, implies

---

[46] Κατὰ ἰατροῦ φαρμακέως, 6-7. Libanius writes in the vein of Cynic and Stoic popular philosophy, probably echoing older traditions. Already to Seneca and his generation, the physician had become " the friend " of the patient (*De beneficiis*, VI, 16, 1) sympathizing with him and loved in return as a friend (*ibid.*, 4-6) ; cf. above, note 43.

[47] Cf. *e. g.* the *Introductio* of Ps. Soranus, *op. cit.*, p. 245, 17; 22; 33. Even the late deontological writings soon became integrated into some of the collections of the Hippocratic works compiled in the Christian era; cf. Fleischer, *op. cit.*, pp. 108 ff.

principles hardly compatible with Scribonius' love of mankind, or Sarapion's belief in the brotherhood of men.[48]

In the short span of time during which ancient medical humanism
was current, once it had finally been formulated in opposition to the
ideals of earlier generations, it most likely remained restricted to a small
minority of physicans. Scribonius himself divined the slim chances for
general acceptance of his belief and put the responsibility for this failure
upon the patients. " Rarely," he says (p. 4, 9 ff.), " does anyone make
an evaluation of the doctor before putting himself and his family under
his care. And yet, if people have their portrait painted, they will first
try to make sure of the artist's qualities on the basis of that which experience can tell, and then select and hire him." It is no wonder, therefore,
he continues (p. 4, 15), that so many physicians rest content with little
effort. Where no intelligent selection is made, where the good and the
bad are held in equal esteem, " everybody will practice medicine as he
sees fit " (p. 4, 24). The true reason for the relative ineffectualness of
Scribonius' programme probably lies in a shortcoming which it shared
with all the other ancient attempts to shape medical practice in accordance
with moral concepts. None of them had the backing of institutions or
organizations that had the power to enforce rules of conduct.[49] Yet,

[48] For Galen's rules concerning treatment of the imperial family and of the rich, cf.
e. g. Opera Omnia (ed. Kühn), vol. 13, pp. 635-38; 14, p. 659; also 12, p. 435. Surely,
the distinctions here made became even more marked when the hierarchic structure of
the empire was consolidated. The importance of the class of city physicians has been
pointed up through Herzog's interpretation of an edict of Vespasian in which their
privileges are set forth (Urkunden zur Hochschulpolitik der römischen Kaiser, Sitz-
berichte Berlin, 1935, pp. 967 ff.; cf. also Below, op. cit., pp. 23 ff.). Following perhaps
the example of Augustus, Vespasian granted to all physicians exemption from taxes and
from the burden of having soldiers billeted in their houses. Antoninus Pius revoked this
edict and introduced a numerus clausus for the privileged physicians in each city (cf.
Below, op. cit., pp. 34 ff.); Galen's rather damning statement on those who practice
medicine in order to be tax-exempt—to my knowledge never quoted in the pertinent
literature—may throw some light on Antoninus' reasons for curtailing the benefits of
Vespasian's edict. The imperial policy, in my opinion, was motivated by the recognition
of the usefulness of medicine to the state, a topic widely discussed at that time (Quintilian, Inst. Orat., VII, 1, 38; 4, 39; also Ps. Quintilian, Declamationes, 268). Herzog
ascribes Vespasian's action to the recognition of medical philanthropy (op. cit., p. 985),
and restores the text accordingly (v. 6). Yet he himself concludes from the passages in
Quintilian and from other statements that Vespasian invested physicians with the right
to form corporations on account of " the usefulness of medicine " (p. 982 f.). It was not
until Byzantine times that the privileges granted were made dependent on sufficient
technical knowledge and on the morally unobjectionable character of the recipient (Below,
op. cit., p. 41).

[49] Throughout antiquity, medicine remained free from supervision by civil authorities.
Even Roman law dealt only with cases of death attributed to the physician's treatment,

this very fact makes the achievement of the individuals who aspired to a medical ethics all the more impressive. It is praiseworthy indeed that under the given circumstances so many—some whose names history has recorded, and others whose identity has been obliterated—heeded Sarapion's appeal "to heal their own minds first " before giving help to their patients; that they were willing to forego material advantage for the law of their own conscience; that they took the initiative in raising and clarifying the moral issue, thereby laying the foundation for all later medical ethics.

It seems safe to add that among the ideals conceived by the ancients none was loftier than that which envisages love of humanity as the professional virtue of the physician. Even the Hippocratic *Oath* assumes full significance and dignity only if interpreted in the way in which it was understood by Scribonius and those who came after him. That this ideal of professional ethics also is the one most difficult to live up to, goes without saying. In fact, one cannot help wondering whether unending failure rather than even momentary success must not be the inevitable fate of those who commit themselves in earnest to such a seemingly utopian doctrine. For does it not essentially amount to the demand that the physician should be a citizen of two states, as it were, the one here and now, where he has obligations to his country, the other " laid up in heaven," where he is obligated to mankind alone? How can such a conflict of duties ever be fully resolved?

No one saw this dilemma more clearly than did Osler, when in his last address, from which I quoted at the very beginning of my lecture, he extolled the ideal of ancient medical humanism and held it up as the ideal to be followed in the future. He spoke after the First World War, after the lights of civilization had gone out over the world. With intrepid honesty he acknowledged the fact that " scientific men, in mufti or in uniform " under the pressure of hostilities, of civic duties rightly or wrongly understood, had compromised their conscience.[50] In the atmosphere of modern nationalism and modern technology it had proved even harder than it may have been in the world of old to distinguish between the role of the physician and that of the citizen. Nevertheless, Osler was not shaken in his belief in the ideal, nay he staked all his hopes on a new effort to realize it.

" Two things are clear," he said, " there must be a very different

---

or with questions of fees and similar contractual problems (cf. Below, *op. cit.*, pp. 108 ff.; also pp. 12 ff.; 63 ff.).

[50] *The Old Humanities and the New Science*, p. 13.

civilization or there will be no civilization at all; and the other is that neither the old religion combined with the old learning, nor both with the new science, suffice to save a nation bent on self-destruction." Reforms are needed. " The so-called Humanists have not enough Science, and Science sadly lacks the Humanities." But even if this defect were remedied, still more remains to be done. What matters is to keep in one's heart and mind " the magic word ' philanthropy ' ", love of mankind. Then, one day " the longings of humanity may find their solution, and Wisdom-Philosophia at last be justified of her children." [51]

Perhaps for those who have lived through the nightmare of another World War, who have witnessed the horrors of Fascism and Communism, an effort still greater than Osler's is required in order to have trust in ideals and in the future. If they seek for encouragement, they will find it ever anew, I think, in the sober appeal to good will and reasonableness which Osler made at the close of his memorable last speech, *The Old Humanities and the New Science*.

[51] *Ibid.*, pp. 19; 34; 64.

MEDICAL ETHICS IN HIPPOCRATIC BONE SURGERY *

THIS ESSAY WAS DEDICATED TO OWSEI TEMKIN
ON HIS SIXTY-FIFTH BIRTHDAY

MARKWART MICHLER

The golden age of Greek medicine is so called not only because of its rôle in the evolution of medical *techne* into a science, but also on account of those ethical precepts on which its medical men based their activities. At an early date this attitude made " deontology an integrant part of medical education," as Neuburger says,[1] and its oldest forms became models for the general moral philosophy of Socrates.[2] Within medicine, however, these ethics continued to have practical goals determined by the tasks of medical workaday routine. And this purpose conditioned their formal expression.

In the Oath and other deontological writings we encounter an almost complete doctrine. Anyone wishing to penetrate further into the ethical

* I am grateful to Mrs. H. Hirst for valuable help in translating and to Professor E. H. Ackerknecht for going over the English text. (The Latin titles appearing in the footnotes have been replaced in the text by the English titles of the Loeb Classical Library in order to facilitate the reading. [Ed.]).

[1] M. Neuburger, *Geschichte der Medizin*, Stuttgart: Enke, 1906-1911, vol. I, p. 189.

[2] W. Jaeger, *Paideia*, Berlin: de Gruyter, 1954, vol. II, p. 11 ff.

beginnings will have to consult the clinical treatises among the older Hippocratic writings. Here he will find scattered ethical rules which spring directly from the daily work of the physician. As maxims (*gnomai*), they are added to the clinical descriptions and are no less expressions of these ethics than the oath or later the precepts. Therefore the praise of a physician " whose mistakes are negligible," the advice " where the physician can do no good, let him do no harm," the remark that a medical man acquires personal sorrow from other people's sufferings, have been interpreted time and again up to recent times.[3] They not only deepened our knowledge of the professional attitudes of ancient physicians but also showed that the beginnings of their moral philosophy were inseparably linked to their practical activities. When Edelstein explained the genesis of these ethics through the social environment, he at the same time brought more strongly to mind their limitations. He showed that it is inadmissible to project modern concepts into these ancient maxims. However, he also made it clear that the development of ethical principles within certain groups of medical men represented " a great achievement " compared to ancient conditions.[4]

At this stage of the discussion it may be useful systematically to scrutinize a single writing for its ethical substance. Although both of the writings on bone surgery, " On Fractures " and " On Joints," tend to deal more with manual activities than do other ancient books, they bear witness at the same time to the fact that surgery contributed extensively to the development of Hippocratic ethics, and that it in turn was bound by the ethical rules of medicine. Although its prime concern was the reliability and improvement of practical methods, surgery has from time to time, through the very mastering of technological problems, developed ethical standards which have become the common property of all medicine.

With regard to the history of medical ethics, special importance must be placed on those doctrines which were apt to undermine the older prin-

---

[3] Cf. Neuburger, *op. cit.*, p. 192; on *ophelein e me blaptein* cf. W. Müri, *Arzt und Patient bei Hippokrates*, Beilage zum Jahresbericht über das Städt. Gymnasium in Bern, Bern, 1936, p. 5 ff.; H. Diller, ed., *Hippokrates Schriften* (Rowohlts Klassiker der Literatur und der Wissenschaft, Vol. 4), Hamburg: Rowohlt, 1962, in his introduction, to Epidemics I and III, p. 14; about *ep' allotriesi te xymphoresin idias karpontai lypas* (De flat. 1; VI 90 Littré [L.] = Corpus Medicorum Graecorum [CMG] I 91) and its consequences to medical ethics see H.-J. Frings, " Aus fremden Leiden eigene Sorgen," *Sudhoffs Arch. f. Gesch. d. Med.*, 1959, *43*: 1 ff. and K. Schubring, Übersehene Zitate," *Hermes*, 1960, *88*: 451 ff.

[4] Cf. L. Edelstein, " The professional ethics of the Greek physician," *Bull. Hist. Med.*, 1956, *30*: 395 f.

ciples of medical practice that placed the protection of the physician above
the welfare of the patient. In " The Art " the medical man is still instructed to avoid patients " overwhelmed by their diseases." Realizing
the limitations of medical art, he was not supposed to concern himself
with incurable maladies. This regulation may be old and go back to
archaic times, when the death of a patient resulted in a loss of reputation
and authority for the medical seer. Later it may have proved a suitable
safeguard against the unfounded suspicions of hostile laymen.[5] The first
to speak out against the inhuman attitude that was apparent in such a
rigid regulation is the author of " On Fractures " and " On Joints." In
his chapter about the deforming consequences of the irreducible luxation
of the hip with a backward dislocation of the caput femoris, he describes
in detail the altered walk of these incurable patients,[6] and in the midst of
the description of the acquired and the congenital forms he suddenly
begins his attack:

Now someone could indeed say such conditions fall outside the medical art for,
after all, why is it necessary to ponder further about diseases which have become
incurable? It is, however, quite wrong to think that this were the case: surely it
is obvious that one should be an expert at those as well, for it is not possible to
separate the one from the other. For one has to apply one's art to the curable
[morbid conditions] lest they become incurable, and this is done by knowing the
best way to prevent them from advancing to incurability. But one has to be
familiar with incurable conditions in order to avoid needless torments. Brilliant
and conclusive predictions [are derived from] recognition of the trend, of the
manner, and time when each [morbid state] will come to an end, and whether it
will take the turn to the curable or to the incurable.[7]

These sentences demand knowledge of incurable conditions and, at
the same time, unite three important ethical objectives which are also
referred to separately in other parts of the book. The statement that the
curable and the incurable morbid states cannot be separated forces the
physician first of all to break through the old taboo and to devote himself
also to incurable patients. Yet, even with this demand, medicine remains
far from the ethics of later times, which require giving medical care to

---

[5] De arte 3; VI 4 L.—Cf. L. Edelstein, *Peri aeron und die Sammlung der hippokratischen Schriften* (Problemata 4), Berlin: Weidmannsche Buchhandlung, 1931,
p. 100 ff. With references to the great age of this principle, see K. Schubring,
op. cit., p. 455, n. 2; cf. also the verdict formula in Egyptian medicine, H. E. Sigerist,
A History of Medicine, New York: Oxford Univ. Press, vol. I, 1951, p. 306, and
H. Grapow, *Grundriss der Medizin der Alten Ägypter*, vol. II: *Von den medizinischen
Texten*, Berlin: Akademie Verlag, 1959, p. 33 f.

[6] De art. 58; IV 248 ff. L. = II 203 ff. Kuehlewein [Kw.].

[7] De art. 58; IV 252 L. = 205 f. Kw.

the end to the patient with no hope of recovery. Even " On Fractures " and " On Joints " give the well-meant advice to avoid treatment as far as possible in two particularly precarious conditions, in compound fracture of the humerus or the thigh bone and in open luxations of fingers or toes.[8]

Yet even at this stage that old maxim is dealt its first blow. Another chapter dealing with ablation in traumatic gangrene of the limbs shows that the author was, in fact, well on his way to abandoning it.[9] The method of amputation described shows all the signs of a primitive operative surgery and was replaced by a much better procedure in the Alexandrian period.[10] The older surgical operation was bound to have an infaust prognosis, especially when it involved the loss of complete limbs. The author himself says that those in whom the injury extends as far as the thigh or the humerus rarely survive. The unusual uncertainty in his prognostic specifications is a sign of the hopeless condition of the patient, and again the reader expects the advice to refuse treatment. Yet the urge to help is so strong here that the author ignores the old restraints with the words: " However, one must attempt such treatment as such cases are more horrible to look at than to treat." [11] Confident in his medical experience, he does not refuse such treatment, and here again he forces his way through the bounds of the old protective regulation.

There can be no doubt that knowledge of incurable conditions is also demanded for the sake of prognosis, as is expressly stated in the last sentence of the passage quoted from chapter 58,[12] and that this question occupies a prominent place in the author's arguments. For besides the confidence in the physician which brilliant prognoses help to win, and besides the reputation (*doxa*) they gain for him, they have yet a third important function to accomplish: Only by an exact prognosis can a physician who is prepared to take care of incurable patients now obtain that protection which before was provided by the refusal of hopeless cases. Only an exact prognosis enables him to satisfy two other ethical demands found in the above quoted passage: not to torment the patient needlessly, and to prevent curable states from turning into incurable ones.[13]

[8] De fract. 36; III 540 L. = II 101 Kw.; De art. 67; IV 280 L. = II 220 Kw.

[9] De art. 69; IV 282 f. L. = II 221 f. Kw.

[10] Cf. Celsus, De med. VII 33; Ed. Spencer (Loeb) III 468 f.

[11] De art. 69; IV 286 L. = II 223 Kw.

[12] See above, ftn. 7.

[13] The all too one-sided interpretation of the Hippocratic prognostic by L. Edelstein, *op. cit.*, ftn. 5 above, p. 97 ff., especially with regard to bone-surgery, to which he refers in his essay, *op. cit.*, ftn. 4 above, p. 396, n. 10 and 11, has already been corrected by W. Müri, *op. cit.*, p. 59 ff., n. 9. Cf. also M. Michler, " Die Krüppelleiden in ' De morbo sacro' und ' De articulis,' " *Sudhoffs Arch. f. Gesch. d. Med.*, 1961, *45*: 312 f., n. 1, and in

As the reduction procedures of these ancient bone surgeons had to be effected without an anaesthetic, the second demand should be easily understandable. It is also found in the case of the compound fracture of the lower leg which could not be treated immediately after the accident. The setting may not be undertaken for seven days after the accident and then only if the patient is free from fever, the wound is not inflamed, and there is reasonable hope that the physician can effect the setting: "Otherwise, however, on no account should one cause needless pain."[14] It seems, therefore, only to be consistent that in the rest of the book the utmost stress is laid upon the avoidance of unnecessary pain. It is stated at the beginning of "On Fractures" that the immobilization of the arm in bowman posture causes more pain than the injury itself,[15] and in the following chapter the same thing is said with reference to its extension and fixation in hyperextension.[16] Whether the shoulder luxation is referred to,[17] or the redressement of a gibbosity,[18] again and again the physician is urged to avoid unnecessary pain.[19] The author recommends treatment for all luxations immediately after the accident, "for reduction can be accomplished more easily and more quickly before the swelling has developed and it is much less painful for the patient."[20] It would seem that the combination of the "much less painful" with the "more easily and quickly" shows clearly that such allusions are not only determined by clinical considerations but also by humane strivings not to aggravate the lot of the patient needlessly. "Painless, easy and quick," this deontological orientation places such endeavour into close affinity with other Hippocratic writings referred to by Knutzen.[21] It represents an attitude which, in addition to its endeavours to achieve technological perfection,

recent times G. H. Knutzen, *Technologie in den hippokratischen Schriften peri diaites oxeon, peri agmon, peri arthron emboles*, Wiesbaden: Steiner, 1964 (Abhandl. d. Akad. d. Wiss. u. d. Lit. Mainz, Geistes- u. sozialwiss.-Kl., Jahrg. 1963, no. 14), p. 50 f. (1360 f.).

[14] De fract. 31; III 530 f. L. = II 96 Kw.

[15] De fract. 2; III 422 L. = II 48 f. Kw.

[16] De fract. 3; III 424 L. = II 50 Kw.

[17] De art. 10; IV 104 L. = II 127 Kw.

[18] De art. 47; IV 206 f. L. = II 179 Kw.

[19] Cf. also De fract. 3; III 426 L. = II 51 Kw.; c. 17; III 478 L. = II 75 Kw.—De art. 50; IV 218 L. = II 185 f. Kw.; c. 69; IV 284 L. = II 222 Kw.

[20] De art. 79; IV 316 L. = II 239 Kw.

[21] Cf. Knutzen, *op. cit.*, ftn. 13 above, p. 11 (1321) f. and p. 12 (1322), n. 1, with reference to the deontological series of equivalent expressions in De offic. med. 4 and 7; III 288 L. and 290 L. = II 33 and 34 Kw.; also reference to passages in which they occur separately in De fract.—De art. and the reference to K. Deichgräber, *Professio medici, Zum Vorwort des Scribonius Largus*, (Abhandl. d. Akad. d. Wiss. u. d. Lit. Mainz, Geistes- u. sozialwiss. Kl. Jahrg. 1950, no. 9), p. 11 (863) about the after effects of this series in the "tuto, cito, iucunde" from Asklepiades of Prusa.—About the parallel in De victu in acutis 2; II 230 f. L. = c. 4; I 110 Kw. cf. in Knutzen, *ibid.*, p. 22 (1332).

pre-supposes definite ethical principles, and here *techne* and ethos can only rarely be clearly separated, for they have formed an almost perfect union.

Only in this context can the third demand, to prevent the curable from becoming incurable, be fully understood. It can be fulfilled only when to a sound prognosis is added an exact mastery of the various methods of operating and of the respective implements. " To help, or at least to do no harm " (*ophelein e me blaptein*), these maxims apply also to bone surgery, and at the end of a description of a leg splint we read: " If the rings are correct, soft, and freshly sewn, and if the tension of the rods is applied in the appropriate manner, as fully described, then the implement can be put to good use. If, however, some part of it is not in order, it will do more harm than good." [22] And immediately following this the author gives the general rule: " One must, however, also use the other mechanical aids either correctly or not at all, as it is disgraceful and contrary to medical art to apply mechanical aids which are incorrectly prepared." [23]

However, successful treatment is not achieved specifically with machines but requires also an exact knowledge of the various methods of reduction: " To know all the methods by which the physician effects the reduction and just how best to use them is a sign of good training," as is stated in the writing about the shoulder joint luxation, " yet, one must employ the most effective method appropriate to the observed degree of urgency." [24] It is obvious that these sentences present a technological rule; [25] at the same time, however, they embody the ethos of sound professional knowledge and mechanical efficiency as a requirement of every medical treatment. The acquisition, on the other hand, of such medical knowledge based on experience called for keeping a conscientious record of all failures: " I have written this down with full intent, for good are also those findings (*mathemata*) whose shortcomings came to light when they were tested, also why they failed," [26] says the author after describing his unsuccessful

[22] Epid. I 5; II 634 f. L. = I 11; I 190 Kw. and De fract. 30; III 524 L. = II 92 f. Kw.—If Knutzen believes that the deontological series could be taken as an indication of the close relation between De fract.—De art. on the one hand and De vict. in acut. on the other, one would be equally justified in claiming connection between the bone-surgical writings and Epid. I/III on the basis of the passage at hand, especially as the observance of this principle is also referred to in other passages of the bone-surgical writing.

[23] De fract. *ibid.*

[24] De art. 1; IV 80 L. = II 113 Kw. Cf. correspondingly De art. 71; IV 292 L. = II 226 f. Kw.

[25] On the technological interpretation of this passage, cf. Knutzen, *op. cit.*, p. 22 (1332).

[26] De art. 47; IV 212 L. = 182 Kw.—On the significance of μάθημα cf. Knutzen, *op. cit.*, p. 30 (1340).

attempt to reduce a spinal gibbus by blowing up a bag placed under the patient's back. The frank admission of professional blunders—the ruthless confession of his own and those of others—characterizes this book and makes even its polemics an ethical accomplishment. The description of the methods of bandaging open fractures is a particularly striking example. Here again the author warns against a method that places the bandages only above and below the actual injury and leaves the area of the fracture unbandaged. Although such a method may in a way have been the forerunner of what later became the fenestral bandage, this technique used only with lint bandages and without albumin, starch, or plaster, was bound to lead to deplorable consequences through inadequate immobilization and swelling of the soft parts above the area of the wound. Thus the author ends his description with the following words: " I would not have dealt in such detail with this problem, were I not absolutely certain that this method of bandaging is unsuitable, although used by many." [27] It is but logical that in the following chapter he should warn against using bandages that are narrower than the wound, as they strangle it like a belt.[28] Subsequently the necessary measures against pressure sores caused by bandages or splints, i. e., through the misuse of machines, are discussed quite openly.[29] In this connection Knutzen speaks with good reason " about reality serving to correct medical knowledge." [30] Indeed, honest observation of reality and objective assessment of the results of treatment are one prerequisite for the success of such endeavours; yet the ethos of pitiless veracity concerning one's own and others' failure can hardly be considered of less importance.

During the early stages of a rationally practiced medicine, certainly in no other sphere than that of bone surgery could there have been such a frank debate on technical errors. The permanent results of faulty treatment, visible to all, must have especially pricked the physician's conscience, and what is written about the tibia fracture is typical: " If the bones have not been placed correctly, it is impossible to conceal this fact, as the tibia is quite visible and completely without flesh," whereas in the sentence which follows it is correctly stated that a fracture of the fibula is easier to conceal, even if the fragments have been incorrectly fitted together.[31] When referring to the thigh fracture, the author talks in the same vein

[27] De fract. 25; III 500 L. = II 83 Kw.
[28] De fract. 26; III 502 L. = II 84 Kw.
[29] De fract. 27; III 506 ff. L. = II 86 ff. Kw.
[30] Cf. Knutzen, op. cit., p. 32 (1342).
[31] De fract. 18; III 480 L. = II 75 Kw.—Cf. also De fract. 4; III 428 L. = II 51 Kw., where correspondingly the same is said about the forearm.

" about the great ignominy and infirmity " of the shortened leg, " for when an arm has become shorter, the fact could be well concealed and would be no great handicap; if, however, a leg has become shorter it causes one to limp; then also the healthy leg shows up humiliatingly longer when held alongside the shorter one." [82] And these sentences are followed by those well-known words which in recent times have once again been one-sidedly interpreted as sarcastic witticisms, that it would have been better for him who has suffered such bad treatment to have broken both legs. Then he would at least have retained his balance. Despite the sarcastic tone of these words it should not be overlooked that such a sentence originates from a primitive way of surgical thinking, which keeps an open mind about the possibilities of correction, even when failure seems already inevitable to the layman. The surgical shortening of a healthy limb to compensate shortening of the other leg is not uncommon today. It represents the eventual realisation of that ancient notion, thanks to the greater possibilities of the modern age; and the history of surgery now indeed knows an era in which a compensatory shortening has been achieved by the bloodless fracture of the healthy limb.[83] The treatment for clubfoot

---

[82] De fract. 19; III 482 L. = II 77 Kw.

[83] M. Pohlenz (*Hippokrates und die Begründung der wissenschaftlichen Medizin*, Berlin: de Gruyter, 1938, p. 80) has regarded this passage as a prominent example of the sarcastic polemics of this book, and Knutzen (*op. cit.*, p. 8 (1318) f.) held the same opinion. However, for surgery this problem has long constituted an object of serious consideration. It has in more recent times made bone resection of the healthy leg in suitable cases of shortening of one leg a fully developed operative method (Cf. M. Lange, *Orthopädisch-chirurgische Operationslehre*, München: Bergmann, 1951, p. 61 f.; also W. Wachsmuth, *Die Operationen an den Extremitäten*, Berlin: Springer, 1956, p. 196, in: M. Kirschner, *Allgemeine und spezielle chirurgische Operationslehre*, ed. by N. Guleke and R. Zenker, Vol. X 2. At first glance the surgical operation may indeed seem to have no connection with the artificial fracture of a healthy leg, but really it also represents nothing but a surgically produced fracture, and one should not overlook the phases of its historical development. For while in the last century operative osteotomy was only occasionally performed, Rizzoli had at the same time developed a method for osteoclasy which realized the idea of the Hippocratic author, and E. Gurlt has already drawn attention to it in this connection (*Geschichte der Chirurgie*, Vol. I, Berlin, 1898, p. 253). Cf. J. Rochard, *Histoire de la chirurgie française au XIXe siècle*, Paris, 1875, p. 696 f.; for the description of the surgical procedure and the auxiliary tools, see: Th. Kocher and F. de Quervain, *Encyklopädie der gesamten Chirurgie*, Vol. II, Leipzig: Vogel, 1903, p. 250. There can be no doubt that such a method was at the same time also empirically inspired by the knowledge of successful refracturing of badly healed bone fractures, and the history of osteoclasy shows indeed that Rizzoli's method emerged from earlier methods which aimed at the refraction of badly healed fractures (cf. B. Valentin, " Die Geschichte der Osteoklasie," *Arch. f. orthop. u. Unfall-Chir.*, 1958, 49: 467 ff.; see also the chapter on osteoclasy in his *Geschichte der Orthopädie*, Stuttgart: Thieme, 1961, p. 141 ff.). This

offers another perfect example of the fact that those ancient physicians were seeking methods of treatment for already existing deformities.[34]

Thus the duty of telling the truth brings about this extreme degree of frankness. Without regard for the physician, each new experience is utilized for the sake of the patient and the improvement of methods. The final test in this matter is the answer to the question how the author will handle injuries for which he himself cannot yet suggest a satisfactory method of treatment; we find an example in his frank admission regarding an injury of the spine with a ventral dislocation of the vertebrae and ensuing paraplegia: " I myself have no method of reducing such a condition unless one or the other case may benefit from vibration on the ladder or any other such method, or possibly from stretching, as has been described earlier in this writing. However, I can cite no drastic procedure to combine with the stretching as, for instance, the board represents the drastic method in the case of kyphosis." [35] Here again, in an unfavorable case, the author does not extenuate his perplexity. Yet what seems more important is the fact that he does not state categorically that there is no method; in both cases he simply says, " I have no method," thus, in this instance also, keeping a door open for new contrivances (epinoemata).

The probity of the writing appears also in the ethical basis of its concept of mathema:[36] the frank discussion of malpractices is used here as a method of instruction and incorporated into the teaching of the correct

artificial refracturing of an incorrectly healed limb is, however, very old. In the Middle Ages evidence of it is already given in Roger of Salerno, and it can also be traced in antiquity in Celsus (cf. Roger, Practica chirurgiae III 16, 17 and Rolando, Libellus de cyrurgia IV 12, 13; quoted from Gurlt, op. cit., p. 714; Celsus, De med. VIII 10, 7 N; Ed. Spencer (Loeb) III 556). The fact that Abulkasim in two passages of the third book of his surgery (ch. 1 and 22) expressly rejects the artificial refracturing of badly healed bone fractures—with the typical argument that the ancients had nowhere mentioned it in their writings—should show all the more clearly that it was also practised in Arabian medicine. (Cf. Gurlt, op. cit., p. 646). Among shepherds it is likely to go back to the oldest times. Since chapter 5 of the Mochlicon (IV 350 L. = II 249 f. Kw.) proves that the Hippocratics also treated large animals, it may be presumed that they knew this method, although it is not specifically mentioned in the book. The refracturing of the afflicted limb, however, can only remove such shortenings as were produced by an axial deviation of the fragments, and it is for these cases that Celsus recommends this method. Shortening by retraction of the fragments without the essential axis-deviation will rather be aggravated than ameliorated by refracturing. The idea to undertake an artificial fracture of the healthy leg in order to adjust the shortening might, therefore, have occurred to the Hippocratic physicians, and for this reason the quotation under consideration should not be seen only as sarcasm.

[34] De art. 62; IV 262 ff. L. = II 211 ff. Kw.

[35] De art. 48; IV 212 f. L. = II 182 f. Kw.

[36] Concerning the μάθημα concept, cf. the comments of Knutzen, op. cit., p. 31 (1341) on ch. 47 of De art. quoted above, p. 302.

treatment of fractures and luxations. Describing a mistake with all its consequences makes it avoidable, and the student is safeguarded against repeating it. Other works from the ancient corpus also warn against diagnostic errors and therapeutic mistakes, but it may be assumed that at that time bone surgery alone made a didactic system (*didagma*) of it which keeps recurring in every discussion of any form of injury. " I must therefore mention which of the physicians' mistakes I want to teach not to do (*apodidaxai*) and which theories about the nature of the arm I want to propagate (*didaxai*) with my teachings." This beginning of " On Fractures " with its *apodidaxai* and *didaxai* constitutes the program of the whole book, " for the following dissertation is also instruction (*didagma*) about other bones in the body." [37] Hence, we find a great number of such *apo-didagmata*—if this word is permissible [38]—in every subdivision of this work, and this *mathema* which obtains its knowledge from experience gained from mistakes can hardly be overrated in the development of surgical instruction. As an integrant part of systematic surgical didactics it has to this day affected the style of textbooks on this subject. [39] The precision which marks the description, for instance, of the mistakes and dangers in the selection of points of cauterization in the treatment of habitual dislocation of the shoulder [40] testifies even today to the splendid beginnings of this methodology. Such realistic ethics can hardly have emerged out of moral speculations, and even now the book clearly demonstrates that here certain spheres of medical ethics combined

[37] De fract. 1; III 414 L. = II 47 Kw.

[38] As examples which have not been mentioned before, the following are quoted: De fract. 2 and 3; III 416 ff. L. = II 47 ff. Kw., c. 6; III 438 L. = II 56 Kw., c. 7; III 440 and 442 L. = II 57 and 58 Kw., c. 11; III 454 L. = II 64 Kw., c. 16; III 474 f. L. = II 73 f. Kw., c. 20; III 484 f. L. = II 78 Kw., c. 21; III 488 f. L. = II 78 f. Kw., c. 22; III 490 f. L. = II 79 Kw., c. 31; III 524 ff. L. = II 93 ff. Kw., c. 43; III 554 L. = II 106 Kw.—De art. 1; IV 78 f. L. = II 111 ff. Kw., c. 13; IV 116 L. = II 133 Kw., c. 14; IV 118 ff. L. = II 134 ff. Kw., c. 32; IV 148 L. = II 150 Kw., c. 33; IV 154 L. = II 152 f. Kw., c. 35; IV 158 f. = II 154 f. Kw., c. 40; IV 172 ff. L. = II 161 ff. Kw., c. 48; IV 214 L. = II 183 Kw., c. 50; IV 220 L. = II 186 Kw., c. 51; IV 224 f. L. = II 189 Kw., c. 52 ff.; IV 226 L. = II 190 ff. Kw. (Description of the consequences of unreduced hip luxations, *passim*), c. 63 ff.; IV 268 ff. L. = II 214 ff. Kw. (Warning against the reduction of open luxations, *passim*), c. 71; IV 294 L. = II 227 Kw., c. 86; IV 324 L. = II 243 Kw.

[39] As an example, one modern surgical work might be mentioned which reflects this inner relationship already in its title: *Fehler und Gefahren bei chirurgischen Operationen*, ed. by R. Stich and K. H. Bauer (3rd ed.), Jena: Fischer, 1954. From the editors' preface, which significantly bears the motto: " Quae nocent, docent," one sentence may suffice: " That is why Makkas and one of us, three decades ago, tried for the first time, with a staff of experienced assistants, using the literature and our own painful experiences, to point out the dangers which are connected with surgical operations." In the meantime, further editions of this work have been published.

[40] De art. 11; IV 104 ff. L. = II 127 ff. Kw.

with certain principles of treatment to reach that admirable level. As already noted, a definite contribution to the development of this surgery was made by both ethos and *techne*; they are still inseparably interwoven and this may also be the reason for the " practical commonsense " of these professional ethics.

Not until such a basis existed, i. e. not until ethics and *techne* had produced a basic stock of proper methods of treatment, could the efforts of the ancient physicians to detach themselves from the charlatan and the impostor [41]—which Edelstein regards as the main impetus in the development of medical ethics in that period—be successful. Only by giving better and more successful treatment were the Hippocratic physicians enabled to set themselves apart. It is therefore understandable that they were interested in not giving any cause for confusion of their methods with those of others. The book bears witness to these efforts in several other passages. The fact alone that a method is used by charlatans and impostors is enough for the author to avoid it when he has others at his command. Thus he writes about the " ladder treatment " for spinal injuries: " The physicians, however, who do use it are unskilful, at any rate as far as I know them. This idea is old, and I pay high tribute to the one who had it first. . . . I myself, however, have shunned treating all [cases] of that kind in this way, because such methods are preferred by charlatans." [42] The description of the complicated and sensational method extends over the next two chapters. It shows what a heavy burden it was for the patient, and the author concludes his statements with the remarkable dictum: " However, in every art, and not least in the medical art, it is disgraceful to cause a lot of trouble, sensation, and palaver, and then be of no use." [43] Like the book as a whole, this sentence demonstrates again that the development of medical ethics in this early bone surgery is not only closely bound to medical practice, but that it is also to be understood as a slow progression that only gradually overcame the older customs dating back to archaic times.

Undoubtedly, from the sociological aspect, the desire to detach oneself from the charlatan and the medical magician will have played an important part, but this alone does not explain the process. " Indeed, not to apply anything at all is sometimes a good remedy for the ear, as well as for many other things." [44] Such an utterance in connection with the fracture of the cartilage of the outer ear would clearly go beyond such desires, for

[41] See ftn. 4 above.
[42] De art. 42; IV 182 f. L. = II 167 f. Kw.
[43] De art. 44; IV 188 L. = II 171 Kw.—Concerning *ophelein* cf. above, ftn. 3, and below.
[44] De art. 40; IV 172 L. = II 162 Kw.

it is by no means the expression of a therapeutic nihilism but results from the experience that in this case any kind of dressing would be bad. But then, as today, every physician risked losing his patient's confidence if he took no action at all. It is this sentence, therefore, that reveals the whole inner meaning of that often quoted sentence from the concluding chapter of this book, the wisdom of which has not been lost to medicine to this day: "The highest value, however," so it says in chapter 78, "must in every case of the art be placed on how to cure the patient. If there are many ways of curing him, the simplest should be chosen, for this is more sincere and more correct as far as the art is concerned for anyone who is not attracted by crude cheating." [45]

[45] De art. 78; IV 312 L. = II 236 f. Kw. This maxim once more shows the close bond between ethos and *techne* without which the Hippocratic physician would have been unable to detach himself from gross fraud. The ethical elements—*andragathikoteron*—should therefore not need any further explanation, but the technological one—*technikoteron*—has given rise to several misunderstandings. Knutzen (*op. cit.*, p. 56 (1366) ff.) was right when he questioned Müri's interpretation, which linked the demand for minimal treatment to the *physis* concept of the writing (*op. cit.*, p. 11). However, this demand is not completely explained by the struggle against overestimation of the means and in favor of attributing importance to the total medical activity. For even if the thinking (*phronein*) of the physician is primarily focussed on the result of his work (*ergon*), in the treatment of the individual case considerable importance should also be attached to the means to which success is due, as this writing points out. For the final state of an injured limb it can, after all, not be immaterial whether it be stretched by the force of a clumsy apparatus or by the more finely gauged measures of the human hand, and wherever the human hand will suffice, the apparatus is to be avoided. Therefore, if for the treatment of an injury there are many ways (*polloi tropoi*), one has to choose the most incomposite way (*aochlotaton tropon*), for it is in the simplest sense of the word more in conformity with the art (*technikoteron*). The deeper sense of this postulate will therefore become much clearer if one considers its content in relation to the last aphorism: "What pharmaceutics don't cure, iron does; what iron doesn't cure, fire does . . ." (Aphor. VII 87; IV 608 L.). The principle of applying always the simplest means seems to have been immanent in Greek medicine from an early age. At any rate, Jamblich already attests to it for the Pythagoreans in the ascending line: Dietary measures, cataplasms, pharmaceuticals, cutting, and burning (Diels-Kranz, *Die Fragmente der Vorsokratiker*, Berlin: Weidmannsche Buchhandlung, 1912, 58 D 1, Vol. I, p. 467), and Scribonius Largus later on, instead of speaking of the "partes," will speak of the "gradus" of medicine (cf. K. Deichgräber, *op. cit.*, ftn. 21 above, p. 10 [862]). In the greater number of cases the more extensive and more complicated method usually not only inflicts greater pain on the patient but also increases the risk he is exposed to, and thus the old principle in medicine has remained alive well past antiquity. Similar passages in Arnald of Villanova are in all probability merely ancient tradition (*Des Meisters Arnald von Villanova Parabeln der Heilkunst*, übersetzt, erklärt und eingeleitet von Paul Diepgen, (Sudhoffs Klassiker der Medizin 26), zweite Doktrin, p. 12 ff.), but to a large extent this principle is still valid in medical practice, and even in the hospital a new and simpler method will usually rapidly replace a complicated older one, provided the results are the same. The corresponding passage in De fract. 15 (III 472 L. = II 72 Kw.) explains this attitude, and there is no need to look for a more profound meaning in its words.

The practical good sense which is once again apparent in these last quotations can be described as the common root to which both ethos and *techne* still remain subordinate. Therefore, a "theoretical knowledge of medical virtues" is nowhere expressly laid down, such as the one that the great philosophers tried to formulate a little later on for general ethics,[46] and which subsequently also appeared in the deontological writings of medicine. Examining just one writing does not allow one to make a final comment on the interpretation of Edelstein, who looks upon the attitude of the Hippocratic physicians as "an ethic of outward achievement rather than of inner intention."[47] The image of the honest ethics of a craft, which he adopts from Ruskin, could well refer to the origins; but just as the surgery described in this book no longer represents a mere craft, so too had its ethics outgrown that stage, even though there is as yet no philosophizing about moral principles. Here *techne* and ethos grow together, and with each other, and are about to awaken a higher moral consciousness in the medical man. No matter how one classifies this process, it would certainly be wrong to restrict its range of values to mere utilitarianism simply because it still lacks the theoretical elaboration of these problems. This ethos cannot be looked upon as an independent moral philosophy superimposed on the practice of medicine, nor is it on the other hand confined to a superficial utilitarian way of thinking: for the "help" (*ophelein*) of the writing already demands more from the physician. Certainly it is in the first place clinical considerations that call for the avoidance of needless pain—so as not to endanger the success of a reduction through muscular tension[48] or in order to guard against a dangerous syncope[49]—but there is also the admonition "to avoid needless torments."[50] If the former always kept the technological purpose in mind, and if a success therefore benefited the physician's reputation, the latter in any case has as its sole object the welfare of the patient.[51]

[46] Cf. Aristotle, Eth. Eudem. 5, Bekker 1216b.

[47] L. Edelstein, *op. cit.*, ftn. 4 above, p. 396 and n. 10.

[48] Cf. the indication in De art. 10; IV 104 L. = II 127 Kw. and, for instance, also in c. 18; IV 132 L. = II 142 Kw., where, in reduction of the elbow joint, the author indeed merely warns against touching the caput of the humerus with the processus coronoideus, but he is concerned above all not only with the danger of fracturing but also with the avoidance of muscular tension caused by pain, which would inevitably complicate the reduction.

[49] Cf. e. g. De art. 68 and 69, IV 282 and 284 L. = II 220 and 222 Kw.

[50] Cf. the initially quoted c. 58 from De art.; IV 252 L. = II 205 f. Kw. or e. g. also: De fract. 31; III 526 f. L. = II 96 Kw.

[51] The fact that Galen in his comments on the bone surgery writings explains pain in each case only objectively from the injury itself without expressing any opinion on the ethical problems must not be allowed to lead to any wrong conclusions. Galen obvi-

This ethos, which is dictated by practical commonsense, may well be responsible for the basic innovation evident in this writing, the medical treatment of congenital cripples.[52] Here again it may be significant of the author's attitude that his attention is not only directed to the curable forms, but to the incurable also, by the handling of which only little reputation was to be gained, particularly according to the opinion held at that time. In the case of the inwards dislocation of the hip which occurs in newborn children or in early childhood, he describes the crawling movement of such children if untreated: "All those, however, who have had proper instruction" attain, with the help of crutches, the ability to walk satisfactorily in an upright position.[53] With regard to another form of hip-dislocation, it is stated a few chapters later that: "The utmost care, however, is needed by those who have met with this accident whilst still quite young children, for if they are neglected in their childhood the whole leg becomes disabled and is retarded in its development." [54] With these sentences the author opposes an environment which mercilessly expelled the cripple from human society, and in this connection Müri has spoken about a "new concept of unfitness for life," relatively good health as opposed to completely good health.[55] Besides the practical results envisaged, this book again and again looks to the care of the patient, care which is not completely explained as a striving for the pleasure of a successful reduction, but which at the same time requires a human sympathy which goes beyond the mere ethics of the craft. As much as this ethic may, in a strictly philosophical sense, still be far removed from a theoretical system of medical moral principles, it might yet be compared with that *arete* which Aristotle later on assigns to the morally noble actions of the statesman as one of the three basic forms of the *eudaimonia*.[56]

ously avoids any comments on the ethical commandments of the writing, on principle. The reasons for his attitude are not clear; nevertheless it should be remembered that in his time philosophical moral doctrine had long since also determined the ethical principles of medical science (cf. Edelstein, *op. cit.*, ftn. 4 above, p. 408), and that Galen, in these questions, gave precedence to philosophy. (Concerning the problem of pain, cf. e. g., in addition to the passages quoted above from De art. 10; 57; 69, his comment I 36; III 101; IV 34; XVIII A 371, 639 f.,. 718 Kühn (K.)—In addition to the ethical maxims quoted above from De art. 42; 44; 58; 78, cf. his comment III 20; 27; 103; IV 60; XVIII A 515; 523; 645; 766 K.; cf. further e. g., in addition to De fract. 30, his comment III 32; XVIII B 583 K.).

[52] Cf. Michler, *op. cit.*, ftn. 13 above, p. 306 ff.
[53] De art. 52; IV 230 f. L. = II 193 Kw.
[54] De art. 55; IV 242 L. = II 200 Kw.—See also c. 60; IV 258 L. = II 209 f. Kw.
[55] Müri, *op. cit.*, ftn. 13 above, p. 9 f.
[56] Aristotle, Eth. Eudem. 4; Bekker 1215[b].

Such a *praxis kale* in a specifically medical guise increases its " help " (*ophelein*) and equates it with the words of the oath, according to which the physician should order what is to the advantage of the patient; [57] it makes it the nucleus of a moral philosophy which later on helped to establish the *humanitas* of the physician.

[57] Jus iur.; IV 630 L.

AN ANCIENT POEM ON THE DUTIES OF A PHYSICIAN
PART I

JAMES H. OLIVER
Columbia University and
The American School of Classical Studies in Athens

GENERAL OBSERVATIONS

In 1927 a Belgian archaeologist, Paul Graindor, assembled twenty-one large fragments of an ancient monument from among the thirteen thousand inscribed stones deposited in the Epigraphical Museum at Athens. The provenience of the fragments indicated that the monument had originally been erected in the sanctuary of Asclepius on the South slope of the Acropolis. Graindor was able to piece together three of the fragments from the top with part of an inscription in simple Attic prose to the effect that a certain Quintus Statius Glaucus had erected the statue of his grandfather and had engraved his grandfather's paean (a hymn to the healing god Asclepius). The other eighteen fragments seemed to belong to the paean, but Graindor made no attempt to extract from them an intelligible text. The stones were too heavy for a man to hold more than two in place, if indeed he discovered any joins between them. Glue alone would not suffice to attach to each other large stones with a small contact surface; and if one had the physical and financial means to undertake the task of rebuilding the monument, he was still uncertain as to what results he would obtain. The letters, being large themselves, were too few on each separate fragment to throw much light on the subject.

Thus in 1935 when J. Kirchner was reediting the Corpus of Attic inscriptions for the Berlin Academy, he followed Graindor's text of the three pieces with part of the heading, and he commented that there were eighteen other unintelligible fragments, of which he did not reproduce a copy.

In the meanwhile the American mission for the excavation of the

120

ancient Athenian Agora had collected several thousand more fragments of Athenian inscriptions, among which one other piece of the
same monument was recognized early in 1935. Thereupon, Dr. T.
Leslie Shear, director of the expedition, decided that the discovery
of our fragment imposed upon the Americans the responsibility for
the publication of the whole monument, and I was commissioned to
undertake the rebuilding of the monument with the assistance provided by the excavation staff and equipment during the summer
vacation.

We began our work with a search for other pieces of the monument among the thirteen thousand stones of the Epigraphical Museum. Here the chief mender of our excavation staff, Iannes
Bakoules, a man of difficult temperament but of extraordinary skill,
gave me most valuable assistance in locating the fragments. We
were able to collect more than double the number hitherto recognized.
Mortar still adhered, not only to most of the new pieces but also to
Graindor's, for they had apparently been built into a late wall after
the monument had been broken up. As soon as we brought the stones
together, we cleaned them carefully and discovered that the monument had been inscribed on more than one surface. We extended our
search to the South slope of the Acropolis, where we were rewarded
with other discoveries but with little that was pertinent to the task
in hand.

When all was ready, the pieces which effected joins, were fastened
with bronze dowels and glued together in the passage of the Epigraphical Museum, the director of which, K. Kourouniotes, extended every facility and made valuable suggestions. A foundation
of brick and plaster was prepared, and a great section consisting of
twenty-nine contiguous fragments was hoisted into an upright position with the help of a crane and made secure by filling the gaps with
plaster. A few other fragments which joined with each other but
not with the main section, were glued together and left on the ground.
Finally, with excellent photographs by H. Wagner and with the
necessary data, I published the results of our work in the periodical
Hesperia, V (1936), 91-122.

It appeared that the monument had been a large triangular base
with slightly concave sides beveled at the edges. This was sur-

mounted by an overlapping cap, on the upper surface of which near the front the cuttings apparently for a bronze tripod are still visible. Such tripods were frequently erected in Athens to commemorate victories in athletic, literary or musical contests. The base was of the white or golden Pentelic marble with which the Parthenon had been built, and it was inscribed on all three sides. Prosopographical evidence enables us to date the monument somewhere in the neighborhood of 220 A. D.

On the front the main inscription had been cut in beautiful letters. The name of the grandfather Sarapion, described as a Stoic philosopher, adorned the cap. Below stood the heading saying that Quintus Statius Glaucus priest of the Savior god had erected the statue of his grandfather and engraved the paean according to the permission of the Council of the Areopagus. Immediately below this the text is chiefly lost but seems to refer to a literary or musical contest. Then follows in large letters the poem, which turned out to be not a paean but a short philosophical work on the duties of a physician. It is composed in a Doric dialect flavored with a few epic forms. The choice of this literary medium may have been due to the example of the Doric poems in the famous Asclepieum at Epidaurus. Well below the philosophical poem and in smaller lettering comes the paean at last, but practically nothing has been preserved of it.

On the left side was engraved a paean composed by the great Athenian tragic poet Sophocles seven centuries earlier. It is actually labeled as his paean, and its fragments were not elsewhere preserved. This side constitutes the most interesting section for classical scholars, but it was not engraved by the ancient stonecutter with the same elegance as the rest of the monument.

On the right side was a list of those who chanted the paean. Among them were members of aristocratic Athenian families and incumbents of important priesthoods.

After the publication of the monument, the difficulties in the philosophical poem on the duties of a physician attracted the attention of Paul Maas, who is familiar to classical scholars among other reasons because of his authoritative edition of the Doric hymns from the Asclepieum at Epidaurus. He attacked the poem in order to recover the sense and to restore the exact words in the lacunae wherever possible. Assisted by other well-known students of Greek metrics, he prepared for the poem a reconstructed text, which he very kindly sent to me. In the meantime, our workman Bakoules stumbled on another fragment of the monument.[1] It bears the inventory number E[pigraphical] M[useum] 5840, and it fits into the very section containing the philosophical poem on the duties of a physician. It is not worth while demolishing and rebuilding the monument to put this one fragment in place; so I content myself with a drawing (Figure 1) to show how this fragment would stand in relation to neighboring pieces, if we did. In regard to the restorations already proposed by Paul Maas, it brought a surprise in one line, but it confirmed his conjectures for two others. He has now prepared a revised edition of the philosophical poem, and of this I present an English translation which the reader may compare with the Greek text in Part II, where the restorations are bracketed.

As a supplement to the following commentary by Paul Maas, I wish to make a few other general observations. The thought reflects the Stoic doctrine of the brotherhood of man but particularly the old philosophy of Hippocratic writings. The Hippocratic Oath is mentioned in line 3, and the command and prohibition appearing in lines 4-6, as Maas also notes, are contained in the Oath: " Into whatever houses I enter, I shall go for the benefit of the sick, and refrain from all voluntary injustice and corruption both in other ways and in the way of erotic actions upon the bodies of women and men both free and slave." [2] But there is more. The words ἀβεβάλοις of line 7 and ὄργια of line 9 almost occur in juxtaposition at the end of the Hippocratic law:[3] τὰ δὲ ἱερὰ ἐόντα πρήγματα ἱεροῖσιν ἀνθρώποισι δείκνυται, βεβήλοισι δὲ οὐ θέμις, πρὶν ἢ τελεσθῶσιν ὀργίοισιν ἐπιστήμης. It was a commonplace in ancient writings to speak of medical work as a divine

---

[1] Still another fragment—but from the right side of the monument—has recently been recognized by W. K. Pritchett, *American Journal of Philology*, LIX (1938), 343-345. It gives us Munatius Themison as the name of the year's archon.

[2] C[orpus] M[edicorum] G[raecorum], I, p. 5, 6. Also in the essay on the physician, *CMG*, I, p. 20: δίκαιον δὲ πρὸς πᾶσαν ὁμιλίην εἶναι· χρὴ γὰρ πολλὰ ἐπικουρέειν δικαιοσύνῃ, πρὸς δὲ ἰητρὸν οὐ μικρὰ συναλλάγματα τοῖσι νοσοῦσίν ἐστι· καὶ γὰρ αὐτοὺς ὑποχειρίους ποιέουσι τοῖς ἰητροῖς, καὶ πᾶσαν ὥρην ἐντυγχάνουσι γυναιξί, παρθένοις καὶ τοῖς ἀξίοις πλείστου κτήμασιν· ἐγκρατέως οὖν δεῖ πρὸς ἅπαντα ἔχειν ταῦτα.

[3] *CMG*; I, p. 8. The thought need not be the same.

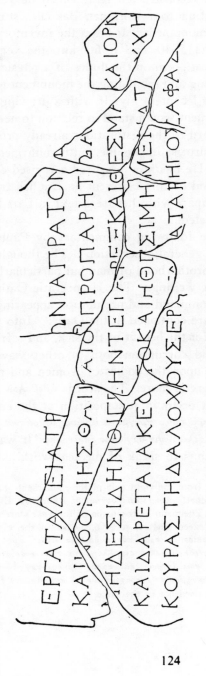

Figure 1. This drawing of the first five lines of the poem shows the relation of the new fragment (EM 5840) to the other pieces. The new fragment appears in the very center and contains parts of lines 2-5. Just to the right of it in line 2 appears an unusual symbol. The latter can now be interpreted as the circumflex accent which partly rests on the vertical hasta of an iota and envelops the sign ⊦ (only partly discernible) which indicates the rough breathing. In antiquity accents and breathings were seldom written, and in the case of a diphthong, they were usually placed over the first vowel. For a few examples and further references see Ad. Wilhelm, *Sitzungsb. Preuss. Akad. Wiss. Phil.-hist. Klasse,* 1933, 845-6.

service and of physicians and their prescriptions as holy and godlike (ἰητρὸς γὰρ φιλόσοφος ἰσόθεος),[4] while the training of a physician was represented as an initiation into sacred rites (ὄργια). On the privileged and sacred character with which physicians were usually invested all through Greek and Roman antiquity, see also the recent essay of R. Herzog, " Urkunden zur Hochschulpolitik der römischen Kaiser," *Sitzungsb. Preuss. Akad. Wiss., Phil.-hist. Klasse*, 1935, 967-1019.[5]

TRANSLATION

These are the duties of a physician: first (to repeat) the Paeonian [6] chants and to heal his mind and to give assistance to himself before giving it to anyone (else), and not to look upon (his patient) or make approaches in a manner contrary to divine laws and to the oath. He would cure with moral courage and with the proper moral attitude. And he would not, (spiritually) unequipped when as helper he handles lovely matrons and maidens, burn in his breast with desire (in a manner unworthy of a true) physician. Therefore I declare to the godly minded and the pure . . . and . . . healers . . . and sacred rites not perchance secretly to . . . this helps . . . child . . . and again art. Having become such a one in his judgment, he would be like God savior equally of slaves, of paupers, of rich men, of princes, and to all a brother, such help he would give. For we are all brothers. Therefore he would not hate anyone, nor would he harbor envy in his mind, nor increase his pretensions . . . not . . . Hygieia but . . . art . . . heart.

---

[4] *CMG*, I, p. 27, 3.

[5] W. Hartke, *Gnomon*, XIV (1938), 507-512, correctly argues that Herzog's thesis that Vespasian created freedom of organization for higher schools of learning is not yet proved; but whether this is true or not, Herzog's article contains an abundance of useful information.

[6] Paeon or Paean was the physician of the gods. I myself reject the " Paeonian chants " and read, Ἔργα τάδε ιατρ[οῦ αἰ]ώνια · πρᾶτον ε[Translate my text: *These are the eternal duties of a physician: first . . . and to heal his mind* (or *first to heal . . . and his mind*), etc.

Part II

PAUL LAZARUS MAAS
Königsberg in Prussia

GREEK TEXT AND ANNOTATIONS

Carmen de officiis medici moralibus

Ἔργα τάδε ἰατρ[οῦ· Παι]ώνια πρᾶτον ε[
καὶ νόον ἰῆσθαι καὶ οἷ πρόπαρ ἤ τῳ ἀ[ρήγην
μηδ᾽ ἐσιδῆν θιγέην τε παρὲξ καὶ θεσμὰ καὶ ὄρκ[ον.
καὶ δ᾽ ἀρεταῖ ἀκέο[ι]το καὶ ἤθεσι, μὴ μὲν ἀτ[ε]υχή[ς
5 κούρας τ᾽ ἠδ᾽ ἀλόχους ἐρατὰ[ς] ἅτ᾽ ἀρηγὸς ἀφάσ[σων
στέρνα πόθωι χλιάοι ετε[5-6 l.]ς ἰ[η]τῆρος.
τοὔνε]κα τοῖς ἀπόφαμι θε[όφροσιν ἠδ᾽] ἀβεβάλοις
11-12 l.]ας τε γαμ[ca. 8 l.   ἰ]ητῆρες
          ο]ιο κα[ὶ] ὄργια μὴ [ταχ]ὺ λάθην
10   ·]αὐτά τοι ἀ[ρή]γει
* * *]ασ[   ]ς τέκος, αὖθ[ι] δὲ τέχνα.
τ]οῖος μὲν [γνώμαν γεγ]αώς, θεὸς οἷα [σ]αωτήρ
δμώων ἀκτ[ε]άνων [τ]ε καὶ ἀφνειῶν καὶ ἀνάκτων
ἶσος [ἔο]ι, πάντεσσι δ᾽ ἀδελφεὸς [ο]ἷά τ᾽ ἀρήγοι.
15 πάν[τες γὰρ πέλομε]ν κάσιες. τ[ῶ μ]ηδέ τιν᾽ ἔχθοι
μηδ[ὲ φρεσὶ ζᾶλον κε]ύθοι ἢ ὄ[γκον] ἀέξο[ι.
μὴ μ[   ]μιν ηλ[
αἰσχ[   ]Ὑγιείας,
ἀλλὰ δ[   ]ε[* *] τέχν[
20 τοίως [   ]αι ἦτορ.

finis carminis.

Notae

De testimonio lapidis

Scriptio plena: τάδε ἰατροῦ (1); sic potius quam τάδ' εἰατροῦ. — iota mutum neglegitur: τῶ — τινί (2). — accentus spiritus interpunctio desunt excepta voce οἱ (2). — litterae quarum mutilatione sensus afficitur: 9 Υ vel Κ, 17 Λ vel Χ. — 15 Η et Τ primus agnovit W. Peek. — suppleverunt W. Dittenberger (*IG* III 3845) 6 η, 8 ι, 12 σ; J. H. Oliver 4 ι, 5 σ et σων, 9 ι, 11 ι, 12 τ, 13 ε et τ; W. Peek 15 μ, 16 ἐ φρεσὶ et γκον; W. Theiler 12 γνώμαν γεγ; cetera ego.

De re metrica

Spondiaci 6. 8. — interpunctio post caesuram septenariam 10. 12. 15. 16. — hiatus 4. 6. 16 (bis). — ceteroquin versus admodum fluenter decurrunt.

De rebus grammaticis

Sermo artificiosus, abstinens pedestribus, remota cupidius appetens. Formis doricis epicae intermiscentur: πρᾶτον, ἰῆσθαι, λάθην (= λήθειν), ἐσιδῆν — ἰητήρ (6. 8, si vera supplementa), χλιάοι, gen. ...ο]ιο (9). mirum illud θιγέην (3) elementa utriusque dialecti copulata offert.

ἀρηγός (5), vox inaudita; quam in ἀρωγός mutare tamen non audeo; cf. ἀρηγών.

ἀρήγω (14, suppl. 2. 10) de medico aegrotum curante aliunde non affertur; de medicamentis iuvantibus adhibet Hippocrates.

ἀτευχής (4) ' inermis,' vocabulum rarum, hic translate dictum.

ἤθεα ' mores boni ' (4), sensu novo.

κάσιες (15); haec forma nondum legebatur.

μέν solitarium (4. 12), adhibetur παραπληρωματικῶς.

πρόπαρ ἤ ' prius quam ' (2), constructione nova.

τις pro ἄλλος τις (2 τῷ) audacter dictum, nisi fallit supplementum.

χλιάω ' tepefio ' (6), vocabulum rarum; hoc exemplo confirmantur duo lectiones Nicandreae adhuc addubitatae (cf. *GEL*).

Hyperbaton τοῖς ἀπόφαμι θε[όφροσιν ἠδ'] ἀβεβάλοις exemplis qualia sunt Il. Λ 831 προτί φασιν 'Αχιλλῆος, Callim. fr. 118, 2 οἵ φασι τεκόντες explicari potest, sed vix excusari; nam ἀπόφαμι non est encliticum. cf. Callim. epigr. 55 Τῷ με Κανωπίτᾳ, fr. 191 Τόν με παλαιστρίταν, Elegia in Telch. 22 ὅ μοι Λύκιος, Rhinton fr. 10 K. ὅ σε Διόνυσος. liberius tamen Theocritus in Aeolicis (29, 24) ἐξ ἐπόησε σιδαρίω.

Ad singulos locos

1: tentavi Παι]ώνια πρᾶτον ἐ[πᾴδην, quod de animo medici firmando accipiebam; nam de curatione aegrotorum sive ad animum sive ad corpus pertinente omnino non agit poeta.

2: cf. evang. Lucae 4, 23 ἰατρέ, θεράπευσον σεαυτόν et Olympiodorum in Plat. Gorg. 513 d, p. 187, 25 Norvin (ed. 1936) οὐ δεῖ ἰατρὸν νοσεῖν· ὀφείλει οὖν πρότερον ἑαυτὸν ὑγιάζειν καὶ οὕτως ἄλλους κτλ. (verba sunt Iacobi Psychristi, celeberrimi medici V. p. Chr. saeculi, de quo vide Gossen, *Real-Enc.* v. Jakobos 3, ubi et hic locus addendus et Malalas 370).

3 et 5 sqq.: cf. Hippocratis Iusiurandum . . . ἐκτὸς ἐὼν πάσης ἀδικίης ἑκουσίης καὶ φθορίης τῆς τε ἄλλης καὶ ἀφροδισίων ἔργων ἐπί τε γυναικείων σωμάτων καὶ ἀνδρῴων.

10 sq.: ars medici in sanandis morbis secundarium locum obtinet, maior quaedam vis (divina scilicet) αὐτὰ ἀρήγει, ipsa per se iuvat. — αὖθι δὲ τέχνῃ notissimum Callimachi versum claudit, Elegia in Telch. 18, sed sensu prorsus diverso.

12 sqq.: color Epicteteus, ne dicam Christianus.

Medical Deontology in Ninth Century Islam[*]

MARTIN LEVEY[**]

HIS discussion is concerned primarily with the work of Isḥāq ibn 'Alī al-Ruhāwī and his deontological treatise, *Adab al-ṭabīb*, "Practical Ethics of the Physician." This work is unusual in that it is the only one known to have considered the aspects of ethics on a broad scale in Arabic medicine. Further, it is of value since it was written in the ninth century, a period of spreading ferment in a renaissance which included the acquisition of older knowledge from widely scattered sources and also rapid strides in translation of scientific and philosophical material into Arabic. In addition, the content is of great interest in its delineation of the manner in which Muslim (and to some extent, Christian) religious ideas were made to harmonize with the older science and in particular with the ethics of the Greeks.

During the ninth century, the flood of translations of the great Greek, and to a lesser extent Indian, mathematicians, physicians, astronomers, geographers, and philosophers reached an unparalleled height. These works, due mainly to Syriac-speaking Christians, were of excellent calibre for the most part. They acted as catalyst for the unprecedented acceleration in the development of Arabic science in the ninth to eleventh centuries in the Near East, the Mahgrib, and in Spain.[1]

It was also in this same ninth century, as a result of these translations, that the Muslims were brought face to face with new and sophisticated ideas of ethics and morality. While the introduction of new concepts was proceeding, the Muslims tried to bring about some kind of understanding of the traditions of the differing elements of Islamic thought.[2]

Ethics, or "practical philosophy" as the Arabs called it, was a product in the pre-Islamic period of a tribal society with a marginal economy. This gave rise to female infanticide; polygamy was accepted and was common; so were drinking and gambling;

[*] This study was conducted with the aid of U.S.P.H.S. Grant 12594.
[**] State University of New York, Albany, New York.

[1] Max Meyerhof, in a chapter "Science and Medicine," in *The Legacy of Islam*, Oxford, 1931, pp. 315ff. J. Schacht and M. Meyerhof, *The Medico-Philosophical Controversy between Ibn Butlan of Baghdad and Ibn Ridwan of Cairo*, Cairo, 1937, pp. 7 ff.
[2] R. Walzer and H. A. R. Gibb, in *Encyclopedia of Islam*, new ed., vol. I, 1960, pp. 325 ff.

generosity, courage, self-control, and hospitality were linked with personal and tribal honor, as was resort to vengeance.

Muhammad and the Koran, on the other hand, preached general principles which did not conform with the needs of a nomadic life but were probably intended to lift his people from their static, culture-hardened ethical system to a new cosmopolitan form, fit for an urban society. This involved new precepts, such as belief in and duty to Allah, forgiveness, moderation, restricted retaliation, honesty, humility, charity, kindness, and the brotherhood of believers,[3] virtues meriting rewards of Allah. In addition to the Koran, other ethical compilations such as the hadith, based on the model actions of Muhammad, assumed a great importance in Muslim life.

Before Arabic writers became acquainted with Greek philosophical literature, they had learned of the Pahlawi and Indian moral literature, which had been translated from the Pahlawi and Sanskrit versions during the reigns of al-Manṣūr (754-775) and Hārūn al-Rashīd (786-809), Abbasid caliphs. Ibn al-Muqaffaʻ (d. 757/8), an Iranian convert to Islam, translated *Hudhāi-namak* (in Arabic, *Siyar mulūk al-ʻajam*) "History of the Kings of Persia," and produced the celebrated translation, *Kalīla wa-dimna.*[4] To ibn Muqaffaʻ is also credited *Adab al-kabīr* and *Adab al-ṣaghrīr,* works on ethics.[5] Later, the integration of pre-Islamic, Koranic, Persian, and hadith ethical thought was brought about by ibn Qutaiba (d. 889/890) in his *ʻUyūn al-akhbār.* Essentially, the Persian and Indian ethics were of a wisdom-literature type but they were, nevertheless, practical contributions in a minor degree to the development of Muslim ethics.

The synthesis of not always compatible ethical values was a very difficult one in Islam since it involved a gradual choice and the blending of widely differing religious and philosophical ideas stemming from cultures of varying and unusually complex content. This provided a good reason for the continuing debate which went on in early medieval Muslim society on the standards of ethical values.

In the ninth century, it was a great trial for the Muslims to become aware of Greek ethics at a time when they were bringing

---

[3] Cf. D. M. Donaldson, *Studies in Muslim Ethics,* London, 1953, chapter 2; al-Shahrastānī's *Nihāyat al-iqdām fī ʻilm al kalām,* A. Guillaume, Ed., Oxford, 1934, pp. 158 ff. in regard to early religious ethics and law; abū al-Qāsim Hibatallāh ibn Salāma, *Al-ñāsikh wa'l-mansūkh,* Cairo, 1310 H., introduction.

[4] L. Cheikho, *La version arabe de Kalilah et Dimnah,* Beyrouth, n.d.

[5] Cf. D. Rescher, *Mitteilungen d. Seminars f. Orientalische Sprachen* (1915 and 1917).

their ethical literature to its utmost in study and organization. It was in this milieu that such early writers of ethical works as al-Jaḥiz (d. 868), ibn Qutaiba, and also the historians abū Ḥanīfa al-Dīnawarī (d. 895), ibn Waḍīḥ al-Yaʻqūbī (d. 897), and al-Ṭabarī (d. 895)—all contemporaries—lived and worked.[6]

From the point of view of medical deontology, the importance of the impingement of Greek ethics on this crucial period lies in the fact that the great Muslim physicians, all of whom were deeply interested in philosophy, had seriously to reconsider the basis of their ethics, both personal and professional. It was essential that they bring their ideas into some kind of working agreement with Greek ethics which had a very different metaphysical foundation. At the same time, in various ways, a tremendous pressure was exerted on the older ideas of the Muslims by the rational medicine, science, and philosophy taught at Jundīshāpūr (established by Khusrau Anūshirwān, 531-579), in other Nestorian centers,[7] and finally among the Arabs. It is of interest, in remembering the fertility of these centers, to recall the fact that by 900, in the case of the works of Galen, for example, 129 of his medical and philosophical treatises were known in Arabic and already much used by the Arabs.[8]

A factor which exerted a two-pronged influence upon the early Muslims is the Aristotelian notion that virtue is embodied in the just mean. Something similar is to be found in the Koran, and since the Islamic tendency is toward conservatism, this determined conciliation of opposites, establishing justice, worked for a time in ethics and became popular. However, one of its accompanying results was that it generated a menace to the orderly growth of science.[9] Other Greek elements influenced the deontological picture of the ninth century. One of the more important was the Stoic philosophy found in Galen. Platonic, peripatetic, and other forms of ethical thought found their paths to the Muslims in different ways.

6 Donaldson (n. 3), p. 97.

7 T. J. de Boer, *The History of Philosophy in Islam*, London, 1961, pp. 11 ff.

8 G. Bergsträsser, *Ḥunain ibn Isḥāq, Ueber die syrischen und arabischen Galen Uebersetzungen*, reprint from *Abhandlungen zur Kunde des Morgenlandes* 1925, *17*; further information on Ḥunain's Galen bibliography by the same author in the Leipzig, 1932 issue of the same journal; K. Deichgräber, *Die Griechische Empirikerschule*, Berlin, 1930, pp. 38-39; R. Walzer, *Mediaevalia, Antike und Orient im Mittelalter*, vol. I, P. Wilpert and W. P. Eckert, Eds. Berlin, 1962, pp. 179-195; Fr. Rosenthal, "On the Knowledge of Plato's Philosophy in the Islamic World," *Islamic Culture*, 1940, *14*, 387-422.

9 de Boer (n. 7), p. 40.

The ninth century, a time of conflict in ethical thought, was the background against which al-Ruhāwī brought out his deontological treatise, *Adab al-ṭabib*, to be described in this article. Unfortunately, not much is known of the author. He was mentioned indirectly by ibn abī Uṣaibi'a (1203/4).[10] Al-Ruhāwī was probably from Ruhā, a city of northwest Mesopotamia. Earlier, it had been called Edessa, a well-known Nestorian center of learning at one time. It is also known that al-Ruhāwī was a Christian and that he compiled two works based on Galen. (Despite his nominal Christianity, his beliefs were essentially Muslim, as will appear below.)

The *Adab al-ṭabib* is to be found only in Istanbul in the Sulemaniye Kutubkhane, number 1658. It comprises 112 folios with seventeen lines to the page. The meaning of the word *adab* in the title, in its pre-Islamic sense,[11] has been defined by Gabrieli[12] as a hereditary norm of conduct or custom derived from ancestors and from others taken as models. This meaning changed in time, paralleling the evolution of the Muslim culture. Especially was this developed in the century of al-Ruhāwī, when those studies came to the fore which centered more on man himself, his psychology and environment, his material and physical culture. In this way, *adab* came to indicate a profane rather than a religious idea. It grew to have a humanistic connotation, turning from *urbanitas* to *humanitas* and, at the same time, enlarging its ethical and practical content. This was the meaning in the ninth century; it was, in brief, "conduct with a strong ethical connotation," or "practical ethics."[13]

In this work, *Practical Ethics of the Physician*, al-Ruhāwī seems to rely much upon Aristotle's *Metaphysics* and on Plato's *On the Soul*. Some of the quotations attributed to these authors are from apocryphal writings which agree more readily with Muslim tenets. Al-Ruhāwī also quoted much from Hippocrates and Galen. Other authorities mentioned are Pythagoras, Epicurus, Democritos, Zeno, al-Kindī, Ḥunain, and Isḥāq.

10 M. Steinschneider, *Die arabischen Uebersetzungen aus dem Griechischen*, reprint, Graz, 1960, p. 31; B. R. Sanguinetti, *J. Asiatique*, 1855, 6, 156; G. Fluegel, *Ḥājji Khalīfa's Lexicon bibliographicon . . .* , Leipzig, 1835-1858, 7 vols., vol. I, p. 234, vol. III, p. 353; M. Steinschneider, *Polemische und apologetische Litteratur in arabischen Sprache*, Leipzig, 1877, pp. 50, 136; ibn abī Uṣaibi'a's (1203/4-1270) *Kitāb 'uyūn al anbā' fi ṭabaqāt al-āṭibbā*, A. Mueller, Ed. Koenigsberg, 1884, 2 vols., chap. 8 on "Syrian physicians at the beginning of the Abbasid dynasty." Cf. also L. Leclerc, *Histoire de la médecine arabe*, Paris, 1876, 2 vols., vol. I, p. 497.

11 I. Goldziher, *Encyclopedia of Islam*, 1st ed., vol. I, p. 122 under *adab*. Cf. C.-A. Nallino, *La Littérature Arabe*, Paris, 1950.

12 *Encyclopedia of Islam*, 2d ed., vol. I, under *adab*.

13 *Adab al-ṭabib* MS, chap. I on fol. 4a.

As a collection of material on medical deontology, the main purpose of the treatise is to elevate the practice of medicine in order to aid the ill and to enlist the aid of God in his support, vocationally and otherwise.

The text is a full and comprehensive one on the relations among physician, patient, visitors, nurse, and servant, together with their directions, injunctions, and moral obligations in the course of medical practice.[14] Together with these practical matters, al-Ruhāwī insisted on the necessary interrelation of spiritual and bodily physic. From very early Greek physicians to the later Arabic medical writers, maladies of the soul were treated by medical procedures.[15] Even in the period of the Muslim mystics, it was quite usual for the spiritual director to be considered as a physician. It is no surprise, therefore, that al-Ruhāwī, in accordance with Galenic medicine, laid much stress on the highest type of humanity as being found in the cultivation of Greek rational ethics to attain man's oneness with God. There was thus a necessity for the development and growth of moral understanding. This was the reason that al-Rāzī wrote his little treatise,[16] "Book on the Spiritual Physick," a work on popular ethics, and a companion, as al-Rāzī called it, to his medical work, *Kitāb al-Manṣūrī*.[17] Before going on with a more detailed discussion of al-Ruhāwī's medical deontology, the contents of *Adab al-ṭabib* should first be described.

In the first chapter, on the loyalty and faith which a physician must possess and the ethics he must follow to improve his soul and moral character, al-Ruhāwī states that the attributes of a physician resemble those of a good governor. Aristotle is quoted to the effect that "a governor must possess four qualities: he must be sensible, learned, pious, and he must act without haste. A governor may embroider his rule or corrupt it. All of these attributes are sound in a physician. Both have similar duties since a physician is the governor of souls and bodies. There can be no doubt that souls and bodies are better than estates. Therefore, a physician must take upon himself proper ethics and science useful for his profession."[18]

---

[14] *Ibid.*, fols. 52a ff.
[15] Carra de Vaux, *Encyclop. of Islam*, 1st ed., vol. I, u. *akhlāq*, p. 233.
[16] This manuscript is to be found in the British Museum, 1530.
[17] Cf. de Boer (n. 7), pp. 77-79. Al-Rāzī's work on moral health has been translated by A. J. Arberry, *The Spiritual Physick of Rhazes*, London, 1950. *Vide* Fr. Dieterici, *Alfārābī's Philosophische Abhandlungen*, Leiden, 1892.
[18] *Adab al-ṭabib* MS, fol. 4b.

According to al-Ruhāwī, the physician must have complete faith in God since all of man's powers come from Him. Again, he stresses the idea of moderation.

Know that with the moderation of these powers in man his moral character may be virtuous and praiseworthy and his soul pure and clean. When these powers come out without having undergone a moderating influence, then his moral character is ruined and evil.[19]

To back up his statements, the author quotes Aristotle, Homer, Galen, and an unknown Socrates. The statements attributed to Aristotle are apocryphal and the Socrates mentioned could not be the well-known figure of philosophy.

Chapter two may be considered as a small treatise on the preventive medicine of the time. It is of interest to note that the health of the physician himself is a subject important enough to follow the chapter on faith in God. The title of chapter two is, "On the means and measures by which a physician treats his own body and limbs. This part includes many duties which must be discussed in detail."[20]

The third chapter concerns the attitude of the physician toward the patient and the method of therapy. The physician should not employ a substitute to treat the ill or to maintain health. What is beneficial in therapy should be continued; otherwise, it is best not to use any therapy. Hippocrates is quoted to show that the therapist must go beyond the necessary action to benefit the patient. However, if a drug is doubtful, it is not to be employed.[21]

This chapter is a mixture of etiquette, bedside manners, religious moralizing, and idealistic ethics as the following paragraph will show:

The physician must not be vengeful, envious, hasty, sad, vexed, or greedy; on the contrary [he must be] forbearing in regard to faults, indulgent with people, steady, erudite, soft, humble, quick to goodness, content, thankful, and with great praise as being far from sin, virtuous, and clean inside and outside. When a physician possesses these meritorious morals, he should not meet with ignorant people, so as not to descend to their ignorant level.[22]

The next two chapters discuss necessary advice to servants of the patient and his visitors. It is the duty of the physician to advise the servant on the care of the patient and also to make known the proper behavior of the visitor toward the ill one.

19 *Ibid.*, fol. 10b.
20 *Ibid.*, fol. 2b.
21 *Ibid.*, fol. 59b.
22 *Ibid.*, fol. 60a.

It is difficult to determine the amount of ethical content in the various duties and responsibilities which the physician may or may not carry out. In the ninth century the practitioner had to be a botanist, pharmacist, and pharmacologist so as to check upon drug remedies.

Since drugs are the most important agents in recovery from illness, the physician must be careful in knowing them first, both the good and the bad.

The remedies are of two types, one simple and one compound. For this reason, the spoilage of compound remedies occurs more often than it does for simples. This is because of error in compounding and insufficiency of skill in the art of composition, mixing, and mingling. Do according to what I mention, O physician, since you are obliged to know it.[23]

In order to learn about simple and compound drugs, the physician is advised by al-Ruhāwī that this cannot be done from books but only by careful attention to the masters who grow the plants and work with them. Not only does al-Ruhāwī place a duty upon the physician in regard to the use of such drugs as opium, scammony, cantharides, euphorbium, and others but this duty is enlarged to include supervision of drug merchants and druggists in their handling of remedies. That this became an impossible task for the physician can readily be seen in the later *hisba* literature where this supervision is described as being taken over by the *muhtasib,* an official whose duty it was to protect public morality, especially in trade, assure the purity of the faith, and protect people from charlatanry and fraud.[24]

In chapters VII to XI, al-Ruhāwī returns to the proper conduct of the physician in regard to his patient and nurse, the behavior of the patient in taking the orders of the physician, and what the patient must do with visitors who interfere with the physician.

Hippocrates is quoted to the effect that the conduct of the medical art involves three factors, the illness, the patient, and the physician. The last two have the obligation to work together against the illness. In the case of some ailments, visiting is prohibited. Should a visitor come, then he must wear clean clothes, have a good odor, and not stay overlong. The conversation should be pleasant and not of disturbing matters.

To cope with visitors and with difficulties which arise during illness, a man should prepare himself during health, "keep him-

[23] *Ibid.,* fol. 64a.
[24] Cf. M. Levey, "Fourteenth Century Muslim Medicine and the Ḥisba," *Med. Hist.,* 1963, 7, 176-182; R. Levy, Ed. *Ma'ālim al-qurba fī aḥkām al-ḥisba by ibn al-Ukhuwwa,* London, 1938.

self from rage and anger, have patience, and acquire good morals. Then he will find these easily in time of illness."[25]

The dignity and honor of the physician are explained in chapters XII and XIII, "On the dignity of the art of medicine," and "On the respect due to a physician according to his skill and the necessity to honor him above royalty and virtuous people."

Since we have mentioned the dignity of the medical art and its priority in rank to other arts and crafts, it encourages people of reason and culture to acquire it. It inspires them to follow its commands and refrain from the things prohibited. It urges them to show regard for practitioners. Therefore, it is necessary for me to mention that which is notable of its dignity, and the best of its virtues.[26]

Further, "It is known that the intention of the physician is to inquire into one's health and his aim is to obtain it. He cannot do this except by the art of medicine, the purpose and aim of which are this. It is given as a gift by the exalted Allah."[27]

All through the treatise of al-Ruhāwī, the author is deeply concerned with the standard of the medicine of the day and the dignity of the physician. He writes that since the dearest possession of man is considered to be health, then those who have acquired the profession of medicine are on the side of the virtuous and rational ones, "the foremost of the people in station, highest in rank, greatest in worth, and most truthful in speech." This, says. the text, is because when this art was bestowed on mankind, God did not consider all persons fit to learn it and so He gave it to some virtuous ones "whose hearts are pure, with a sharp intellect, who love the good, have mercy, sympathy, and chastity."[28]

As to the Hippocratic oath, this was not required of a physician by al-Ruhāwī. Since the profession was given only by God to those who qualified, an oath would hardly have been necessary.[29]

He who blames the physician discloses his ignorance; he is from the lowest class of people. The evidence for this is that he should not ask for

25 *Adab al-ṭabib* MS, fol 7.7b.
26 *Ibid.,* fol. 77b.
27 *Ibid.,* fol. 78b.
28 *Ibid.,* fols. 70b-71a.
29 The Prophet said that God did not send down any disease without also sending down the remedy. The Prophet called in a physician when he needed one. "From abū Harīra comes the following story. One of the Anṣārī fell ill one day. The Prophet called in two physicians who were in Medina and said to them, 'Cure this man.' In another version of the same tradition, they put this question to the Prophet, 'O Prophet, is the science of medicine any good?' And he replied, 'Yes.'" (Cyril Elgood. "Ṭibb-ul-Nabbī or Medicine of the Prophet," *Osiris*, 1962, *14*, 33-192 [p. 126].) These are from a collection of traditions of the Prophet and his Companions gathered by al-Bukhārī (809-869). It is called *Saḥīḥ.* The Koran (1.4) reads, "Thee do we serve and Thee do we beseech for help," on the question of curing one.

help from his people and his friends when an illness occurs, but only from the physician. His intention is clear and his ignorance obvious.

We have also previously said that the exalted Allah is health-giving and maintains the well-being of the healthy. He is the real physician and He taught the people that by which they keep their health and treat their illness. Then he who blames the art of medicine blames the acts of Allah, the exalted Creator.[30]

The argument thus went full circle in that the physician was simply an agent of Allah and could bear no blame. The ethic of the physician was an extension of that of a religious man serving his Creator.

In chapter XIV the physician is admonished not to confine himself only to the regulations but to pay attention to what the patient needs in his treatment from among useful things, following the precepts of Hippocrates.

The worst misfortune to both the physician and patient is when the latter and his servant are of low breeding. Because some people have little knowledge, and even in health do not understand what is said to them, then how can they cooperate in the case of disease? For this reason, the physician, before he gives advice to the patient, must know the latter's reasoning and his culture, and also the reasoning of his nursing aide. If he can rely upon their soundness, then he may advise what he thinks about remedies and treatments. If he does not trust their reasonableness, then he withholds information so that there will be no slip in the names of remedies, in their measures, in their improvement, and in the times of using them. This is because the patient may die by error and the physician will attract to himself a bad name and win blame together with his fatigue. It is the same as when one has sown good, pure seeds in bad soil, and then his seed dies and his fatigue is for nought.[31]

The next five chapters concern those who are fitted to study medicine, how it should be practised, the conduct of quacks and charlatans, how the government should do away with these frauds, and the type of examination which one must pass to become an accepted physician.

With regard to the oath of Hippocrates, al-Ruhāwī explains why there were only a few physicians who were accepted by those who knew the art. It was Galen's opinion that the physician should hand down his art only to his son since "it was not fit to make a statue from any stone and not useful to go hunting with any dog."[32] Al-Ruhāwī has an answer for this assertion.

As to the soul which is not fit to receive the medical art [i.e., a worthless son of a physician], the belief which decrees it is only a permissive one. In the opposite case, it is understood that he is fit to receive it. However,

---

[30] *Adab al-ṭabib* MS, fol. 80a. [31] *Ibid.*, fol. 86a. [32] *Ibid.*, fol. 89b.

when he is from those who cannot preserve what is in the oath, then he should not study the medical art. Galen said that one of the reasons for which Hippocrates composed the book *On Belief* [i.e., the oath] is what we have mentioned about the examination of one who seeks to study the medical art in his body and in his soul.[33]

The virtuous soul is then emphasized as an excellent criterion by which to choose those aspiring to the practice of medicine. Al-Ruhāwī writes that Hippocrates realized that the number of physicians was decreasing and so he made up the oath in place of the necessity of the hereditary transmission of the art so that all those who qualified might study medicine. "Hippocrates hung this oath on the neck of the physician and made him swear that when he treated the ill, he must try to benefit, not to harm them."[34] In this way, all physicians became sons of Hippocrates.

In the ninth century, there were many substandard physicians. Some of these practitioners were fairly skilful and shrewd, as al-Ruhāwī describes them. He writes that they butter up the Sultan with electuaries, select pretty women good for one's health, give remedies for digestion, make one's hair beautiful, and incite sexual desire.

Others claim to prescribe lovers' charms, write books which incite to passion, and remove treasures from mounds. The author relates that "they travel like flies, roam the roads and streets, prefer that homes be free of the men [when they] show up for their dastardly acts. It is necessary that authorities protect the public and all subjects from these flies and thieves. They hide themselves from the eyes of people with the appearance of their dress and the grossness of their claims."[35]

The non-virtuous and untrustworthy practitioner cannot be relied upon to treat the ill or, more important, to maintain the health of anyone. For not teaching some people the medical art, al-Ruhāwī gives four reasons. One is that the complexion of the body of the student may be immoderate, i.e., there is a change in the morals and acts of the soul. Two, the candidate is not familiar with good and bad habits, to pursue them when they are good. Three, there are times when these two reasons come together in their bad aspects to increase corruption. Last, a reason not to teach a student medicine is when he will pursue it only for worldly wealth and power. The physician's son must also meet these conditions.[36]

[33] *Ibid.*, fol. 90a.
[34] *Ibid.*, fol. 90a.
[35] *Ibid.*, fol. 106a; H. Sigerist, *A History of Medicine*, 1961, vol. II, p. 304.
[36] *Adab al-ṭabib* MS, fol. 89a; Sigerist (n. 35), p. 305.

The text relates that, in ancient times, the profession and the study of medicine carried dignity. Various reasons are given for later decline. The first is that those who entered the profession "because of covetousness thought that trust in them could not be lost either in their science or in their practice. Thus, they turned to what came easily; they abandoned care, reading, and service, and became inclined to flattery . . . so that the truth was lost." Second is the reason that "the physician, in addition to his medicine, needed to use deceit in other avenues of earning a living, as in trade or in a shop. . . . As a result of this, there is a scorning of the art. . . ." Third, many have entered the art who do not know its principles, its values, and its obligations.[37]

Many have been led into medicine, according to al-Ruhāwī, through the widely held opinion that it is God who is the cause of all, so that no matter how medicine is practised or remedies prescribed, the decree of God will prevail. This fatalism was common among the poorer classes of society, but al-Ruhāwī did not share this belief *in toto*.

In order to control and to eradicate the quacks and similar inferior practitioners of medicine, al-Ruhāwī advocated the examination of physicians. In his plan, al-Ruhāwī claimed to fall back on Galen and Hippocrates. Its purpose, he wrote, was to follow the pattern of ancient Greece to raise the level and nobility of medical practice. He believed that it was up to the ruler to "make the truth clear, to make the benefits common, and the good to be general."[38]

The proposed examination was planned and fully discussed by al-Ruhāwī. It was meant to cover the entire spectrum of medical knowledge, including the candidate's moral ideas and background. To pass this severe test, a man had to spend a long time with books, be in the companionship of practitioners in the service of the ill, and have experience in the care of the details affecting the treatment of souls and bodies.[39]

[37] *Adab al-ṭabib* MS, fol. 91a. In "Medical Table Talk," *Da'wat al-aṭibbā'*, ibn Buṭlān (twelfth century) discusses with others in the medical profession the decline of the dignity of their vocation and the lack of knowledge of it. The manuscript is in Istanbul, Aya Sofya 3626, especially fols. 4a, 4b: "The seekers [of science] are decreased in number and those who desire it are few. Their books have been sold to druggists to meet the need of the few. By God, as an art, it [i.e., medicine] has perished and its fire has died out. Those who aim for it are interested in it only for the coin and not in the physician's art. It is said that by wisdom is bodily medicine practised, and by money are medical men diseased. When you see a physician attract diseases to himself, how can he nurse another? A poem says, 'Can an ill one recover if it was the physician who made him sick?'"

[38] *Adab al-ṭabib* MS, fol. 99b.

[39] *Ibid.*, fol. 92a.

A man was first given a test on Galen's *On the Sects of Physicians*. Those which are considered to be independent divisions of medicine, according to Galen, are treatment of viscera, treatment of the eye, setting of broken bones, use of the iron cautery, lancing, clystering, bleeding, and others.

He who claims one of them must know the object of his practice, which part it is of the bodily parts, what it is composed of, the location of its parts, the illnesses which affect these parts, the causes of these illnesses, the symptomatology, and the therapy. In short, it is necessary for him to know all kinds of therapy applicable to these illnesses, the preservation of health, and the periods for this. For this reason, it is necessary to examine the applicant in every aspect of the art, from the general problems to the specific in detail.

An example of this is if someone came and claimed that he was an ophthalmologist. It is necessary to test him on the simple anatomy of the eye, why each one of its parts is necessary. If he does not know these, then he does not know which parts make sight possible or by which parts it is possible to preserve and cover the eye, etc.

When he does not know the complexion of a part, i.e., one of the simple parts of the eye, together with what we have mentioned, the positions of these parts and their relationships, then he does not know the various types of their ailments. When he does not know these, he does not understand the symptoms and so does not know the causes. In that event, he cannot point to the indicator which denotes the kind of illness. When the symptoms are not understood, then it is impossible to determine its treatment.

After that which has been mentioned, he must know the properties of the simple and compound drugs used to treat ailments of the eye. Each property of a remedy has a function and one simple may have several functions; a compound remedy has many more functions. It is not fair to the patient if the physician does not know about them. It is also necessary to know how to improve remedies. . . .

If he treats the eye with the iron, then he must know the forms of the instruments . . . and why they are so shaped. He must have experience with them as, for example, the instrument used for the socket of the eye for tears coming from it. If he knows this, then he knows where tears come from and how it is possible for its three ducts to pierce the front side. . . .[40]

This is an example of the examination area covered by the test for one practising in a limited field only. The general practitioner was the man who knew all branches of medicine; his examination was based on an edition of Galen which consisted of only sixteen books. Their titles are listed in order:[41] *The Sects*

40 *Ibid.*, fols. 92b-93b.

41 Al-Ruhāwī writes that it was the learned physicians of Alexandria who realized that they could not read all of Galen's books. They therefore organized them as sixteen books. These were gathered in an abridged form (*Adab al-ṭabib* MS, fol. 97b). The order of the books as given by the text is different from the arrangement of the Alexandrians, from that of Ḥunain ibn Isḥāq (d. 873), and from the one of Thābit ibn Qūrra (834-91) (*Adab al-ṭabib* MS, fols. 97b, 98a).

in Medicine, The Small Art, The Pulse, Summing Up of Therapy, The Elements, The Complexion, The Faculties of Nature, Anatomy, The Value of the Organs, The Crisis, The Days of the Crisis, The Large Book on the Pulse, Simple Remedies, Compound Remedies, Art of the Cure, The Argument.

The next step in the examination, after the divisions of medicine, was to investigate the man as to his soul, his education, his culture from childhood on, his associations, his attention to his physical concerns, and his ambitions. He must be concerned with people and must employ justice in his associations. "He must treat people as he would like to be treated himself, with sympathy."[42]

Al-Ruhāwī writes that the ancient Greeks guarded the level of medical practice in another way, by checking on the treatment.

When the physician visits and treats the patients, upon entering, he first asks for white paper, and after considering the patient's case, he writes, "I have visited this particular patient on such and such a day. It is the first day of his illness, and the second, and the third, . . . according to whatever it is, and I found the illness of such and such a patient to be so and so. The diagnosis was made by his urine, by his pulse, etc. The symptoms are so and so. I have prescribed such and such a remedy for him, and such and such a food." Then he leaves what he has written with the relatives of the patient. When he returns, he examines what has changed and what has happened, and he writes it down on what we have mentioned. He does this on every visit. If he sees any warning sign of a crisis, he mentions it. When the crisis of which he warned is encountered, he writes it down at the end of the patient's case and illnesses.

If the patient recovers, then he takes the chart with him as a reminder for another case which may affect that man. Should the patient die and they say that it is due to an error of the physician, then the physician accompanied by authorities goes to the relatives and explains the chart. The learned physicians study the entries on the chart. If the illness is according to what he described and the symptoms fit the symptoms of the diagnosis of that illness, etc., and it is shown that the remedy and therapy were proper, then he departs with thanks. If the facts are contrary to what he thought, then he gets what he deserves; he will not return to the art of medicine. If there was an error, then he must be killed.[43]

The final chapter of the book is entitled, "On matters which a physician must observe and be careful about during periods of health to prepare for the periods of illness, and at the time of his youth for his old age."[44] This is a further extension of the preventive medicine related earlier in the book by the author. To

42 *Adab al-ṭabib* MS, fol. 73b. This is a kind of castrated Golden Rule.
43 *Ibid.*, fols. 101a-101b.
44 *Ibid.*, fol. 112a.

al-Ruhāwī, preventive medicine was a practical extension of his belief in the necessity for moderation in all aspects of life.[45]

The notion of the Godhead as an all-embracing concept in which man finds his model and oneness, with minor exceptions, is fully elucidated in al-Fārābī, who lived in the early tenth century and devoted himself to the healing art of the spirit. In the belief that philosophy was the broadest science in whose acquisition man comes to resemble the Godhead, the ultimate of desires is found.[46] In al-Fārābī's work, therefore, the First Being is the end in philosophy, so that the practical efforts of men must be directed toward likeness with God. The means or methods among Muslim thinkers, as in al-Ruhāwī,[47] did not include any doctrine of humanism. According to Donaldson, Muslim ethics on a neo-Platonic model came partly from the Enneads of Plotinus wherein is described the movement from God to man and vice versa. Al-Fārābī could not transcend this idea nor could ibn Sīnā successfully.[48]

It was abū 'Alī ibn Miskawaih (d. 1030), physician and one of the greatest Muslim authorities on ethics, who believed that it is only among other human beings that individual man attains perfection. Instead of Aristotle's friendship as the expansion of self-love, ibn Miskawaih stated that it was a kind of love for one's neighbor.[49] His beliefs, however, were conditioned by many and varied subtleties.

In the autobiography, Kitāb al-sīra al-falsafa, of al-Rāzī (c. 865-925), Islam's greatest physician, who took for himself the values of the philosophers, some of his philosophical principles

---

[45] de Boer (n. 7), p. 110.

[46] Maqāla fī ma'āni al-'aql, Ed. in Fr. Dieterici (n. 17), p. 39, R. fī al-akhlāq, Suppl. Aligarh 81, 46.

[47] Donaldson (n. 3), p. 109.

[48] R. fī al-akhlāq, MS Leiden 1464,6 and 2143. Cf. Kitāb al-shifā, Bib. Nat. Paris fonds arabes 6829. S. Salim, Ed., Fī ma'āni kitāb reṭorīqa, Cairo, 1950. H. Ghoraba, Ibn Sina's Bain al-dīn wa'l-falsafa, Cairo, 1948.

He had an important influence upon al-Ghazālī (1058-1111), one of the most successful philosophers of Islam in his ethical writings; cf. H. Bauer, Ueber Intention, Reine Absicht und Wahrhaftigkeit das 37. Buch von al-Ghazālī's Hauptwerk, Halle, 1916, as part of Islamische Ethik; H. Bauer, Von der Ehe das 12. Buch von al-Ghazālī's Neubelebung der Religionswissenschaften, Halle, 1917, in Islamische Ethik II; H. Bauer, Erlaubtes und verbotenes Gut das 14. Buch von al-Ghazālī's Hauptwerk der Religionswissenschaften, Halle, 1922, in Islamische Ethik III; H. Wehr, Al-Ghazālī's Buch vom Gottvertrauen das 35. Buch des Ihyā' 'ulūm al-dīn, Halle, 1940, in Islamische Ethik IV; W. M. Watt, Muslim Intellectual: A Study of Al-Ghazālī, Edinburgh, 1963. For the therapeutic value of hope for sinful men, cf. Wm. McKane, Al-Ghazālī's Book of Fear and Hope, Leiden, 1962, pp. 45-46, 51-63. For Sufism as a resolution of conflicting ethics, cf. the brief account of A. J. Arberry, Sufism, An Account of the Mystics of Islam, London, 1950.

[49] de Boer (n. 7), p. 130; Tadhīb al-akhlāq wa'taḥrīr al-a'rāq in the British Museum. Vide Leclerc (n. 10), p. 482.

concerning the ideal may be discerned. These include the concepts that the goal of life is not usefulness but knowledge and justice, that Allah is the judge who punishes and gives, that one's state in after-death depends on the state when the soul and the body were united, that one's differentiation between good and evil depends on reason, that one must not assume needless pain, and that it is not necessary to be ascetic since Allah has given the means to maintain life, not pain. The basis of al-Rāzī's moral idealism is, therefore, a monotheism with some free will of the individual. He displays a feeling of religiosity which is primarily of a Hellenistic tradition rather than that to be found in the Muslim traditions of the Sunna. In his account, al-Rāzī accepts the Aristotelian differentiation between theoretical and practical philosophy.

As to the physician, al-Ruhāwī states that the primary requisite is to have faith in God. He must also be devoted to Him "with all his reason, soul, and free will." A physician must also possess the faith that God sent His Apostles to mankind to teach what the mind alone could not.[50] This is, by the way, the only passage in the treatise which would tend to indicate that the author was a Christian. This did not affect his total immersion in Muslim culture. Al-Ruhāwī saw fit to derive much of his practical ethics from Galen's *Commentary on the Epidemics of Hippocrates,* thus proving his dependence upon Greek sources also.

In view of the fact that many of the medical and philosophical works until about 900, whether in Arabic, Persian, Greek, or Syriac, have not yet been published, it is difficult to assess the influence of early writers upon al-Ruhāwī with a proper perspective. A more complete understanding of early Arabic medical deontology within a suitable framework must, therefore, await further detailed study.

It is significant that in the *Adab al-ṭabib,* in spite of the attempt. of Isḥāq ibn 'Alī al-Ruhāwī to credit all authorities from whom he derived ideas, mention is never made of an earlier Arabic or Syriac or Persian work devoted to medical ethics. So far as is known, then, the treatise of al-Ruhāwī is the earliest full study extant in Arabic in its field.[51]

50 *Adab al-ṭabib* MS, fol. 5b.

51 Cf. the Hebrew *Manhij ha-rōfe'ūn* in very brief sentences which outline a medical savoir faire by Isaac Israeli (*c.* 832-*c.* 932). The work was originally written in Arabic but this is lost (cf. ibn Juljul, "Generations of Physicians," Fuat Sayyid, Ed. Cairo, 1955, p. 87); David Kaufmann, *Magaz. Wissenschaft Judentums,* 1884, *11,* 97-112. It is composed of fifty propaedeutic aphorisms. Some of these are to be found in Joannes Damascenus (Mesue the Elder (d. 857); Leclerc (n. 10), vol. I, p. 110. Al-Rāzī's aphorisms

Later medical deontology did not stray far from the path trodden by the author; he had amalgamated his sources so well that his work agreed very well with the practical ethics of later physicians. Whether later deontology was due to al-Ruhāwī is uncertain. His ideas, based to a large extent on the revered Hippocrates and Galen, were assured of a ready acceptance by the author's contemporaries. There is no doubt of the primary importance of the thoughts of Galen in al-Ruhāwī's work. One example will suffice. Three tenets from Galen's *Passions of the Soul* were emphasized by al-Ruhāwī. These are: 1. Stress on the Aristotelian mean, i.e., moderation and temperance. 2. Liberation from passions by training and practice. 3. Nature, or the temperament of the body, as an ethic-forming factor.[52]

The ancestry of these is Platonic, Aristotelian, Pythagorean, and mainly Stoic, according to van der Elst.[53] The treatment of the passions as a part of moral philosophy continued over a long period until the time of the French encyclopedia of Diderot and d'Alembert and still later. In Descartes, for example, the mastery of passions through reason is fully discussed as part of a moral system.[54]

In dealing with the ancients, Islamic thinkers attempted to resolve all ethical difficulties as a rearrangement of the pieces in a puzzle. It would have been far more satisfactory if the pieces had not been forced into a mold, and if the conflict, with more facts and increased discussion, had continued. Nevertheless, al-Ruhāwī's text is unique in that it represents the consensus of thought on deontology in his century so well that the reader has much to study in its various contradictions and resolutions.

are described by M. Steinschneider, *Virchows Arch.* 1866, *37*, 378. Cf. also reference to medical ethics by al-Zahrāwī in S. K. Hamarneh and G. Sonnedecker, *A Pharmaceutical View of Abulcasis . . .*, Leiden, 1963, p. 49.

52 P. W. Harkins and W. Riese, *Galen on the passions and errors of the soul*, Columbus, 1963, pp. 123-124; I. Mueller, *Ueber Galens Werk vom wissenschaftlichen Beweis*, Muenchen, 1895.

In regard to training in moderation and control of emotions, so important in treatment, evil passions are controlled by the help of God (and the physician, of course). In the ethics of the medieval Muslims and similar religious groups, it is generally the fear of God which serves to restrain man, not his fellow human being. Cf. a good but late description in Bar Hebraeus' *Book of the Dove*, A. J. Wensinck, Tr., Leiden, 1919, pp. 32-43. Further elaboration is in Bar Hebraeus' *Ethicon* where he discusses the love of God (Wensinck, pp. 85-117). Bar Hebraeus, a mystic, wrote his *Ethicon* in 1590 in Syriac. It is very similar to al-Ghazālī's *Iḥyā' 'ulūm al-dīn*.

Emotions in "The Medicine of the Prophet," *Ṭibb al-nabbī*, (n. 29), p. 63, were considered to have an effect upon the body.

53 Robert v.d. Elst, *Traité des passions de l'âme et de ses erreurs par Galen*, Paris, 1914, p. 43.

54 Harkins and Riese (n. 52), p. 112; K. Sprengel, *Vortraege zur Gesch. der Medizin*, Halle, 1794-96.

Isaac Israeli's
Fifty Admonitions to the Physicians†

ARIEL BAR-SELA* and HEBBEL E. HOFF*

INTRODUCTION

Last summer, while reading in the Universitätsbibliothek of Tubingen, we chanced upon a work of unique character bound between Maimonides' treatises on Asthma and Coitus in Ms. Orient. 4°836 of that library. This work, entitled "Şefer Muşar Harofi'm"—The Book of Admonitions to the Physicians— and attributed by the scribe to "Isaac Israeli of blessed memory," struck us as being of unusual interest and quite different from most ancient works on medicine in that it is not a text of medicine but rather a compilation of personal advice and counsel to the physician. In particular, we were moved by the unusual mixture of idealism and practicality which makes this work strikingly applicable to our own time. We thought it therefore desirable to render it into English in order to make available this interesting work to the English-speaking physicians and medical historians of today.

Isaac son of Solomon, known in the West as Isaac Israeli or Isaac Judeus, was born in Egypt in the first half of the ninth century; neither the date of his birth nor that of his death are known with certainty, but they are generally taken to be 840 and 950 respectively. He started his medical career as an oculist in Cairo, then migrated west to Qayrawan (Tunisia), where he first served Zyadat Allah, the last of the Aghlabite rulers of Tunisia, and later the conquering Fatimid Imam of Egypt at whose behest he wrote most of his medical compositions.

In the introduction to the English translation of Roger Bacon's *The Cure of Old Age and the Preservation of Youth,* published in London in 1683 by Richard Brown, the translator counts Isaac among the foremost Arabic physicians and states: "Isaac Beimiram, the son of Solomon the Physician. He flourished about the Year of Christ 1070. After Johannes Serapio's time. He writ much in Physick, as of Fevers, of Urine, of Diet, of the Stomach, beside several Tracts in Philosophy." Though inaccurate, this brief de-

† Supported by Office of Vocational Rehabilitation Grant No. 463.
* Department of Physiology, Baylor University College of Medicine, Houston, Texas.

scription reflects the measure of prominence attained by Isaac Israeli.

Since most of the available information about Isaac is drawn from the biographical dictionary of Arabic physicians of ibn abi Usaybia,[5] we have included a translation of the entire biographical sketch of Isaac contained in that work.

(I'sḥaq bin Sulyman) al I'sraili was an eminent physician; eloquent, learned, famous in skill and knowledge, a good author, of excelling mind, and he was surnamed abu Y'aqub. He is the one whose renown has spread and whose knowledge has become known by 'al I'sraili'. He was of the people of Egypt; he first practised as an oculist, then he settled in al Qayrawan and was a follower of I'sḥaq bin 'Amran who taught him. He attended the Imam abu Muḥammad 'Ubaid Allah al Mahdi, ruler of Africa, in the art of medicine.

Just as I'sḥaq ibn Sulyman was excellent in the art of medicine, so was he a keen master of eloquence, and dextrous in the disputations of the sciences. He lived a long life, dying at over a hundred years, and he had not taken wives, nor begotten a son.

It was said to him: "Would you not be more fortunate if you would have had a child?" And he said: "Since I have the Book on Fevers—No!" meaning that the propagation of his memory by the Book on Fevers is more enduring than its propagation by a child. It is related that he said: "I have four books that will perpetuate my memory more than a son, and they are the Book on Fevers, the Book on the Nutrients and on the Drugs, the Book on Urine, and the Book on the Elements." He died about the year twenty and three hundreds [i.e., 932 A.D.].

A'ḥmad bin I'brahim bin abu Khalid, known as ibn al Jazar, said in the Book of the Histories of the Kingdom, that is, at the commencement of the reign of the Imam abu Muḥammad 'Ubaid Allah al Mahdi who appeared from the West: "I was told by the practitioner I'sḥaq bin Sulyman who said: 'When I came from Egypt to Zyadat Allah bin al Aghlab, I found him dwelling with the troops in al A'rbas. I rode over to him, and when he was informed of my approach, for he had already asked for me, he dispatched to me five hundred dinars, which encouraged me on the journey. I was summoned before him on the hour of my arrival, and I salaamed in obedience and performed the obeisance, as is required to be made to kings. And I saw his council, void of veneration, with an overpowering desire for amusement, and as the laughter rose, I was first addressed by bin Ḥunbash, known as al Yawnani, who said to me: 'Would you say that the salty would exhilarate?'

"I said: 'Yes.'

"Said he: 'And would you say that the sweet would exhilarate?'

"I said: 'Yes.'

"He said to me: 'Lo, the sweet is the salty, and the salty is the sweet?!'

"I said that the sweet would exhilarate by its lightness and pleasantness, and the salty would exhilarate by its harshness, and he persevered in his obstinacy, as he was fond of sophistry.

"As I saw this, I said to him: 'Would you say you are alive?'

"He said: 'Yes.'

"Said I: 'And is the dog alive?'

"He said: 'Yes.'

"I said: 'Lo, you are the dog and the dog is you?!'

"And Zyadat Allah laughed with intense laughter, and I realized that his zest for a jest was greater than his desire for decorum.

"Said I'sḥaq: 'When abu 'Ubaid Allah, called al Mahdi, came to Riqadah (?), he drew me near and advanced my rank. He had a stone in the kidney and I was treating him with remedies, among which were the cauterizing tongs. I sat on a certain day with a group from the Privy Council and they asked me about various forms of infirmities, and whatever I explained to them, they could not understand my words. I said to them: 'Lo, you are cattle, and there is nothing human in you except the name.' The story reached abu 'Ubaid Allah, and when I visited him he said to me: 'You confront our brethren, The Believers, of the Privy Council as is not allowed. By Allah the Compassionate, if you were not excused by being ignorant of their rights, regarding what is theirs from the knowledge of truth, the men of the Law would have beheaded you.

"Said I'sḥaq to me: 'And there I saw a man who would pursue decorum in whatever came his way, and a jest has no market with him.' "

The books (of I'sḥaq bin Sulyman) are: The Book of Fevers, five treatises, and there cannot be found on this subject a better book; I quote from the writings of abu al Ḥasan 'Ali bin Riḍwan his statement about it: "Say I, 'Ali bin Riḍwan the physician, that this useful book was compiled by an excellent man, and I have applied much of what is in it and I found it unsurpassed; from Allah is guidance and aid"; the Book of Simple Drugs and Nutrients; the Book of Urine; the Extracts of his Book on Urine; the Book of the Elements; the Book of Definitions and Forms; the Book of the Garden of Philosophy and in it questions on Theology; the Book of the Introduction to Logic; the Book of the Introduction to the Art of Medicine; a Book on Pulsation; a Book on Theriac; a Book on Philosophy; these are eleven dissertations.

A contemporary of Rhazes and Haly Abbas, Isaac Israeli was the first truly great physician of the Western part of the great Arab Empire. The tribute of Meyerhof,[8] who called Isaac "the greatest Jewish medical man in the Middle Ages," is only slightly exaggerated. His popularity and influence are attested to by the numerous old copies of his major compositions found in European libraries today. His works were translated into Hebrew and Latin and were widely used by medieval physicians. According to Sarton,[10] Isaac's treatise on urine in its various translations, summaries, and elaborations constituted the basis of European urological practice throughout the Middle Ages. Just as Isaac himself had predicted, his books on fevers, urine, drugs, and nutrients propagated his name for generations after his death.

Of the six medical works listed above, Friedenwald[2] and Steinschneider[11] report that only three are still to be found in European libraries, namely, the treatises on Simple Drugs and Nutrients, Urine, and Fevers. The subject of the present work exists only in Hebrew and only in one manuscript—Cod. Orient. 4°836 (fol. 93r-95v) —at the Universitätsbibliothek, Tubingen. Ibn abi Usaybia does not list it under its present title, but it could have been a part of the Introduction to Medicine mentioned above. According to Berliner,[1] it was first discovered by Moise Soave of Venice who published an Italian translation in the *Giornale Veneto di Scienze Mediche* in 1861. Kaufmann[7] considered it premature to attribute this work to Isaac Israeli; he believed it to be an original Hebrew composition of a much later date and not a translation from the Arabic as suggested by Steinschneider.[11]

A similar opinion was advanced by Guttmann[4] who posited several objections to the attribution of this work to Isaac Israeli. Of these objections, two appear to us to have validity, namely, that the statement made in Chapter 35 that "the urine informs only on matters in the liver and urinary pathways" contradicts Isaac's views expressed in his famous treatise on the Urine, and that the abundance of Biblical and Talmudic phrases in this work suggests a Hebraic origin rather than an Arabic one. Guttmann's claim that it is unlikely that a work of so famous an author would be forgotten is unacceptable in view of the fact that of the eleven works of Isaac listed by ibn abi Usaybia only a few have survived. Nor can we accept Guttmann's claim that this work is too witty to be ascribed to Isaac in view of the anecdotes related about Isaac's wit by Ibn Abi Usaybia.

In the absence of other manuscripts of the same work, and because this work is not mentioned by ibn abi Usaybia, it is difficult to establish its authenticity. It appears to us, however, that the vocabulary and the syntax strongly suggest that this is indeed a translation from the Arabic, and the Biblical and Talmudic phrases might well have been a translator's substitution for similar Arabic idioms, if not the phrases of the author himself. It is significant that the term for "enema" employed in the text (Chap. 48) is the Arabic *al ḥuqna* and not the term *clyster* which was commonly used by European Jewish writers of the Middle Ages . Furthermore, the disputations mentioned in the same chapter were considered vital in the era of Isaac and thereafter but not in Europe of the late Middle Ages. These considerations suggest a much earlier origin than the dates proposed by Guttmann and Berliner.

Another striking feature is the absence of references to any well-known authories other than Hippocrates and Galen. This, too, strongly suggests the era of Isaac which was at the beginning of the rise of Arabic medicine and before the emergence of the great masters who were so abundantly quoted in mediaeval Europe.

At the end of this work there appears an obscure Hebrew phrase—written in *a'btsr*. Kaufmann considers the possibility that this is a date—"in the month of Ab in the year 290"—and concludes that this is inadmissible since the year 290 (1530 A.D.), is later than the date of the writing of this particular manuscript, let alone the composition of the work itself. If, however, we assume this date to be 290 of the Hijrah (903 A.D.), then the year falls well within the life span of Isaac Israeli and could perhaps be the year in which this work was composed.

In our enthusiasm, and owing perhaps to differences in titles, we overlooked the fact that an English translation of this work was made in 1944 by Jarcho[6] from the edited Hebrew text[12] which was published in 1884 by Kaufmann together with a German translation.[7] Although some excerpts of this work have been published earlier by Friedenwald[2,3] and Morrison,[9] it is to Jarcho that the credit is due for first offering the entire work in English. However, since our translation was independently prepared, and since it is based upon the original manuscript and accompanied by the translation of ibn abi Usaybia's biographical sketch of the author, we believe it nonetheless advisable to offer our version for publication.

In preparing the translation from the Hebrew, we have attempted to adhere to the text as closely as possible—often at the expense of linguistic fluency—in order to provide the reader with the author's own words rather than our interpretation. References to the edited Hebrew text[12] and to Kaufmann's translation[7] have been added only where differences were substantial.

We are indebted to the Universitätsbibliothek of Tubingen for the microfilm copy of the manuscript, to the New York Public Library for the microfilm copy of the printed Hebrew edition of the text,[12] and to the Library of Columbia University for the microfilm copies of the articles of Berliner,[1] Guttmann,[4] and Kaufmann.[7]

150

REFERENCES

1. Berliner, A. Isak Israeli's Propädeutik für Aerzte. Vorbemerkung, *Magazin für die Wissenschaft des Judentums*, 1884, *11*, 93-96.
2. Friedenwald, H. The ethics of the practice of medicine from the Jewish point of view. *Johns Hopk. Hosp. Bull.*, 1917, *28*, 256-261.
3. Friedenwald, H. Manuscripts copies of the medical works of Isaac Israeli. In: *The Jews and medicine*. Baltimore, The Johns Hopkins Press, 1944, Vol. 1, pp. 185-192.
4. Guttmann, J. Über die Unechtheit der dem Isaak ben Salomo Israeli Beigelegten Schrift "Sitte der Arzte," *Monatsschrift für Geschichte und Wissenschaft des Judentums*, 1919, *63*, 156-164.
5. Ibn Abi Usaybia. U'yun al Anba' fi Tabaqat al Atibba', A. Muller, Ed., Koenigsberg, 1884, Book 11, pp. 36.
6. Jarcho, S. Guide for physicians (Musar Harofim) by Isaac Judaeus (880?-932?). *Bull. Hist. Med.*, 1944, *15*, 180-188.
7. Kaufmann, D. Isak Israeli's Propädeutik für Aerzte, *Magazin für die Wissenschaft des Judentums*, 1884, *11*, 97-112.
8. Meyerhof, M. Medieval Jewish physicians in the Near East. *Isis*, 1938, *28*, 432-460.
9. Morrison, H. Isaac Judaeus and his times. *N. Engl. J. Med.*, 1932, *206*, 1094-1099.
10. Sarton, G. *Introduction to the history of science*. Baltimore, Williams and Wilkins Co., 1931. Vol. 11, p. 75.
11. Steinschneider, M. *Die Hebraeischen Übersetzungen des Mittelalters und die Juden als Dolmetscher, Akademische Druk-U.* Graz, Verlagsanstalt, 1956 (reprint), pp. 388-395, 755-761.
12. Yitshaq Hayisraeli. Sefer Musar Harofi'm (Book of admonitions to the physicians) *Ozar Tov*, 1884, *11*, 11-16.

Sefer Musar Harofi'm

THE BOOK OF ADMONITIONS TO THE PHYSICIANS

Therein are fifty chapters

1.   It is the nature of living creatures to seek their livelihood and attend to things that sustain their existence. Even man, whose image is like the image of God, is necessarily obliged to endeavor and engage in matters which will sustain his existence, his survival, and the salvation of his soul, before engaging in the rest of the studies and affairs in which others, beside himself, participate, because a man is close unto himself.[1] And therefore, the value of the art of medicine is very great, and a man is always obliged and compelled to learn it at the commencement of his studies.

2.   Whereas the knowledge of medicine is very extensive, and the days of men are too short to attain its perfection,[2] the accomplished physicians are set apart, and refined, and purged of the ignoramuses, by their constant occupation in the study of books and their meditation over them day and night, and their dedication to it apart from other men, before they are needed in their profession.

3.   The quickness of action in an artisan's performance, or his slowness, or his deliberateness, is according to the importance of the object on which he acts, or its triviality and unimportance. Thus, it behooves him

[1] The expression "a man is close unto himself" is a Talmudic legal presupposition that a man, by nature, tends to do the best he can for himself (Sanhedrin 9b).
[2] Compare with the first aphorism of Hippocrates: "Life is short, the Art is long; the occasion fleeting; experience fallacious, and judgment difficult."

who bores a crystal[3] to contemplate, and attend to his labour, so that he will not ruin by his haste the beauty of that work, which is not the case when dealing with the mire of the streets. And therefore, it behooves him who is occupied with the curing of the bodies of men, who are the noblest of the lower creatures,[4] to consider, to contemplate, and to be very precise with their diseases, and to perform his actions with a thoughtful mind and with deliberation, lest he err in something he cannot correct. And therefore has the Sage[5] said, that when you see a physician hastening to answer regarding any disease you inquire upon, and boasting of his treatment, consider him a fool. And said the Lord of Physicians: "I have never administered a laxative potion to a man, that my thoughts were not disturbed, and my sleep wandered from my eyes, before I administered it, and thereafter, for four nights."[6]

4.   Just as I have mentioned that it behooves not the physician to be hasty in his actions, so also it behooves him not to be lazy and very tardy since most of the diseases will not await him. Rather, he must stay between the opposites; neither rash and hasty, nor lazy and tardy. Only when acute[7] ailments develop must he be quick to form his ideas and to act because they press him.

5.   If you examine the books of the ancient physicians, you will find in them subjects the understanding of which is perplexing, and others that will be difficult for you, so that it might come to your mind to deny them. You have no right to speak up and dispute them, because of the great stature of those people in the eyes of man.[8] Should you have lived in their lifetime, you would have disputed with them, and come to terms with them regarding these matters. Now you must trouble yourself, and search for various interpretations for them, or deviate from the texts until, many times, certain matters in those discourses would be resolved in your mind in a way not intended by him who composed them. Indeed[9] it is possible that the author did not speak correctly, for there is not a man who errs not.[10]

---

3 The text employs an obscure Biblical word—*bdolaḥ*—(Gen. 2:12, Num. 11:7) from which the similarly obscure English term *bdelium* is derived. Kaufmann renders it *pearl*.

4 This conforms to the philosophical concept of the time which divided creatures into various orders of existence and ascribed to man the highest order of the lower creatures but ranked him below such higher forms as angels. Kaufmann renders it "the noblest of all creatures of this lower world."

5 Similar statements are to be found in the aphorisms of Rhazes and Mesue Sr. who were contemporaries of Isaac: Liber Almansoris Rasis: Dubitabilis est doctor qui iudicat facile; Aphorismi Jo. Damasceni: Si interrogatur semper velociter respondeas: dubitandus est. (Ref. Stillwell R 170, Venice 1497, fol. 98a and 150a respectively).

6 The Lord of Physicians, here, is Galen (see Chap. 6). Interestingly enough, Maimonides, in his Regimen of Health, attributes an identical statement to Ibn Zuhr (Avenzoar).

7 The Ms. employs an abbreviation—*ḥḥdi*—which we read *haḥadim*—sharp, acute, as does Kaufmann.

8 Compare with the Rabbinical edict "It is not permissible to dispute the lion after his death" (Gitin, 83b).

9 Kaufmann reads *veu'lai;* we read the more emphatic *veu'lam.*

10 This phrase is commonly translated to read *sin* rather than *err;* see Kings I, 8:46; Ch. II, 6:36; Eccl. 7:20.

152

And the books in which this occurrence happens mostly are those composed and expressed without argument or proof, but as adjudged edicts, like the books of Hippocrates.

6.   Best among physicians is he who is occupied with, reads, and reviews the many books of the ancient physicians, and especially the books of the Lord of Physicians, Galen, who spoke at length, strove, and always labored over the treatment of ailments.

Therefore, they are mistaken who say that you should not go to the physician but to the empiricist, because the ignoramus knows not what he tries and kills a thousand before curing one. And should he say "rely on me because I have experience," harken not unto his voice, because life is too short to attempt the recognition of a single disease or the nature of one herb. Therefore, we[11] must have recourse to what the ancients have tested in the thousands of years past, who, in the magnanimous charity of their heart and their mercy upon us, have written and rendered unto us all that they have tested.

7.   Should the knowledge of the physician or his wisdom be visible and revealed in the appearance of his face and frame, most men would not have erred in recognizing them and gaining the measure of their knowledge as it really is. And indeed, most of the common people would not consider, in evaluating them, anything except the magnitude of their words and talk, their self-praise, and the magnitude of their body,[12] their belly, and their beard. And therefore it was said that the ignorant see with the eyes and the enlightened see with the heart.[13]

8.   If the physician but comes from a distant land, and speaks in a foreign tongue, not understood, the multitude will think him enlightened and gather unto him and take counsel from him.

9.   It is to the discredit of this art,[14] and its fault, that it is joined by ignoramuses and fools who speak in its name, and there is no one to protest though all its affairs are hidden, deep, and most difficult for the wise and the enlightened.

10.   Most of the ignorant physicians may at times benefit you, because they will fail, fall silent,[15] and ask you to rectify that which they have corrupted.

11.   The physician does not effect the cure, but only prepares, and clears the stones from the path for Nature to act, for it is she who acts.

12.   In most of the prolonged ailments men become confused, despair of their cure and say that the physician is unable to cure them, because

11 Kaufmann omits we.
12 The Hebrew gulmam could be read to mean either body or robe.
13 Compare with Samuel I, 16:7—"for the Lord sees not as man sees; man looks on the outward appearance, but the Lord looks on the heart."
14 Surprisingly, Kaufmann reads here adamah—land.
15 fall silent. The word is most difficult to read. We read vyishtqu—and they will fall silent. Kaufmann reads vyishahatu—destroy—but since he is in doubt, he adds a question marks and "corrects" the word to read vyashhitu.

cure to them is the removal of the disease all of a sudden, and they know not that when the humors become unripened or dry, as they are in quartan fever, ripening is delayed, and then months or years in that long ailment become the measure of its days.

13.   Because attainment of the goal in the art of medicine is a possibility, not a certainty, while death is decreed and inevitable, it is impossible for a good and skilled physician to suffice for all men.

14.   Just as you need to read all the books composed on the art of medicine, so you will need to understand their contents in terms of the fundamentals of natural science, because medicine stems from it, and also become proficient in the rules of logic, so that you will be wise in refuting the ignoramuses who walk in the guise of physician, and frighten them from before you, and they shall fear you.

15.   The need for the physician to preserve health—for he is needed in the preservation of health—is not less than the need for him to remove diseases, because it is better for man not to sicken than to sicken and recover.[16]

16.   The physician should not take the healing of a patient by another physician as a proof that he is an expert in the Art unless he be examined first by the various criteria that I have mentioned,[17] because Nature is the healer in most times without a physician.

17.   How very guilty is the physician who promises to remove a disease because thus he alters the status of what actually exists, a possibility, and represents it as a certainty.[18]

18.   If you can nourish the sick with nutrients that are related and similar to his foods in health, you will manage him in the right manner. And you should also aim to feed him at his accustomed time; thus you will strengthen his Nature.

19.   Endeavour all you can to render the concoctions and the various potions pleasant to the palate of the sick, because then they will be drawn into and benefit the members; therefore sugar and honey are added and mixed with them.

20.   The more you know and understand the temperament[19] of the patient and his characteristics at the time of health, and accustom yourself to palpate his pulse and observe his urine, the easier will his cure be for you.

21.   If you can perform and fulfill your task with nutrients or nourishing medicaments, do it not with drugs, because most of them are enemies and foes of Nature, and especially the purgatives among them.

[16] This chapter in the Ms. is confusing, self-contradictory, and meaningless unless the negative *e'in*—is not—with which the paragraph begins is applied to the entire chapter and the repetition of the first phrase is taken as an affirmative repetition.
[17] Some of these criteria are detailed in Chap. 2.
[18] See Chap. 13.
[19] Temperament and complexion, in their archaic connotation, denote constitution and predisposition.

22.   He who consults many physicians, if all do not visit him together and consent to one agreement, endangers his life, because if the one should come alone the others might try to alter or add to what the first had ordered.

23.   Endeavour always to treat with simple drugs because knowing their power is easier for you than understanding the compounded.

24.   Be not contemptuous of any cure of which you hear, because at times there can be attained by simple means that which you could not effect by multiple actions and drugs.

25.   Rely not in your treatment upon drugs that act as nostrums, because most of these are nonsense and deceitful follies.

26.   Hasten not to treat the mild illnesses by altering the temperament[19] or by evacuation, because for most of them Nature alone will suffice, with the help of a good regimen.

27.   Among the virtues of the physician are, to be satisfied in his own regimen with the good nutrients in moderate quantities, to be neither a glutton nor a drunkard, and also to be disgraced and shamed by becoming ill with a protracted illness, lest the populace ask how he who cures not himself can cure others.

28.   Muzzle your mouth from prognosticating[20] or proclaiming edicts; most of your utterances should be with qualifications.

29.   Allow not your mouth to transgress[21] by disparaging any physician; lo, you find no man who has not his hour.[22] Let only your actions praise you, and glory not in the disgrace of others.

30.   Make an effort to visit the sick of the destitute and the poor and to cure them, for you find no righteousness greater than this.

31.   Reassure the patient and declare his safety even though you may not be certain of it, for by this you will strengthen his Nature.

32.   Trust not in the peddlers and the producers of compounded drugs because at times they will omit a drug,[23] due to its high cost, or use one old and weak of power and ruin your labor. Therefore, limit your treatment with the compounded drugs which they peddle.

33.   There are diseases the cure of which lies only in your preventing the patient from conducting himself in the evil manner in which he does, yet they always request the physician to act, and should he not act, they consider it a defect in him.

34.   (Missing)

20 Prognosticating. The word in the manuscript is *mlndba* or *mlgdba*. The former could be an erroneous spelling of *milehinabe'*—to prophesize or to prognosticate, as we have rendered it, while the latter could well be a carry-over from the Arabic *gdb*—to dispraise, to disapprove; Kaufmann reads *milehinabe'*.

21 An identical Hebrew phrase is to be found in Ecclesiastes 5:6.

22 Compare with Ethics of the Father (Avoth) 4:3—("Ben 'Azai). He used to say: 'do not be contemptuous of any man nor count anything as improbable, for you have not a man who has not his hour, nor a thing which has not its place.' "

23 Or "reduce a drug."

35.   The urine informs only on matters in the liver and the urinary pathways, and this when it is considered in all its circumstances, yet most of the ignoramuses of our generation seek to prognosticate over it, without seeing the patient, and to say what ails him, whether he will die or live and other stupidities.

36.   It is a good quality[24] in the physician to come early to the patient while the illness is increasing and reaching its fullness, not at the arrest and decline of the illness, because then will people rejoice in him and praise his action.

37.   Flee, oh physician, from endeavoring to cure the very difficult diseases because they cannot be cured, or those who harbor them might tire from the burden, or from expending their possessions, and suspect your treatment.

38.   Should the patient not submit to your discipline, and should his servants and members of his household not be diligent in following your command quickly, nor honor you as is proper, do not persevere in the treatment.

39.   State your fee to the patient when the illness is mighty and strong, lest after his cure he should forget your labor over him.

40.   The more you increase the fee for your labor, and make dear the price of your treatment, the more your actions will be respected in the eyes of men; only in the eyes of people for whom you labor without charge will your work be belittled.[25]

41.   The physician cannot pay attention and deliberate properly while treating a patient without charge, and his feet will not lead him to his house, and the treatment will not prosper.

42.   Exceed not in visiting the sick and prolong not sitting with him unless necessary in the process of treating the disease, because new faces are those that gladden.

43.   Attending to numerous patients[26] is the cause of confusing the mind of the physician and deranging his actions.

44.   Most ignoramuses will ask you not to advise regarding your treatment of the sick, but to tell them if the patient will live from that disease or will die. For, they say in their hearts, being wise in their own eyes, that if he is to live, he will not need the physician, and if death is to be victorious, the physician could not prevent it. The fools know not, that when he says that he is to live, it is on the condition that they treat him and manage him properly.

45.   Most of the ignorant physicians persist in every disease to let blood and purge, even if its cause be the thinness and diminution of heat. And

[24] We read *midat*—quality. Kaufmann reads *hovat*—duty.
[25] Compare with the Talmudic statement: "A physician who treats without charge is worth nothing" (Baba qama 85a).
[26] Or 'diseases.'

they will inform those who consult them, that should these humors remain in their bodies, they would suffocate them, and they will describe to them, to frighten and scare them, that the white humor on the surface of the blood is pus, and that they are full of putridity, and they will order them bled again until they dry all their humors. May God return all their reward upon their heads, dry their strength like clay, and turn their juice into summer's drought, Selah.

46.　　Persevere in the treatment of princes and the noble among the people, because they will reward you from their wealth, and praise you always, and love you after their recovery. But the worthless triflers will hate you, once they are safe, remembering the price which you have taken from them, for it is as a portion of their soul.[27]

47.　　It is a widespread custom, and a well-known folly, that men gather and come to let their blood, even though they do not need it. Some tell others that a certain day is good for blood-letting, and that one whose blood is let on it will be safe from such and such a disease. They gather by the hundreds in the house of the blood-letter, and after he sheds their blood he will expound to them, in order to take from them another portion, that he sees in the blood that they need to repeat the blood-letting, and the fools will return to be bled as before, until he would pour of the blood[28] into all his vessels, and the full he will set aside.

48.　　Also there is a folly spreading among the multitudes, that they fancy themselves as physicians in some ailments. They believe that it is not proper for him who has an internal abscess to eat a thing or to partake of even the very thin nutrients, thinking that the food would obstruct the trachea and prevent cough, until they cause Nature to stumble and weaken her vigor. They also believe that there is no need to administer any drink in this disease, and some of them withhold bread from all who harbor fever.

And I have seen in this country that a physician ordered an enema given to a sick person to soften his nature,[29] and as he rose to leave with it he became weak, his heart fainted, and his soul departed. From that day on, all the people of that city refrained from administering enemas to any sick person, thinking that it slays like a sword, and they made it into a law, and the physician is not permitted to administer it there.

And there are descriptions of treatments thought to be right and true, while they are a clear fallacy, such as their thinking that the young of the cocks are cooler than their females,[30] and that vinegar, since its origin

27 This somewhat obscure phrase is translated differently in Proverbs 23:7.

28 This could be a play on words since the word 'blood' could be read to mean "his money."

29 "Nature" here is a euphemism for feces.

30 This statement can be understood only in terms of the Galenical concept of the four temperaments. A century or so after Isaac, a similar subject gave rise to the vivid and pugnacious dispute between Ibn Butlan of Baghdad and Ibn Ridwan of Cairo (Schacht, J. and Meyerhof, M. *The medico-philosophical controversy between Ibn Butlan of Baghdad and Ibn Ridwan of Cairo.* Cairo, The Egyptian University Press, 1937).

is from wine, is not proper to be mixed with the nourishments of the sick. They also believe women to be warmer than men, and that sneezing marks the crisis in disease.[31] When they see that upon walking barefoot and when they cool from the outside with the chill of the air their belly softens, due to the cold and the recoil of decaying matter into the body and the intestines, they think that all that cools is laxating, according to the intensity of the coolness, and many similar follies.

49.   The skilled physician need not predetermine the time for blood-letting, purging, and his other actions, because speculation is useless and diseases are compelling.[32]

50.   Much work and practice weaken the vigor of the physician and constrict his soul, because he always reflects and worries over each patient, desires his health and prays for him, as he would do for the kin who is related to him.

> Finished is the Book on the Physicians' Conduct
> And praised be the Lord who protects the ignorant.
> (Written in a'btsr) [33]

[31] See Kings II, 4:35.
[32] Kaufmann renders this paragraph quite differently; where we read "predetermine" he reads "determine experimentally," and where we read "speculation" he reads "experiment." We do not find his rendition justified either linguistically or with respect to the meaning of this paragraph which appears to us to be both clear and meaningful.
[33] See introduction.

THE PHYSICIAN'S PRAYER ATTRIBUTED TO
MOSES MAIMONIDES *

FRED ROSNER

The Physician's Prayer attributed to Moses Maimonides (1135-1204) is a lofty and beautiful prayer which first appeared in print in a German periodical in 1783 (1). The editor of this journal, Heinrich Christian Boie, and his associate, Christian Wilhelm Dohm, provide no notes or commentaries nor any indication as to who the author is. The prayer bears only the title, " Daily prayer of a physician before he visits his patients: From the Hebrew manuscript of a renowned Jewish physician in Egypt from the twelfth century." A photostatic reproduction of this earliest version of the prayer appeared recently in a Hebrew medical journal (2). Since the 1783 German edition, numerous versions, abbreviations, or excerpts thereof have been presented in English (3-16), German (17-23), Hebrew (2; 23-24), French (25-27), Dutch (28), and Spanish (29). There are undoubtedly others. Much heated debate exists among the various writers concerning the true authorship of the prayer. This controversy will be presented chronologically and an attempt will be made to arrive at a reasonable conclusion as to whether or not Moses Maimonides actually wrote the " Prayer of Maimonides."

The first Hebrew version of the prayer was published by Isaac Euchel, editor of the Hebrew periodical *Ha-Meassef*, in 1790 (24). The title indicates that Marcus Herz was its author and that it was translated at his request from German into Hebrew. Half a century later, in 1841, the London newspaper, *The Voice of Jacob*, published the first English rendition from the Hebrew, under the title " Daily prayer of a physician " (3). The writer, using the pen name of " Medicus," states,

The composition of this prayer has erroneously been attributed to Maimonides, but it is the production of the late Dr. Marcus Herz, a celebrated physician of Berlin. It was published by him in the German language, and the Hebrew version, which is to be found in the (Ha) maasef (24), owes its existence to the prolific pen of Itzig Eichel.

We next find the prayer, again in German, in a German Jewish newspaper, the *Allgemeine Zeitung des Judenthums* for 1863 (17). The

* From the Division of Hematology, Department of Medicine, Maimonides Hospital, Brooklyn, New York.

editor, Ludwig Philippson, makes no mention of authorship at all, but the title reads, " Daily prayer of a physician before the visits to his patients. From the Hebrew manuscript of a celebrated Jewish physician from the twelfth century." This title is nearly identical with that of the first German version, which appeared eighty years earlier (1). Philippson again reprinted the German version six years later (1869) in his voluminous book, *Weltbewegende Fragen in Politik und Religion aus den letzten dreissig Jahren* (18). In 1892, yet another German version appeared in the *Allgemeine Zeitung des Judenthums* (19), this time by Julius Pagel and entitled " The prayer of the physician."

In the last year of the nineteenth century Reverend Madison C. Peters, Pastor of the Bloomingdale Church in New York City, published a short English version of the prayer (4) in his book, *Justice to the Jew*. This English version, in which authorship is not mentioned at all, later initiated heated debates among Jewish scholars.

In the same year, Moïse Schwab, the celebrated bibliographer, published his *Répertoire* (30), in which he states that Marcus Herz authored the prayer published over a century earlier in *Ha-Meassef* (24). At the turn of the century, Golden published excerpts of the prayer in English in an American medical journal (5). His article, entitled " Maimonides' prayer for physicians," states that Maimonides composed the prayer. A later letter addressed to the *American Israelite* is evidence that he extracted the prayer from Peters' book (4).

In 1902, the prayer appeared again in German (20) under the title, " Prayer of a Jewish physician in the twelfth century." The writer, Dr. Theodor Distel, specifically states that the prayer was published originally in 1783 in the *Deutsches Museum* (1) and that its importance prompted him to reprint it verbatim. Another quarter century was to pass before this 1783 version was again mentioned, in spite of the rather widespread interest in the prayer and its authorship, manifested by numerous articles on the subject during this period.

In 1902, the same year that Distel reprinted (20) the original German version of the prayer (1), it was again copied in German in a Swiss newspaper (21), using Distel's title, " Prayer of a Jewish physician in the twelfth century." No commentary or discussion of authorship is to be found in this Swiss version. Rabbi Jules Wolff of La Chaux-de-Fonds, reading the prayer in the Swiss newspaper, was so impressed that he promptly translated it into French. In a letter, dated February 26, 1903, to the editor of the periodical *L'univers israélite*, which was published the following day (25), Wolff provides the first, and excellent, French version of the prayer. He states that it is a "prayer composed by a famous Jewish physician from Egypt in the twelfth century (Maimonides?)." Thus Wolff seems to assume, perhaps with a little doubt, that Maimonides is the true author of the prayer; Moïse Schwab, however, is quick to reply three weeks later, in another letter to the editor of the same periodical (31), that the prayer could have been written by any Parisian physician. He further states that the prayer is definitely the work of Marcus Herz, friend and physician of Moses Mendelssohn, that Herz wrote it in German in Berlin, and that a Hebrew translation was published by Isaac Euchel in the *Ha-Meassef* in 1790 (24).

Although later authors state that German versions of the prayer appeared in the February 4 and August 21, 1904, issues of the periodical *Israelitisches Familienblatt*, this writer has been unable to locate copies of these journals in numerous libraries in the United States. I cannot, therefore, verify this for myself and must leave it in doubt, since numerous errors in bibliography have crept into various subsequent papers published on this subject.

In 1908, Dr. Gotthard Deutsch, Professor of Jewish History and Literature at the Hebrew Union College of Cincinnati, wrote a letter to the editor of the journal *The American Israelite* (32), vehemently denouncing those who believe Maimonides actually wrote the famous prayer. The first part of his letter, tracing the prayer from 1790 (24) to 1903 (25; 31), was reproduced in the miscellany section of the *Journal of the American Medical Association* in 1929 (33). The letter continues as follows:

God only knows into how many medical journals, textbooks of medicine, etc., this prayer found its way. The first source of the error is evidently Philippson. How he could commit this blunder is inconceivable to me. He could not have quoted from memory, for he gives a fairly accurate translation and he could not have translated from the original without seeing in his text that the prayer was written by Marcus Herz in German and translated into Hebrew by Euchel. Philippson, however, does not give Maimonides as the author, and I would like to know who was the author of this additional piece of historic information which I notice is stated by Wolff with a question mark. To me, this wandering hoax was a valuable piece of illustration of historic criticism. . . .

Six years later, William W. Golden, Superintendent of the Davis Memorial Hospital in Elkins, West Virginia, wrote a letter to the editor of *The American Israelite*. It was published in the June 25, 1914, issue as follows:

Sir: Reverend Madison C. Peters in one of the editions of his book " Justice to the Jew " quotes a prayer for physicians by Maimonides. Can you tell me where the original can be found, or at least in what authoritative work on history, literature or medicine can it be found, and oblige?

Yours very truly . . .

Golden, who in 1900 had published excerpts of the prayer (5) and, in no uncertain terms, had attributed authorship to Maimonides, as described earlier in this paper, now seems to have had second thoughts on the matter. The reply to his letter came from Dr. Gotthard Deutsch in the same June 25, 1914, issue of *The American Israelite* and was subsequently reprinted in chapter 6 (The Maimonides Prayer Myth) of Deutsch's *Scrolls* (34).

Deutsch's reply begins as follows: "This so called prayer of Maimonides is an old hoax. It was actually written by Marcus Herz, a prominent physician of Berlin (1747-1803) who attended Moses Mendelssohn in his last illness. . . ." Deutsch thus reiterates all the arguments expounded in his earlier letter of 1908 (32). He further states that

. . . Haeser embodied it in his "Geschichte der Medizin" 1, p. 837, Jena 1875. Having thus been recognized by a standard publication, it was accepted by Julius Pagel, professor of the history of medicine at the Berlin University (1851-1912), also a Jew, in his essay on Maimonides as physician, which forms part of the memorial volume " Moses Ben Maimon," edited by the Gesellschaft Zur Foerderung der Wissenschaft des Judentums, I, p. 244, Leipzic, 1908. Following all this, its authenticity could no more be doubted than the authenticity of the gospel of St. John. The Israelite (March 12, 1908) gave it its seal of approval, although I contested it in the subsequent issue, but repeatedly since it has been proclaimed as being written in distinctly Maimonidean spirit. Recently I wrote a letter to the editor of " Ost und West," who had published it as Maimonidean. He thanked me, but preferred not to publish it. As the very popular " Medizinische Wochenschrift " of Berlin published it in 1902, and any number of medical journals reprinted it, no amount of argument will rob Maimonides of the credit for having written this typically sweet-lemonade prayer, characteristic of the rationalistic tendencies of the era of " Aufklaerung," and I still have hopes that one hundred years hence, somebody will credit Herodotus or at least Rabbi Jose Ben Halafta, the genuine author of Seder Olam, with my " Foreign Notes."

It seems quite evident that Deutsch was unaware of the 1783 edition of the prayer (1), and thus he attributes the authorship of the prayer to Marcus Herz, whose version did not appear until 1790 (24). This ignorance of the 1783 edition of the prayer must have been shared by Schwab (30; 31) and numerous later writers who also ascribe the prayer to Marcus Herz in spite of the specific mention by Distel in 1902 (20) of the existence of the 1783 edition antedating Herz by seven years.

Thus, Deutsch's criticism of Philippson seems unfounded. Philippson was probably aware of the *Deutsches Museum* edition of 1783, and in his own 1863 (17) and 1869 (18) versions of the prayer, he used the same title as in the 1783 original, namely " Daily prayer of a physician before he visits his patients: From a Hebrew manuscript of a renowned Jewish physician of the twelfth century." Deutsch further perpetuates the misconception (32; 34) later quoted by Friedenwald (14) that the prayer was embodied in Haeser's textbook of the history of medicine (35, p. 837). In actuality, only a brief footnote exists in Haeser's text, which, translated from the German, states: " Compare the beautiful morning prayer of a Jewish physician from the twelfth century in L. Philippson's Weltbewegende Fragen. . . ." In Haeser's discussion of Maimonides in the same work (pp. 595-597), no mention is made of the prayer. Nor is there any mention of the prayer in the two earlier editions of Haeser's textbook in 1845 and 1859 respectively. This indicates that Haeser, too, was unaware of the 1783 edition and first saw the prayer printed in Philippson's paper in 1863 (17).

Seeligmann in Holland (28) writes in 1928 that, in response to an inquiry regarding a Hebrew version of Maimonides' prayer, he remembers that it was probably not composed by Maimonides. He then states that Marcus Herz wrote it and traces its history from the Ha-Meassef in 1790 (24), through Philippson (17; 18) and Haeser (35). Seeligmann further writes that the first Dutch version is by Hektor Treub, which Dr. M. J. Premsela published in his brochure Medische Fastoensleer (Amsterdam 1903, pp. 52-53).

Emil Bogen (7), in response to the reprinting of part of one of Gotthard Deutsch's letters (32) in the Journal of the American Medical Association (33), correctly points out the existence of the 1783 version, which was not known to Deutsch. Bogen agrees with Kroner (36), who shows the harmony that exists between the other writings of Maimonides and the so-called " Prayer of Maimonides " in both form and spirit.

Bennigson and his colleagues (22) reprinted the German version in Leipzig in 1931; they briefly trace the history of the prayer from its origin in the Deutsches Museum (1). They erroneously state that it was reprinted in German by Distel in the Deutsche medizinische Wochenschrift in August 1904, when they probably mean 1902 (20). This error has been perpetuated by Kagan (13) and Muntner (23), neither of whom probably had access to the periodical in question. Another, probably typographical, error in Bennigson's paper (22) is the June 1893 date given for Pagel's (19) version of the prayer, an error again perpetuated by Kagan (13). The correct date is June 1892.

Keller (8), in 1931, in an essay entitled, " The Ideal Practice of

Medicine from the Rabbinical Point of View," compares the Prayer of Maimonides to the Hippocratic Oath and quotes excerpts from both. Maimonides, he says, considers the patient important because he is the creation of the Almighty, so that the responsibility for the outcome of our treatment rests partly with us as an instrument of the Almighty. Hippocrates, on the other hand, considers the preciousness of a human being from the sociological viewpoint.

To commemorate the 800th anniversary of the birth of Maimonides, in 1935, numerous publications on all aspects of Maimonides appeared in various periodicals, newspapers, journals, and books around the world. Among these are several references to the Prayer. Gershenfeld (10) provides excerpts of the English version. Illevitz (37) and Meyerhof (38) emphatically state that Maimonides did not write the prayer. A Spanish version of the prayer (29) also appeared in 1935. The author, E. Singer, states that it was previously published in the *Allgemeine Zeitung des Judenthums* in 1863 (17), in *Sulamit* in 1842, in *Abend Zeitung* in 1840, and in the *Medizinischer Almanach*.

An interesting inquiry by Sir William Osler concerning the authorship of the prayer was answered by the Chief Rabbi of the British Empire, Dr. Joseph H. Hertz, in a letter dated May 23, 1917, but published in the *Canadian Jewish Chronicle* in 1935 (39). The letter reads as follows:

Dear Sir William:

Some 2 years ago you inquired of me as to the "Physician's Prayer" attributed to Maimonides. I can now give you the following information on the subject:

This prayer is the production of Dr. Markus Herz (1747-1802), a friend and pupil of Immanuel Kant and of Moses Mendelssohn. He was a physician to the Jewish Hospital in Berlin. The prayer was composed by him in the German language and was published in a Hebrew translation in the Periodical Ha-Meassef. The current English version seems to be from this Hebrew translation and first appeared in the London paper "Voice of Jacob" on the 24th December, 1841.

Sincerely yours,
J. H. Hertz.

Also in 1935, Münz, in his book on Maimonides (40), ascribes the prayer to the great medieval physician, although the earlier German edition of his book (41) questions the true authorship.

In 1938, Kagan reprinted excerpts of the English version of the prayer (13) and traced its history. He based his article mainly on two previous papers, those of Bogen (7) and Bennigson *et al.* (22), as evidenced by Kagan's incorporation of the bibliographical errors in Bennigson's article into his own paper as described above. Kagan concludes with six argu-

ments favoring Maimonides as the true author of the prayer. These
arguments can be summarized as follows:

1. The medieval form and style of the prayer conform with Maimonides' other writings.

2. If Marcus Herz was the author, he would have laid claim to its
authorship.

3. Dr. Herz, a master of the German language, would have published
the original prayer in German and would only later have arranged for a
Hebrew translation.

4. If the later German version omitted Herz's name at his request,
he would not have requested Euchel, editor of the *Ha-Meassef*, to mention his name in the Hebrew translation.

5. Herz probably knew of the 1783 German version and sent the
document for Hebrew translation to Euchel, who erroneously ascribed
the German text to Herz. Herz did not know Hebrew since he didn't
translate it himself and probably was unaware of the Hebrew editor's note
making him the author.

6. All the professional ethics expressed in the prayer are also expressed
in some of Maimonides' letters and books.

In 1939, Levinson reprinted the prayer in English (12) as part of a
larger review of Maimonides' medical contributions. In 1944, Friedenwald, in his two volume classic *The Jews and Medicine* (14), also reprinted the prayer in English.

A most interesting booklet comparing the prayer of Maimonides to
the Oath of Asaph (42) and the physician's prayer of Jacob Zahalon
(43; 44; 14, pp. 268-279) was published by Muntner in 1946 (23). In
addition to publishing both Hebrew and German versions, Muntner provides us with a brief bibliographical sketch tracing the background of the
prayer, a sketch which he found in a 1928 Berlin version of the prayer
by Professor Heinrich Levy. The August 1904 date quoted for Distel's
version in the *Deutsche medizinische Wochenschrift* is incorrect and
should properly be August 1902 (20). Muntner calls attention to the
existence of a Hebrew manuscript in the Bibliothèque Nationale de Paris
which is entitled " The Prayer of Moses Maimonides." It is Hebrew
manuscript #873, part 7, fol. 98V°, described in the catalog (45) as
follows: " Prayer of Rabbi Moses Maimonides, beginning with Tefila
Lisegulas Eeshim and terminating by the piece of verse Galgal Soveiv."
The great bibliographer Moritz Steinschneider (46) describes an identical Hebrew work as manuscript Warner #41, part 11, folio 150 and

refers to the Paris Hebrew Manuscript as #285 (perhaps an error or perhaps an earlier different numbering system). In addition, this medieval Hebrew manuscript version of the " Prayer of Maimonides " was published in 1867 in the weekly Hebrew newspaper *Hacarmel* (47).

Muntner (23) correctly points out that this manuscript version of the prayer is a forgery and could not possibly have been written by Maimonides, since numerous references to astrology are not in keeping with Maimonides' vehement opposition to the " pseudoscience " of astrology (48). Muntner further claims that the versions of the prayer beginning with the 1783 German edition (1), although written in the spirit and form of Maimonides, omitting any reference to astrology, are also forgeries and can all be traced back to Marcus Herz.

Probably the most comprehensive review of the subject to date is the one published in Hebrew by Leibowitz in 1954 (2). A photocopy of the 1783 original German version (1) is presented, as well as the first page of the 1790 Hebrew version (24). Leibowitz must have consulted the original sources, since the bibliographical errors described above first made by Bennigson *et al.* (22) and later perpetuated by Kagan (13) and others are absent from Leibowitz's paper. A new Hebrew translation, made directly from the 1783 German version, is also provided in this article.

A second French edition of the prayer appeared in 1956 (26) and a short English version was reprinted in 1957 (16). A brief version of " The oath and prayer of Maimonides " was published in the *Journal of the American Medical Association* in 1955 (15), in which Maimonides is falsely called an Islamic philosopher, an error that was corrected by Lanzkron and Berner in two separate letters to the editor (49).

The most recent version of the prayer that I have been able to find is a 1962 French one (27). Only parts of the prayer are translated into French, according to the author Dr. J. Pines, from the Paris Hebrew manuscript #837 (45) described above.

I have been fortunate in being able to obtain copies of every reference enumerated in the bibliography of this paper. There are undoubtedly other versions, editions, and printings of the prayer in numerous languages in various newspapers, periodicals, and books throughout the world. The popularity of the prayer is attested to by its frequent quotation and publication. Whether Maimonides actually wrote the prayer or not remains an open question. Certainly most of those who are of the opinion that Maimonides did not write it, including Illevitz (37), Meyerhof (38), Simon (26), Hertz (39), Seeligmann (28), and others, base their remarks on the statements of Deutsch (32; 34) and Schwab (30; 31), although " Medicus " had already attributed authorship of the prayer to Marcus Herz in 1841 (3). As has already been pointed out, both Deutsch and Schwab were probably unaware of the 1783 German version of the prayer, which antedated Herz by seven years, and thus they have perpetuated the concept that Marcus Herz authored the prayer. This thesis may or may not be valid.

Other writers such as Bogen (7), Kagan (13), and perhaps Wolff (25) agree with Kroner (36) that the prayer was probably truly composed by Maimonides, since it conforms completely with the ideals, medical ethics, and spirit of Maimonides; they believe that the original will yet be found. Pagel (50) also supports this viewpoint. Certainly, at this point in history, this suggestion is no more than wishful thinking. However, it is conceivable that Marcus Herz saw an original manuscript in Hebrew; he may have based his version, in which he does not claim authorship, on such an original. This proposal seems unlikely. Alternatively, Herz may have seen the 1783 German version and asked his friend Isaac Euchel to translate it into Hebrew. The latter may have erroneously ascribed the German to Herz, as Kagan postulates (13). This theory, too, seems unlikely. It is also possible that neither Maimonides nor Herz wrote the prayer, but that a twelfth century astrologer wrote it in what became the Paris Hebrew manuscript, from which was extracted an abbreviated German version. A further possibility is that Maimonides did indeed write the prayer, but that an astrologer amended it and only the amended versions are extant today. These two latter possibilities are extremely remote.

It seems clear that the manuscript version of the prayer in Paris (45-46) and Oxford (47) mentioned above is a forgery and was not written by Maimonides. This is proved by Muntner (23), who states that the numerous references to astrology in this work make it impossible to ascribe authorship to Maimonides, who was vehemently opposed to this " pseudoscience " (48).

The question remains whether the 1783 *Deutsches Museum* edition (1) of the prayer, upon which many versions in numerous languages (1-29) are based, was truly written by Maimonides or not. As already mentioned, Kroner (36), Pagel (50), Wolff (25), Bogen (7), and Kagan (13) support the former view, whereas Leibowitz (2), Muntner (23), Schwab (30; 31), Deutsch (32; 34), Illevitz (37), Meyerhof (38), Seeligmann (28), " Medicus " (3), and Hertz (39) believe the prayer to be spurious.

The most potent arguments favoring the rejection of Maimonides as the author come from Professor Leibowitz (2), who states that no prominent medical historian supports the view of Maimonides' authorship. Furthermore, in Euchel's Hebrew version of 1790 (24), it is specifically stated that the prayer was composed by Marcus Herz and translated from German into Hebrew at his request. The confusion arose from the discovery of an earlier German edition (1) bearing the unfortunate title ". . . From the Hebrew manuscript of a renowned Jewish physician in Egypt from the twelfth century." This title leads logically to the supposition that Maimonides is the renowned physician referred to. However, if one carefully reads the text of 1783, one notes that contrary to what Kagan states (13), style, phrasing, and concepts are not compatible with a medieval dating. A phrase such as ". . . art is great, but the mind of man is ever expanding . . ." is typical and characteristic of eighteenth century Europe and is at variance with Maimonidean medieval thinking. Here, according to Leibowitz (51), is the idea of progress, which became even more popular in the nineteenth century.

Further evidence for an eighteenth century author lies in the phrase ". . . that act unceasingly and harmoniously to preserve the whole in all its beauty. . . ." This concept of " beauty " or " das Schöne " is characteristic of German literature of the Enlightenment. Moreover, a phrase such as ". . . ten thousand times ten thousand organs hast thou combined . . ." presupposes knowledge of the newer sciences of anatomy, biology, and microscopy. The tensions between colleagues discussed in the prayer are also products of a more modern period and dictated by the new academic hierarchy.

Leibowitz further writes (51) that:

Markus Herz probably wrote the Prayer as a contribution to medical ethics and as a comment on prevailing low standards of the practice. It was usual to insert in almanachs anonymous short contributions. Markus Herz was a warm Jew, proud of the history of his people; he clad his literary piece into the colorful frame indicated in the caption, probably indeed meaning Maimonides, but not based on a manuscript, which did not exist, but as belonging to the belles-lettres. Editions of Hebrew medical manuscripts began only in 1867 (Steinschneider's Donnolo). . . .

Probably the greatest living authority on the medical writings of Maimonides is Süssman Muntner. His book on the subject of Maimonides' prayer (23) has already been mentioned earlier in this paper. Muntner also believes strongly (52) that Marcus Herz composed this prayer in beautiful German and that a very poor translation into Hebrew was produced by Euchel (24). Furthermore, an anonymous or unknown

168

writer added the confusing caption to this earliest (1790) Hebrew version. Muntner further states that Herz based his version of the prayer on the earlier Prayer of Jacob Zahalon (43; 44; 14, pp. 268-279), which was written in the seventeenth century, and was greatly influenced and stimulated by it.

From all the foregoing discussion, the evidence overwhelmingly favors the concept that the physician's prayer attributed to Maimonides is a spurious work, not written by Maimonides but composed by an eighteenth century writer, probably Marcus Herz. Absolute proof that this is so is, however, lacking and may never be discovered.

Recently, in a comparative and historical study of the Jewish religious attitude to medicine and its practice (53), Dr. Immanuel Jakobovits, newly appointed Chief Rabbi of the British Commonwealth, emphasized the ethical and moral responsibilities of the physician as a divine agent in the alleviation of human suffering. Deeply pious and moving prayers of gratitude for divine help, such as those of Asaph (42), Judah Halevy (14, p. 27), Jacob Zahalon (43; 44; 14, pp. 268-279), and Abraham Zacutus (14, pp. 295-321), as well as the physician's prayer attributed to Maimonides (1-29), says Jakobovits, all recognize God as the ultimate healer of disease, while also asserting " the indispensable part played by the physician, his art and his medicines " in the preservation of health.

The Physician's Prayer attributed to Maimonides contains moral and ethical standards by which a physician should conduct his professional life. The daily recitation of this prayer serves to remind the physician of these standards which have been set up for him and which he should attempt to live up to. Physicians should constantly carry with them the highest code of medical philanthropy and professional ethics. Such noble philosophy and high aspirations of the profession are embodied in the Physician's Prayer.

Acknowledgments: The author is indebted to Professor Joshua O. Leibowitz and Professor Süssman Muntner for reading the manuscript and for helpful suggestions. Bibliographical material was obtained through the courtesy of numerous librarians throughout the United States and for this I am grateful. Thanks are also due Mrs. Frances Rose for typing the manuscript.

There follows below the English version of the " Daily Prayer of a Physician " by Dr. Harry Friedenwald, reprinted from the *Bulletin of the Johns Hopkins Hospital*, 1917, *28*: 256-261, with kind permission from the editors and publishers.

DAILY PRAYER OF A PHYSICIAN

Almighty God, Thou hast created the human body with infinite wisdom. Ten thousand times ten thousand organs hast Thou combined in it that act unceasingly and harmoniously to preserve the whole in all its beauty— the body which is the envelope of the immortal soul. They are ever acting in perfect order, agreement and accord. Yet, when the frailty of matter or the unbridling of passions deranges this order or interrupts this accord, then forces clash and the body crumbles into the primal dust from which it came. Thou sendest to man diseases as beneficent messengers to foretell approaching danger and to urge him to avert it.

Thou hast blest Thine earth, Thy rivers and Thy mountains with healing substances; they enable Thy creatures to alleviate their sufferings and to heal their illnesses. Thou hast endowed man with the wisdom to relieve the suffering of his brother, to recognize his disorders, to extract the healing substances, to discover their powers and to prepare and to apply them to suit every ill. In Thine Eternal Providence Thou hast chosen me to watch over the life and health of Thy creatures. I am now about to apply myself to the duties of my profession. Support me, Almighty God, in these great labors that they may benefit mankind, for without Thy help not even the least thing will succeed.

Inspire me with love for my art and for Thy creatures. Do not allow thirst for profit, ambition for renown and admiration, to interfere with my profession, for these are the enemies of truth and of love for mankind and they can lead astray in the great task of attending to the welfare of Thy creatures. Preserve the strength of my body and of my soul that they ever be ready to cheerfully help and support rich and poor, good and bad, enemy as well as friend. In the sufferer let me see only the human being. Illumine my mind that it recognize what presents itself and that it may comprehend what is absent or hidden. Let it not fail to see what is visible, but do not permit it to arrogate to itself the power to see what cannot be seen, for delicate and indefinite are the bounds of the great art of caring for the lives and health of Thy creatures. Let me never be absent-minded. May no strange thoughts divert my attention at the bedside of the sick, or disturb my mind in its silent labors, for great and sacred are the thoughtful deliberations required to preserve the lives and health of Thy creatures.

Grant that my patients have confidence in me and my art and follow my directions and my counsel. Remove from their midst all charlatans and the whole host of officious relatives and know-all nurses, cruel people

170

who arrogantly frustrate the wisest purposes of our art and often lead Thy creatures to their death.

Should those who are wiser than I wish to improve and instruct me, let my soul gratefully follow their guidance; for vast is the extent of our art. Should conceited fools, however, censure me, then let love for my profession steel me against them, so that I remain steadfast without regard for age, for reputation, or for honor, because surrender would bring to Thy creatures sickness and death.

Imbue my soul with gentleness and calmness when older colleagues, proud of their age, wish to displace me or to scorn me or disdainfully to teach me. May even this be of advantage to me, for they know many things of which I am ignorant, but let not their arrogance give me pain. For they are old and old age is not master of the passions. I also hope to attain old age upon this earth, before Thee, Almighty God!

Let me be contented in everything except in the great science of my profession. Never allow the thought to arise in me that I have attained to sufficient knowledge, but vouchsafe to me the strength, the leisure and the ambition ever to extend my knowledge. For art is great, but the mind of man is ever expanding.

Almighty God! Thou hast chosen me in Thy mercy to watch over the life and death of Thy creatures. I now apply myself to my profession. Support me in this great task so that it may benefit mankind, for without Thy help not even the least thing will succeed.

REFERENCES

(Hebrew titles have been translated into English.)

1. Tägliches Gebet eines Arztes bevor er seine Kranken besucht—Aus der hebräischen Handschrift eines berühmten jüdischen Arztes in Egypten aus dem zwölften Jahrhundert. *Deutsches Museum*, 1783, *1*: 43-45.
2. Leibowitz, J. O., "The physician's prayer ascribed to Maimonides." *Dapim Refuiim*, 1954, *13*: 77-81.
3. Medicus, "Daily prayer of a physician." *Voice of Jacob* (London), 1841, *1* (7): 49-50.
4. Peters, M. C., *Justice to the Jew*. The story of what he has done for the world. London and New York: Neely, 1899, pp. 173-175.
5. Golden, W. W., "Maimonides' prayer for physicians." *Tr. M. Soc. West Virginia*, 1900, *33*: 414-415.
6. Friedenwald, H., "The ethics of the practice of medicine from the Jewish point of view." *Bull. Johns Hopkins Hosp.*, 1917, *28*: 256-261.
7. Bogen, E., "The daily prayer of a physician." *J. A. M. A.*, 1929, *92*: 2128.
8. Keller, H., Comparison between Hippocratic Oath and Maimonides' Prayer, in The Ideal Practice of Medicine from the Rabbinical Point of View, in

Modern Hebrew Orthopedic Terminology and Jewish Medical Essays. Boston: Stratford Co., 1931, pp. 142-146.

9. Roman, D., "Maimonides' prayer." *Hahneman. Monthly,* 1932, *67*: 244-250.

10. Gershenfeld, L., "The medical works of Maimonides and his Treatise on personal hygiene and dietetics." *Am. J. Pharm.,* 1935, *107*: 14-28.

11. "Physician's prayer by Maimonides." *M. Leaves,* 1937, *1*: 9.

12. Levinson, A., "Maimonides, the physician." *M. Leaves,* 1939, *2*: 96-105.

13. Kagan, S. R., "Maimonides' prayer." *Ann. M. Hist.,* 1938, *10*: 429-432.

14. Friedenwald, H., *The Jews and Medicine.* Baltimore: Johns Hopkins Press, 1944, vol. I, pp. 28-30.

15. "The oath and prayer of Maimonides." *J. A. M. A.,* 1955, *157*: 1158.

16. Minkin, J. S., *The World of Moses Maimonides with Selections from his Writings.* New York: Yoseloff, 1957, pp. 149-150.

17. Philippson, L., "Tägliches Gebet eines Arztes vor dem Besuch seiner Kranken. (Aus der hebr. Handschrift eines berühmten jüdischen Arztes aus dem zwölften Jahrhundert.)" *Allg. Ztg. d. Judent.,* 1863, *27* (4): 49-50.

18. Philippson, L., *Weltbewegende Fragen in Politik und Religion aus den letzten dreissig Jahren.* Zweiter Theil: Religion. Leipzig: Baumgärtner, 1869, pp. 159-160.

19. Pagel, J. "Das Gebet des Arztes." *Allg. Ztg. d. Judent.,* 1892, *56* (25): 294-295.

20. Distel, Th., "Gebet eines jüdischen Arztes im 12. Jahrhundert." *Deutsche med. Wchschr.,* 1902, *28* (32): 580.

21. "Gebet eines jüdischen Arztes im 12. Jahrhundert." *Cor.-Bl. f. schweiz. Aerzte,* 1902, *32* (19): 611-613.

22. Bennigson, W., Eitingon, M., Graetz, M., Holzer, P., Schiff, A., Schiller, E., and Wolfstein, H., *Des Moses Maimonides Morgengebet bevor er seine Kranken besuchte.* Leipzig, 1931, p. 6.

23. Muntner, S., *The Deutero Prayer of Moses;* with an Introduction about the history of the prayer, attributed to the physician Maimonides and a contemplation on the state of the praying and on the valour of the prayer in general. Jerusalem: Geniza, 1946, p. 57.

24. Euchel, I., "Prayer for the physician as he pours out his anxieties before G-d prior to visiting the sick. Composed by Sir Hofrat Professor Herz." *Ha-Meassef,* 1790, *6*: 242-244.

25. Wolff, J., "Prière d'un médecin juif à l'usage de ses confrères." *Univers israélite,* 1903, *58*: 753-755.

26. Simon, I., "L'oeuvre médicale de Maïmonide." *Rev. hist. méd. hébr.,* 1956, no. 31: 107-120.

27. Pines, J., "La contribution juive à la médecine arabe au moyen âge." *Scalpel* (Bruxelles), 1962, *115*: 207-218.

28. Seeligmann, S., "Morgengebed van den arts naar Maimonides." *Vrijdagavond,* 1928, *5* (1): 404-406.

29. Singer, E., "Maimonides, medico." *Semana méd.,* 1935, *2*: 1960-1965.

30. Schwab, M., *Répertoire des articles relatifs à l'histoire et à la littérature juives parus dans les périodiques de 1783 à 1898.* Paris: Durlacher, 1899, p. 167.

31. Schwab, M., "La prière d'un médecin juif." *Univers israélite,* 1903, *58*: 818-819.

32. Deutsch, G., " Maimonides prayer." *Am. Israelite*, March 19, 1908, p. 5, cols. 5, 6.
33. " The ' Prayer of Maimonides ' and its true author." *J. A. M. A.*, 1929, *92* : 836.
34. Deutsch, G., *Scrolls*, vol. III : *Jew and Gentile*. Essays on Jewish apologetics and kindred historical subjects. Boston : Stratford Co., 1920, pp. 93-95.
35. Haeser, H., *Lehrbuch der Geschichte der Medicin und der epidemischen Krankheiten*. 3rd ed. Jena : Dufft, 1875, vol. I.
36. Kroner, H., " Arzt und Patient in der Medizin des Maimonides." *Ost u. West, Illus. Monatsschr. f. modernes Judent.*, 1912, *12* : 745-750.
37. Illevitz, A. B., " Maimonides the physician." *Canad. M. A. J.*, 1935, *32* : 440-442.
38. Meyerhof, M., The Medical Work of Maimonides, in *Essays on Maimonides*, An Octocentennial Volume, ed. S. W. Baron. New York : Columbia Univ. Press, 1941, pp. 265-299.
39. Hertz, J. H., Letter to Sir William Osler. *Canad. Jewish Chron.*, 1935, *22* : 7 (April 12).
40. Münz, I., *Maimonides (The Rambam)*. The story of his life and genius. Trans. from German, Introduction by H. T. Schnittkind. Boston : Winchell-Thomas, 1935, p. 191.
41. Münz, I., *Moses ben Maimon (Maimonides)* ; sein Leben und seine Werke. Frankfurt a. M. : Kauffmann, 1812, pp. 267-268.
42. Rosner, F. and Muntner, S., " The oath of Asaph." *Ann. Int. Med.*, 1965, *63* : 317-320.
43. Savitz, H., " Jacob Zahalon and his Book, ' The Treasure of Life,' " *New England J. Med.*, 1935, *213* : 167-176.
44. Simon, I., " La prière des médecins. ' Tephilat Harofim,' de Jacob Zahalon, médecin et rabbin en Italie (1630-1693)." *Rev. hist. méd. hébr.*, 1955, no. 8 : 38-51.
45. Bibliothèque nationale—Catalogues des manuscrits hébreux et samaritains de la Bibliothèque impériale. Paris, 1866, p. 142.
46. Steinschneider, M., *Catologus codicum hebraeorum Bibliothecae academiae Lugduno Batavae*. [Leiden :] E. J. Brill, 1858, p. 188.
47. Meshash, R., " The prayer of Rabbi Moses attributed to Rabbi Moses ben Maimon (Maimonides)." *Hacarmel*, 1867, *6* : 350.
48. Marx, A., " The correspondence between the rabbis of southern France and Maimonides about astrology." *Hebrew Union Coll. Annual*, 1926, *3* : 311-358, and 1927, *4* : 493-494.
49. Lanzkron, J. and Berner, H., " Maimonides—physician, astronomer, philosopher, Talmudist." *J. A. M. A.*, 1955, *157* : 1637.
50. Pagel, J., *Maimuni als medizinischer Schriftsteller*. Frankfurt a. M. : Kauffmann, 1908, p. 17.
51. Leibowitz, J. O., Personal communication.
52. Muntner, S., Personal communication.
53. Jakobovits, I., *Jewish Medical Ethics*. New York : Bloch, 1959, pp. 15-18.

MEDICAL ETHICS AND ETIQUETTE IN THE EARLY MIDDLE AGES: THE PERSISTENCE OF HIPPOCRATIC IDEALS *

LOREN C. MacKINNEY

A prevailing tendency of the reading public is its ready acceptance of derogatory generalizations concerning medieval civilization. There is, for example, the traditional generalization that tends to degrade the medieval physician to the position of quack, charlatan, faith healer, medicine man, barber surgeon. Often he is contrasted with the ancient Greek physician, to whom there have been attributed the superlative ideals which the modern age associates with the Hippocratic Oath.

As a result of the historical researches of twentieth-century scholarship, we are beginning to recognize the inaccuracies and exaggerations imbedded in such generalizations concerning the high medical standards of the ancient Greeks and the degradation of the profession during the Middle Ages. So far as the Greek world is concerned, W. H. S. Jones' *The Doctor's Oath* (Cambridge University, 1924) and the introductions

* Much of the research on this topic, in distant libraries, was made possible by grants from the Smith Fund of the University of North Carolina, and from the Carnegie Foundation. Valuable suggestions and assistance on problems of paleography and translation were generously given by Professor Elias Lowe of the Princeton University Institute of Advanced Studies, Miss Dorothy Schullian and William Jerome Wilson of the Cleveland Branch of the Army Medical Library, and Professor B. L. Ullman of the University of North Carolina.

(especially in vol. II) to his *Hippocrates* (New York, 1923 ff.), and Ludwig Edelstein's *The Hippocratic Oath; Text, Translation and Interpretation* (Baltimore, 1943) indicate the necessity of drastic modifications of the traditionally optimistic picture of the Greek medical profession as a band of high minded healers dedicated to the holy ideals of the Sacred Oath.

With regard to the Middle Ages, much has been done to correct the historical astigmatism of tradition,[1] but it has been confined almost entirely to the later medieval centuries, and especially to the supposed influence of Salerno, reputed center of a revived Hippocratic idealism and scientific Greek practice.[2] It is our purpose to show that the preceding period, from about 400 to 1100 A. D., comprising the so-called Dark Ages, had medical ideals that are worthy of a place in the historical record alongside the Hippocratic and Salernitan " codes." Like most of the institutions of Western Civilization, the regulated conduct of physicians in the early Middle Ages seems to have evolved in normally diverse fashion; also without benefit of Salerno, and with much more borrowing from Hippocrates than from Biblical or clerical authorities.

We present a number of treatises, based for the most part on the original manuscript texts. In general, we propose to let them speak for themselves as to the prevailing medieval ideals concerning the training, character, qualifications, dress, and deportment of physicians. Marked resemblances to passages from Hippocratic works, as well as from the Bible and the Church Fathers, indicate a fusion of classical antiquity with Christianity during these early centuries. Equally impressive are the

---

[1] Especially Mary Welborn's " The Long Tradition: A Study in Fourteenth-Century Medical Deontology" in *Medieval and Historiographical Essays in Honor of James Westfall Thompson,* edited by James Cate and Eugene Anderson (Chicago, 1938). See also Henry Sigerist's " Sidelights on the Practice of Medieval Surgeons " (Henri de Mondeville), in *Proceedings of the Annual Congress on Medical Education, Hospitals and Licensure* (Chicago, Feb. 18-19, 1935) ; Pearl Kibre's " Hippocratic Writings in the Middle Ages " (*Bull. Hist. Med.,* 1945, 18, 371-412, especially 402) ; Owsei Temkin's "Geschichte des Hippokratismus im ausgehenden Altertum " (*Kyklos,* 1932, vol. 4) ; and Paul Diepgen, *Die Theologie und der ärztliche Stand* (Berlin, 1922).

[2] S. De Renzi, *Collectio Salernitana* (Naples, 1852 ff.), II, 73 ff., V, 102 f., 333 ff., gives descriptions of MSS and of the Latin texts. Paul Meyer in *Romania* (1903, 32, 86 f. and 1915-1917, 44, 196 f.) describes similar texts in French from MSS in England. Leopold Delisle, *Le Cabinet des Manuscripts de la Bibliothèque Nationale* (Paris, 1874), II, 533; and M. R. James, *The Ancient Libraries of Canterbury and Dover* (Cambridge, 1903), p. 333, cite MSS. R. Cantarella, in *Archeion* (1933, 15, 305-320) cites a few evidences of the Hippocratic Oath in a " civitas Hippocratica " at Salerno before Frederick II. P. Kristeller's " The School of Salerno " (*Bull. Hist. Med.,* 1945, 17, 138-194) presents a broader and more reliable picture of early Salernitan history.

variations and miscellaneous inclusions, factors that show the constant influence of contemporary conditions and of practical experience. It should be remembered that most of these medieval ideals, like the earlier Hippocratic dicta, reflect merely the highest standards of the medical profession. We trust that the evidence presented will not only serve to correct the extremes of generalization now prevalent concerning Greek and Medieval physicians, but also will help fill a gap in modern knowledge of the development of medical ideals.

From the non-medical viewpoint of lay historians who are interested in pre-Renaissance classicism, the evidence presented is noteworthy. It corroborates the thesis of the persistence of Hippocratic ideas in an unbroken line through the early, as well as late, Middle Ages, and in non-Salernitan centers. This factor has been ably discussed in Owsei Temkin's "Geschichte des Hippokratismus im ausgehenden Altertum" and Pearl Kibre's "Hippocratic Writings in the Middle Ages" (cited in footnote 1).

Original source material for the early Middle Ages is scanty, especially for the period prior to the ninth century. However, from these early Christian centuries come three bits of evidence concerned especially with medical ethics and etiquette. A letter of advice written by St. Jerome (late in the fourth century) to a priest in Northern Italy named Nepotian reveals a vague familiarity with the Hippocratic Oath. The young clergyman was cautioned, among other things, to observe secrecy and chastity with regard to the households in which he visited the sick. He also was reminded of certain qualifications which Hippocrates had laid down for secular physicians.

A. [JEROME], TO NEPOTIAN, PRIEST. [A CLERGYMAN'S DUTIES].

It is a part of your [clerical] duty to visit the sick, to be acquainted with people's households, with matrons, and with their children, and to be entrusted with the secrets of the great. Let it therefore be your duty to keep your tongue chaste as well as your eyes. Never discuss a woman's looks, nor let one house know what is going on in another. Hippocrates, before he will instruct his pupils, makes them take an oath and compels them to swear obedience to him. That oath exacts from them silence, and prescribes for them their language, gait, dress, and manners. How much greater an obligation is laid on us [clergymen]. . . .[3] –

Jerome's reference to the Hippocratic Oath as a rule prescribing "language, gait, dress, and manners" indicates either that he was not aware of

[3] F. A. Wright's translation, in *Select Letters of St. Jerome* (London and New York, 1933), Letter 52, p. 225. Nepotian, an ex-soldier and nephew of a bishop in Venetia, had asked Jerome for advice as to a young cleric's duties.

the contents of the actual Oath (which has nothing concerning these matters, with the exception of *sex*-manners), or that he interpreted the Oath very loosely to include precepts found in other Hippocratic works such as *Physician, Law,* and *Decorum.* On the other hand, his warning against immorality and the revealing of household secrets corresponds to the last two admonitions of the Hippocratic Oath. Apparently, Christians of Jerome's day had a rather vague idea of Hippocratic ideals, but had considerable respect for them.

Within a century after Jerome, the Germanic law codes of the Visigoths were taking shape in Spain. In these, and later revisions thereof, there is a regulation concerning women patients that reflects the same age-old sex problem of which the Hippocratic Oath and Jerome's letter gave warning. The Visigothic code reads as follows:

B. No physician shall presume to bleed a [freeborn] woman in the absence of [some of] her relatives . . .; the father, mother, brother, son, uncle or some neighbor. . . . X solidi [penalty]. . . . On such occasions scandals multiply. . . .[4]

About two centuries after Jerome, in the Ostrogothic kingdom of Italy, Cassiodorus in writing to the supervising physician of the royal household referred to " certain sacred oaths of a priestly nature " by which medical students were obligated, and also to the standards of practice set up for a governmentally regulated profession.

C. [He stressed the merits of the healing art as a worthy calling in that it concerns both the present and future well being of patients and aids them when other (i. e., spiritual) means fail. He warned physicians to avoid quarrels, envy, all forms of wickedness, and artifices of healing. He exhorted them to ever seek knowledge, to read the works of the ancients and to manifest zeal and cheerfulness in treating the sick, and also purity in their personal lives. For an effective bedside manner, the following advice was given] : Let your visits bring healing to the sick, new strength to the weak, certain hope to the weary. Leave it to clumsy [practicioners] to ask the patients they are visiting whether the pain has ceased and if they have slept well. Let the patient ask you about his ailment and hear from you the truth about it. Use the surest possible informants. To a skillful physician the pulsing of the veins [*venarum*] reveals the patient's ailment while the urine analysis indicates it to his eye. To make things easier, do not tell the clamoring inquirer what these symptoms signify. . . .[5]

Somewhat different from the governmental regulations of Visigothic

[4] Visigothic code, book XI, 1 (*MGH, Leges,* Sect. I, vol. I, 400).

[5] The original Latin text can be found in *MGH, Auct. Antiq.,* XII, 191 f.; also in M. Neuburger, *Geschichte der Medizin* (Stuttgart, 1911), II, part i, 246 f.; and L. MacKinney, *Early Medieval Medicine* (Baltimore, 1937), p. 163 ff. There is a free translation into English in T. Hodgkin, *Letters of Cassiodorus* (London, 1886), p. 313 f.

Spain and Ostrogothic Italy are the medical ideals expressed in numerous epistolary treatises that appear in the earliest medical manuscripts of the Middle Ages. Most of these manuscripts were written in North-European monasteries during the eight, ninth, and tenth centuries, an era that is often referred to derogatorily as the age of monastic medicine. To be sure, the monastic spirit dominated the compiling of the medical handbooks of the period, but as we shall see, the result was classical as well as pious, and secular as well as ascetic.

Very few of these monastic treatises subordinated Hippocrates and classical medicine to Christ and clerical ministrations in a manner as marked as that manifested in Jerome's letter, or in the sixth-century writings of Cassiodorus, notably the chapter " Concerning Monks Entrusted with the Care of the Sick " in his *De Institutione Divinarum Litterarum* (chapter 31).

One of the most pious expressions of the monastic ideal of medicine is found in the introduction to a manuscript handbook that was compiled probably in a German monastery, late in the eighth century, was recopied about a century later in its present manuscript form (Bamberg MS L III 8), only to be taken to Bamberg Cathedral somewhere around the year 1000 and kept there even to the present day. The author of the introduction was intent on reconciling the late classical medical works, which comprised most of the manuscript, with Christian monastic ideals. In even more detailed and pious fashion than either Jerome or Cassiodorus, he cited the Holy Scriptures, Pope Gregory I, Isidore of Seville, Bede, etc., to show the divine purpose in human medicine.[6]

D. . . . Wherefore one ought not to spurn earthly medicine since he knows it is advantageous rather than harmful and since it has not been held in contempt by holy men. . . . [St. Luke, St. Cosmas, and St. Damian were physicians]. Wherefore let us honor the physicians so that they will help us when sick, remembering [the word of] that wise one [Ecclesiasticus 38: 1. Vulgate] : " Honor the physician of necessity for the Most High created him." And do not hesitate to take what potions he gives you. That same wise one [Ecclesiasticus 38: 4] said " The Most High created medicine from the earth, and the prudent man will not reject it." Therefore he who does not seek medicine in time of necessity deserves the name stupid and imprudent. I say that it is wise to do well by the physician while you are well so that you will have his services in time of illness. . . . God wishes to be honored by his miracles performed through man. According to Isaiah [26: 12] whatever good is done by man is effected by God; he said " The Lord does all of our works through us." [Christ] himself in the Gospel [Luke 18: 27 ?] said

---

[6] The text was described and edited by Sudhoff in *Archiv Gesch. Med.,* 1914, 7, 223-237.

" Without me you can do nothing." . . . [The treatise closes with a lengthy exhortation for physicians to serve ailing humans, whether rich or poor, and with a view to eternal rather than earthly rewards.[7] This admonition, derived from the above mentioned passage of Cassiodorus' " Concerning Monks Entrusted with the Care of the Sick," is accompanied by his list of recommended readings and his warning that monastic healers should put their trust in the Lord rather than in herbs and human counsels. The exhortation ends on the following note of Christian idealism:] Aid the sick, your reward coming from Christ, for whoever gives a cup of cold water in His name is assured of the eternal kingdom where with Father and Holy Spirit He lives and reigns for eternity. Amen.

The remainder of the Bamberg manuscript, which is our earliest manuscript source, exemplifies the more practically secular and classical aspects of monastic medicine. Like most early medical manuscripts it contains Latin translations or condensations of Graeco-Roman works on remedies, diet, monthly regimen, substitute medicines, and other miscellaneous bits of information. Among the last mentioned items is a fragment of treatise K(a) (quoted below) which reiterates the chief points in the Hippocratic Oath. This manuscript with its combination of Christian piety and classical idealism typifies the more conservative aspects of monastic medical literature during the early Middle Ages. So far as medical ethics and etiquette are concerned, there are more important manuscript sources.

Somewhat later than the Bamberg manuscript, in Central France a much more detailed medical handbook was compiled (Paris, Bibliothèque Nationale, MS 11219).[8] In it are found many treatises, including a commentary on Hippocrates' Aphorisms (in Latin), a book (attributed to him) on various medical topics, another on diseases and cures, gynecology and herbs, also an antidotary and a miscellany of epistolary treatises attributed to Hippocrates and Galen. The epistolary treatises appear immediately after Hippocrates' Aphorisms, under the title *Liber Epistolarum*. The first seven, which are actually brief treatises concerning medical training, ethics, and etiquette, constitute one of the most complete cover-

[7] Similar warnings are given elsewhere in the manuscript, on a folio (5) of verses entitled " Cosmas, Damian, Hippocrates, Galen." They read in part as follows : " Sick one, pay the physician what you owe lest when ills return no one will visit you. Physician, care for the poor as well as the powerful. If the patient is rich you have a just occasion for profit; if poor, let one reward [spiritual] suffice. . . ."

[8] A few scholars have dated the manuscript 9-10th century. Professor Lowe was so kind as to check it recently and assures me as to the 9th century dating. It once belonged to a monastery in Luxemburg. Professor Lowe believes that it originated in the Loire region and that it may have been one of the manuscripts used by the humanistic cleric, Lupus of Ferrieres.

ages of these subjects in early manuscript literature. Strange to say, this part of the manuscript has been neglected, even by specialists in medieval medical history.[9] The collection is especially important in that, in combination with similar treatises in other early manuscripts, it reveals a North-European literature which, amidst monastic influences, reflected the classical ideology of Hippocrates. A parallel collection, also strangely neglected, is found in a slightly later manuscript at Chartres (MS 62). This literature, stemming from transalpine monasteries, antedates the earliest examples from Salerno, the much publicized center of Hippocratic ideas, once referred to by Fielding Garrison as "the isolated outpost of Greek medical tradition in the Middle Ages."

The chronological list (below) of manuscripts which contain the treatises under consideration serves to indicate the importance of non-Salernitan, North-European centers. Obviously the present location of manuscripts (almost all of them in the North) and their datings (all subsequent to 800 A. D) do not eliminate the possibility of pre-ninth-century, Italian, sources for the material found therein. In fact, scholars are convinced that most of the classical element in early Medieval medical literature was derived from compilations and translations (from the Greek) that antedate the ninth-century activities in Northern Europe commonly referred to as the Carolingian Renaissance. The earliest centers of translating are thought to have been in Byzantine Italy, in and about Ravenna, during the fifth, sixth and seventh centuries. Medical works in both Greek and Latin were also current in Southern Italy in Cassiodorus' day (ca. 550). It is possible therefore that we are concerned with a Graeco-Latin medical literature that was originally a product of the Byzantine classicism of Ravenna and the monasticism stemming from the Vivarium and Monte Cassino.

---

[9] Hirschfeld's otherwise excellent survey of "Deontologische Texte des frühen Mittelalters" (*Archiv Gesch. Med.*, 1928, 20, 353-371) fails even to cite the manuscript, though he presents the texts of some of the treatises contained therein, from later manuscripts. He also omits (perforce) treatises that are unique to this manuscript. The manuscript is likewise unmentioned in Laux's article on "Ars medicinae" (*Kyklos*, 1930, 3, 417-434) save for the citation of a list of surgical instruments, contained therein. The manuscript is cited, but not for the texts with which we are concerned, in H. Diels, *Die Handschriften der antiken Aerzte* (Berlin, 1905) I, 53.

Manuscripts and Editions of the Treatises.[10]

Bamberg, L III 8, 9th century, folios 1-6 (Sudhoff, Hirschfeld, Laux)
Paris, BN, 11219, 9th century, folios 12-15
St. Gall, 751, 9-10th century, pp. 337-339, 354-359 (Hirschfeld, Laux)
Glasgow, Hunter, V. 3. 2, early 10th century, folio 27
Karlsruhe, 120, 10th century, folios 182-184 (Rose)
Chartres, 62, 10th century folios 1-2
Brussels, 3701-15, 10th century, folios 5-7
Monte Cassino, 97, 10th century, p. 4 (De Renzi, II, 73)
Rome, Vat. Barberini, 160, 11th century, folio 286
Montpellier, 185, 11th century, folio 100 (Sigerist)
Copenhagen, 1653, 11th century, folio 72 (Laux)
Zurich, C 128/32, 11th century, folios 103-104 (Hirschfeld, Laux)
Brussels, 1342-50, 12th century, folios 1-2 (Hirschfeld, Laux)
Rome, Angelica, 1502, 12th century, folio 1 (Giacosa, Hirschfeld)
Breslau, 1302, 12th century, folio 184 (De Renzi, II, 74)
Edinburgh, A. 5. 42, 12th century, last folio
Rome, Vat. Regina, 1443, 12-13th century, folio 39
Rome, Vat. 2376 folio 209 (cited by Diels, I, 123)
Rome, Vat. 2417 folio 275 (cited by Diels, I, 123)
Carpentras, 318, 13th century, folio 79 (Sigerist)
Paris, BN, 15456, 13th century, folio 186
Paris, BN, 7091, 14th century, folio 1 (De Renzi, V, 333)
London, BM, Cotton, Galba, E. IV, 14th century, folio 238 (Rose)
Escorial, a IV 6, 14-15th century, folio 197 (Hirschfeld)
Paris, BN, 6988A, 15th century, folio 121

Using the ninth-century Paris manuscript (BN 11219) as a sort of master copy, we present the translated texts in topical groups; first the more idealistic ones concerning Spiritual Aspects of Medicine and Qualifi-

---

[10] In practically all cases the dating of the listed manuscripts is based on personal examination (either of the original or of photoreproductions), and also on the opinions of specialists such as Elias Lowe and B. L. Ullman. Where there are printed versions of the manuscript text, the editor's name appears in parenthesis after the manuscript listing; viz., (Sudhoff) for Sudhoff's article cited above in note 6; (Hirschfeld) for Hirschfeld's article cited above in note 9; (Laux) for Laux's article cited above in note 9; (De Renzi) for De Renzi's *Collectio* cited above in note 2; (Sigerist) for Sigerist's article "Early Mediaeval Medical Texts in Manuscripts of Montpellier" (*Bull. Hist. Med.*, 1941, 10, 31 f.); (Giacosa) for P. Giacosa's *Magistri Salernitani nondum editi* (Turin, 1901), p. 360; (Diels) for Diels' *Die Handschriften* cited above in note 9; and (Rose) for V. Rose's *Anecdota Graeca et Graecolatina* (Berlin, 1870), II, 275 f.

cations and Training of the Physician; then those of a more practical nature concerning Etiquette, Women Patients, Pulse Taking, Sick Calls, and other aspects of the " Bedside Manner." [11]

I. SPIRITUAL ASPECTS OF MEDICINE

The first treatise to be presented is similar to the Bamberg introduction (above, treatise D), in that it is predominantly religious in its approach to the subject. Although the Paris treatise is the briefer of the two, it is more emphatic with regard to the divine aspects of healing. From beginning to end the healing of the body is subordinated to the healing of the soul.

E. FOR ALL HEALING DIVINE MEDICATIONS ARE TO BE USED.[12]

For all healing divine medications are to be used because divine power is the proper agent for restoring mortal bodies. It is proper to call such an one physician who is responsible for the health of the soul and the well being of the body . . . [the text continues concerning Christ's ordaining of illness for man's good, also food and drink for his bodily welfare, and ointments, herbs, and medical practitioners for his bodily ills. It ends on a spiritual note, viz.,] He who provides for the healing of soul and body, being made immortal by every divine potentiality, merits pristine health and also security from his own guilt.

In addition to treatises of this sort, occasionally one finds brief passages of an other-worldly nature in otherwise secularly-minded treatises. For example, in a minor, anonymous text which Sigerist edited from the eleventh-century Montpellier manuscript (185), and which exists in at least three other manuscripts (Glasgow, Hunter V. 3. 2, folio 27; Rome, Vat. Barberini, 160, folio 286; Codex Fritz Paneth, folio 175) there is the following: " Medicine was created by the Most High [Ecclesiasticus, 38 : 1, 4. Vulgate]. He who fears not God will seek out the physician and not find healing, whereas many of whom physicians have despaired, have been healed by God."

[11] In some cases we have checked or amplified the Paris master text by collation with later manuscripts or editions, notably Chartres MS 62, Rose's version (*op. cit.*, p. 243 ff.) and a late B. M. MS. Furthermore, a few of the treatises presented do not appear in the Paris manuscript. All such variations are indicated in the footnotes. Brackets are used throughout the translations to enclose words or phrases (not in the original text) which have been added in order to clarify the meaning. However, we have not pressed this procedure meticulously since the translations are somewhat free renderings of the original Latin texts; this is not only for purposes of clarification, but also because of numerous variants and uncertainties in the manuscript versions.

[12] This treatise is also found in Brussels MS 3701-15, in similar but not identical wording.

The same Biblical text was cited in support of physicians by other monastic compilers. We have already noted (above, treatise D) that as early as the eighth century this, and other Scriptural passages were quoted to prove that those who refused the God-given ministrations of physicians were " stupid and improvident." A century later, Rabanus Maurus, in the medical section of his *De Universo* (xviii, 5), followed the same line of thought. It seems likely that his section entitled " Medical Healing is not to be Spurned" was borrowed from the eighth-century, Bamberg treatise, though in condensed form.[13]

A briefer, but similarly pious, defense of physicians occurs in a Brussels manuscript (3701-15, f. 5). The author, after a brief discussion of the four parts of the body and the four humors, added the following post-script: " Now let us speak of the minister of nature; the physician, the minister of nature who fights against illness. The physician ought to know the past, to perceive the present, to recognize the future.[14] Luke said in the Bible that it is given to physicians to be the Lord's workers.[15] Like-

[13] This pious factor in much of Rabanus *De Universo*, both in the medical and non-medical portions, was brought to my attention years ago by Edward K. Graham in the course of his graduate research. The point is noteworthy in connection with the generalization frequently made, to the effect that Rabanus Maurus' treatment of medicine is more extensive than that of his chief source, Isidore of Seville's *Etymologies*. Rabanus' work, as a matter of fact, is much *less* extensive in actual medical information. As stated by Mr. Graham in his thesis on Rabanus Maurus: " By far the greater part of Rabanus . . . is made up of fragmentary portions of Isidore's material supplemented by exegesis. . . . Rabanus copies part of Isidore, omits part, and substitutes exegesis for the part omitted." Mr. Graham's dictum applies to the passage in question, " Medical Healing is not to be Spurned." Up to this point Rabanus seems to have copied his medical data from Isidore's *Etymologies* (iv. ch. 1 ff.). Omitting chapters 6 (last part), 7-8 of Isidore, he copied only the title of chapter 9, S. 1 (" Medical Healing is not to be Spurned "). In place of Isidore's text he substituted a highly moralistic and Scripture-laden treatment of the topic. This material is so similar to the Bamberg introduction (above, treatise D) that one is tempted to assume that Rabanus, realizing that his Isidorean borrowings were conspicuously un-Christian, decided to shift the emphasis to the religious aspects of healing. For this, the Bamberg treatise was an ideal source.

[14] This past-present-future theme, which appears in modified form in treatises C (above) and F (below), stems from chapter I of the Hippocratic *Book of Prognostics*, of which there were Latin versions in Italy as early as the fifth century, and of which there are extant copies in ninth-tenth century manuscripts (See Kibre, " Hippocratic Writings . . ." p. 387 f.). The theme was repeated in Galen's commentaries on the Hippocratic *Epidemics* (Kühn edition, XVII, part I, 147), in Isidore's *Etymologies* (iv, 10) and in pseudo-Soranus *Quaestiones Medicinales*, alias *Horus Ysagoge* (Chartres MS 62, folio 1; also edited from late-medieval MSS by Rose, *op. cit.*, II, 243 ff., see esp. 246).

[15] Although the sense of the Biblical quotation vaguely resembles several passages in Luke, the Latin wording (*datur medicis ubi operatus dominus*) is closer to the text of

wise, Hippocrates said that the physician achieves just as much as God permits." [16]

The second of the Paris treatises is all-inclusive in scope and highly idealistic in tone. The absence of any reference to classical medicine is noteworthy. On the other hand, when compared with the Bamberg Introduction (treatise D, above) and the first Paris treatise (E, above), it is decidedly mundane in that it reflects little or no concern for the monastic ideal of spiritual healing. It is an excellent expression of the secular qualifications of early medieval physicians.

II. QUALIFICATIONS AND TRAINING OF THE PHYSICIAN

F. Arsenius to Nepotian,[17] his sweetest son, greeting . . . [several lines of polite, inconsequential matter]. I shall point out what you earnestly desire to know as to what sort of person a physician ought to be. First, he should test his personality to see that he is of a gracious and innately good character, apt and inclined to learn, sober and modest; a good conversationalist, charming, conscientious, intelligent, vigilant and affable, in all detailed affairs adept and skillful. Our art also requires that one be amiable, humble, and benevolent. Humility ever seeks knowledge, ever accumulates, and never goes to excess or offends. Good will restores sweetness, inspires sagacity, maintains remembrances in the heart, love in the soul, discipline in obeying, wisdom imbued with fear and diligence, and respect, for he who loves not honors not and will not be skillful or sure in his work. [The physician should] not be hesitant or timid, turbulent or proud, scornful or lascivious, or garrulous, a publican, or a woman-lover; but rather full of counsel, learned, and chaste. He should not be drunken or lewd, fraudulent, vulgar, criminal or disgraceful; it is not right for a physician to be taken in a fault or to blush for shame in the presence of his people. Even as love of wisdom reveals itself in manners, so let him be irreproachable for he is chosen to a higher honor. Medicine is not to be scorned, but invoked. Inasmuch as the physician has high honors he should not have faults, but instead discretion, taciturnity, patience, tranquility, and refinement; not greed but more of restraint and subtilty, rationality, diligence, and dignity. One of the virtues of this art is zeal in the acquisition of wisdom, long

---

Isaiah 26 : 12 (*omnia opera nostra operatus est nobis dominus*), as it is cited in treatise D above).

[16] The Hippocratic *Decorum* (ch. vi) reads as follows: " The Gods are the real physicians. . . ."

[17] There is no means of surely identifying either Arsenius or Nepotian, though both names appear in records from the early Christian centuries (e. g., note Jerome's correspondent, above, treatise A; and see Hirschfeld's suggestions *op. cit.*, p. 358 f.). Medieval writers were very free in their attribution of epistolary treatises to various authors, famous or otherwise. The letter in question appears in three early manuscripts; the Paris master manuscript and also Brussels MS 3701-15 and St. Gall MS 751. Hirschfeld's edition is based on the Brussels and St. Gall MSS; our translation is based on all three. There are frequent variants in the readings.

sufferance, and mildness. [The physician should strive for] a cheerful pleasant approach; for even as light illuminates a home and makes men see in dark shadows, so a cheerful physician turns sorrow and sadness into joy, and comforts all of the members of his patient, and restores his spirits. According to the secret teachings which should be pursued in medical instruction, let the physician be cheerful because he is the gentle helper [of his patients]. Enlivening the body, checking illnesses, drying up humors, he prescribes diet, eliminates fevers, warms the marrow, gives remedies, recreates the vital power. He notes the symptoms of ailments and applies beneficial medicines. He shows himself an expert in the varieties of herbs and a healing practitioner who prepares intelligent remedies for the reviving of men's strength. He clarifies the present, reveals the eternal future and senses inner factors. The physician is said to be the preceptor of healing, the liberator, the opportune worker who renders aid in time of need.

The opening lines of still another Paris epistle indicate the existence of an additional letter on the same subject, with however a somewhat more practical approach. Although the folio of the Paris manuscript is badly mutilated, a Chartres manuscript of slightly later date (MS 62, 10th century), along with a fourteenth-century London manuscript (BM, Cotton, Galba, F. IV, folio 239) provides the complete text.

G. WHAT SORT OF PERSON A PHYSICIAN SHOULD BE

Let us now explain what sort of person a physician should be. He should be gentle in manners and modest, with the proper amount of reliability.[18] He should be neither lacking in knowledge, nor proud; he should take care of rich and poor, slave and free, equally for among all such people medicines are needed. Moreover, if certain compensation is offered, let him accept rather than refuse. If however it is not offered, do not demand it because, however much each one pays, the compensation for medical services cannot be equated with the benefits. Moreover, enter the homes you visit in such a manner as to have eyes only for the healing of the sick. Be mindful of the Hippocratic Oath, and abstain from all guilt and especially from immorality and acts of seduction. Keep secret everything that goes on or is spoken in the home. Thus the physician himself, and the art, will acquire greater praise. The physician should have slender, fine fingers so as to be agreeable to all and to be subtle in his touch. Hippocrates himself [*Physician*, ch. I] said this. The physician should be no less agreeable in conversation, and not wanting in philosophy. He should be unassuming in manners so that both perfection in the art and good manners may be harmonized insofar as is possible.

Still another of the Paris epistles (found in the Chartres and London, MSS, also in Edinburgh MS A. 5.42) deals at greater length with the practical aspects of the subject, introducing the question of the specific qualifications necessary for those who plan to study medicine. The im-

---

[18] This and the four succeeding sentences, are also found in a garbled treatise in St. Gall MS 571 (edited by Hirschfeld, p. 363).

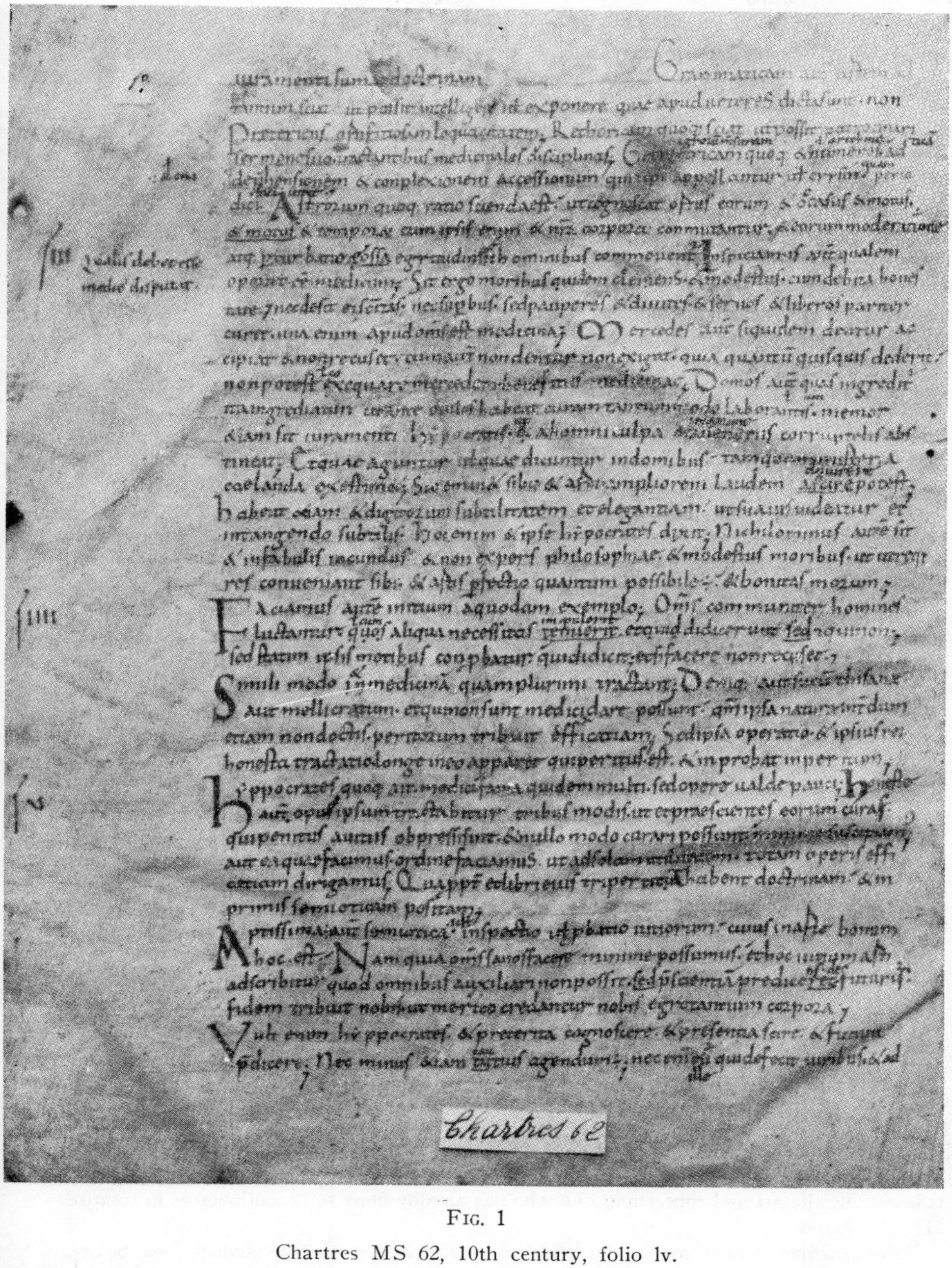

FIG. 1

Chartres MS 62, 10th century, folio 1v.

Portion of a series of letters including the text of treatises G and I which occur in mutilated form in Paris BN MS 11219.

2

portance of hard study is emphasized and it is advised that students start early, at the age of fifteen. The author of the treatise showed no apparent aversion to the classics; Erasistratus was cited in support of the doctrine of a well balanced education.

H. Concerning Those Who are Starting in the Art of Medicine.[19]

We begin concerning him who is starting training in the art of medicine. Let him be of that transitional age, between boyhood and manhood, that is a youth of fifteen which is an apt age for taking up the sacred art of medicine. Let him be neither very large nor very small in size, and such that he may live his youth freely and his old age usefully and easily.[20] In character and spirit let him be zealous and talented, indeed keen so that he may understand readily and be teachable; also strong so that he may be able to endure the recurring labor and the terrible sights that he encounters. He should make the cases of others his own sorrow. Let him be less concerned with other disciplines, but careful about his manners. According to Erasistratus, the greatest felicity is to keep things in balance so that one is both accomplished in the art [of medicine] and also endowed with the best of manners. If either one is lacking, better to be a good man without learning than a skillful practitioner with depraved manners. If indeed the lack of good manners in the art seems to be compensated by [professional] reputation, greater is the blame, for professional knowledge can be corrupted by blameful manners. But if both of these are faulty, I adjure you who are aware of it to withdraw from the art. He who takes up the art of medicine ought also to have knowledge of the nature of things so that he will not seem to be inexperienced therein. And he should be well endowed and wise, indeed adorned with all good characteristics.

The torn folio of the Paris manuscript has a fragment of another treatise (duplicated in the Chartres and London MSS already cited, and also in Edinburgh A. 5. 42) which deals with the training of the physician, but

[19] In the Paris manuscript the treatise is preceded by an exhortation to hard study, viz.: "If one wishes to acquire a knowledge of medicine, first of all let him preserve what he learns by committing it to memory. Then he will be able more frequently to warn disciples that by such gradual acquisition of knowledge they may acquire skill in the art." In the later manuscripts (Chartres, Edinburgh, London) the treatise (H) is the first of a series of letters, and is preceded by an introduction concerning the traditional Greek founders of medicine and methods of training young physicians. The latter section reads as follows: "I begin to tell of the best teaching method for those who are beginning to study the art of medicine. First we shall take up the physician himself, then the art, and afterward medicine itself. Plato, speaking of everything that comes into a course of study, said that the one who has a knowledge of the thing concerning which he is questioned is best able to talk. Since in all things which come under consideration it is necessary to be obliging and helpful to attentive listeners, the following proceedure is best. A middle ground is necessary because of the double problem, concerning him who is beginning the art and concerning him who has already done so. [continues as in treatise H] We begin. . . ."

[20] For further details as to the physical qualifications of the student, see below, treatise K.

in somewhat more academic fashion, reminiscent of Isidore of Seville's *Etymologies* (iv, 13).

I. On Giving the Sacred Oath and What Sort of Books One Should Read.

He who wishes to begin the art of medicine and the science of nature ought to take the oath and not shrink in any way whatsoever from the consequences. And then by this process of oath taking let him take up the teachings. Let him learn the art of grammar to the point where he can understand and expound the sayings of the ancients, omitting all artificialities of speech. Also let him learn rhetoric so as to be able to defend with his own words those who are carrying on medical teaching; also geometry so that, just as one knows the measuring and numbering of fields, so also he may recognize the ailments called *typi* [fevers] and the crises which are produced by *periodici* [fevers]. He must also know the science of the stars so as to recognize their rising, setting, and other movemonts, and the seasons of the year, since our bodies change along with these, and since human illnesses are affected by their normality and abnormality.

The above quotations make it clear that a wide range of material concerning the qualifications and training of physicians was available to the North-French compilers of the Paris and Chartres manuscripts. There are also two additional treatises, not found in these manuscripts, but occurring in four later manuscripts (only one of which is earlier than the eleventh century): St. Gall, 751; Zurich 128/32; Copenhagen 1653; and Brussels 1342-50. The Copenhagen manuscript (late eleventh century), of South-Italian origin, is one of our three earliest traces of Salernitan influence. The subject matter of the two treatises contained in the four manuscripts is much like that already presented; a mingling of high ideals with practical advice, apparently descriptive of secular physicians.

J.[21] Before the physician takes the Hippocratic Oath, and before he attempts surgery, he ought to heed words of wisdom. If he is apt at learning he will heed what his preceptor says. By its very nature this oath is an acceptable work. Even as the entire earth is not suitable for growing seed, but only that part which receives it and brings forth fruit, so also not all of the earth is suitable to receive teaching, but only that part which by a good determination is able fully to retain it. Once there was an ancient. He was not very chaste. When in due order he instituted the canon of medicine, everything he contributed was good.[22] Certain of his disciples who surrendered themselves wholeheartedly to their teachers, remained there and persisted to the end in the art which they wished to learn. Those

---

[21] The treatise appears, with many variants, in all except the Zurich manuscript. The Latin text has been edited by both Laux and Hirschfeld (cited above, note 9).

[22] The Brussels manuscript (1342-50) amplifies the passage concerning "the ancient" with references to Hippocrates, the Empiricists, Julius alias Ceron, and "the citizen of Larissa" who "instituted all philosophy and dialectic and geometry and music."

who changed from one teacher to another, when new ones appeared, not only acquired nothing, but even went unenlightened. To the wise this seemed useful, but to the foolish a joke and a laughing matter.

K,[23] Therefore, before expounding the Hippocratic Oath it is necessary to explain what sort of person a student of medicine should be. First he should be a freeman by birth, noble in character, youthful in age,[24] of medium size, sturdy, apt in all things; indeed, as in body, so in spirit; cognizant of good counsel, benign, virile, benevolent, chaste, endowed with unusual diligence of mind, audacious without being wrathful, not hardheaded, quick to perceive and understand what is taught, one who knows how to speak with brevity, elegant, with a good memory and not indolent. First of all he should be taught grammar, dialectic, astronomy, arithmetic, geometry and music. He should avoid rhetoric lest he become talkative. He should be taught philosophy along with medicine . . . [to be continued below as treatise K(a), on dress and deportment].

The last of our treatises on Qualifications and Training, is another of the Paris epistles; so far as I know, the only extant copy. It is probably the most important of the collection in that manuscript. Outstandingly practical and classical in tone, at the outset it purports to be " Admonitions of Hippocrates " and references are made to other classical authors such as Epicurus. It is broadly all-inclusive in subject matter, taking up successively the qualifications of the physician, medical training, dress and the bedside manner, even to such matters as the method of taking the pulse and the necessity of making three calls each day. Due to its wide scope the treatise serves as a recapitulation of most of the topics already presented, and as an introduction to various aspects of medical etiquette.

L. LETTER ESPECIALLY TO BE READ CONCERNING THE LEARNING OF THE ART OF MEDICINE.
[Qualifications and Training]

Let us begin to expound the admonitions of Hippocrates. Whoever wishes to become proficient in this art ought to be capable of unbounded literary effort, so that by longstanding perusal of various volumes his perception and discernment

---

[23] The treatise appears in all except the Brussels manuscript (1342-50). The title and text vary considerably in the three manuscripts.

[24] The expression "youthful in age" occurs in only two of the manuscripts (Zurich C 128/32, and Copenhagen 1653). The Latin term used, *puerum*, usually applies to boys up to the age of about 16. An earlier example of emphasis on youthfulness is found in section 7 of Charlemagne's Thionville Capitulary (805), where it was urged "that *infantes* be sent to learn [medicine]." (*MGH, Leges,* Sect. II, I, 121). "Instruction from childhood" is also stressed in the Hippocratic *Oath* and *Law* (ch. II). See also treatise H (above) for a reference to youthful students of medicine.

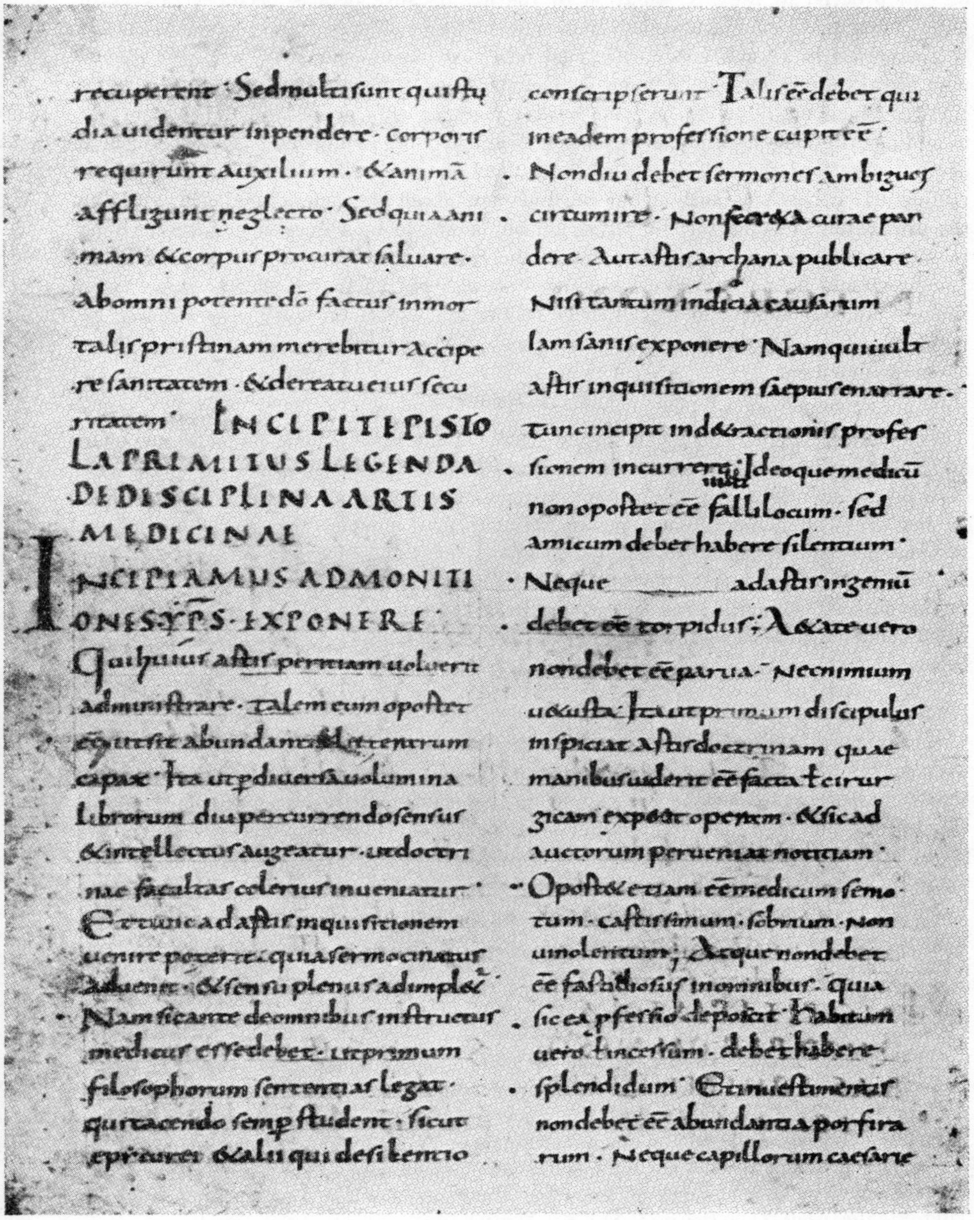

recuperent · Sed multi sunt qui stu
dia uidentur inpendere · corporis
requirunt auxilium · & animam
affligunt neglecto · Sed qui animam
& corpus procurat saluare ·
ab omni potente do factus inmor-
talis pristinam merebitur accipe
re sanitatem · & de reatu eius secu
ritatem · INCIPIT EPISTO
LA PRIMITUS LEGENDA
DE DISCIPLINA ARTIS
MEDICINAE
INCIPIAMUS ADMONITI
ONES YPS EXPONERE ·
Qui huius artis peritiam uoluerit
administrare · talem eum oportet
esse ut sit abundantia litterarum
capax · ita ut p diuersa uolumina
librorum diu percurrendo sensus
& intellectus augeatur · ut doctri-
nae facultas celerius inueniatur ·
Et tunc ad artis inquisitionem
uenire poterit quia sermocinatur
aduenit · & sensu plenus adimple
Nam si ante de omnibus instructus
medicus esse debet · ut primum
filosoforum sententias legat ·
qui tacendo semp student · sicut
epicurei & alii qui de silentio

conscripserunt · Talis ee debet qui
in eadem professione cupit ee ·
Non diu debet sermones ambiguos
circumire · Non secreta curae pan
dere · Aut artis archana publicare
Nisi tantum indicia causarum
iam sanis exponere · Nam qui uult
artis inquisitionem saepius enarrare ·
tunc incipit inde tractionis profes
sionem incurrere · Ideoque medicum
non oportet ee fallilocum · sed
amicum debet habere silentium ·
Neque _____ ad artis ingenium
debet ee torpidus · Ad arte uero
non debet ee parua · Nec nimium
uocusta · ita ut primum discipulus
inspiciat artis doctrinam quae
manibus uidere ee facta t eirus
zicam exposita operam · & sic ad
auctorum perueniat notitiam ·
Oportet ee etiam ee medicum femo
tum · castissimum · sobrium · non
uinolentum · Atque non debet
ee fastidiosus in omnibus · quia
sic ex p ferro deponat · Habitum
uero tincessum · debet habere
splendidum · Crinies tamen ut
non debet ee abundantia por fira
rum · Neque capillorum caesarie

FIG. 2

Paris, Bibliothèque Nationale, MS 11219, 9th century, folio 12v.

Text of treatise L, "Admonitions of Hippocrates. . . ."

increase to the point where facility in teaching is more readily acquired.[25] Then he can proceed to the investigation of the art because he has become conversant with it and understands it fully. Before [studying medicine] the physician should be instructed in all subjects.[26] First let him read the opinions of the philosophers, who always study in silence, even as Epicurus and others who have written about silence. Such ought he to be who wishes to enter this profession. He ought not to indulge in long ambiguous discourses, nor to spread abroad his private cures or the secrets of the art, excepting only data on cases already cured. He who is willing to repeat constantly what he finds out about the art of medicine tends to the profession of detractor. A physician ought not to be a deceiver. Like a friend he should maintain silence. Nor should the candidate for the art be a dullard. In age he should be neither too young nor too old, but such that at the outset, as a learner, he may look into the theories of the art which he will see performed by hand, or may seek the practice of surgery. Thus he may arrive at a knowledge of the authorities.

[Medical Etiquette]

The physician ought also to be confidential, very chaste, sober, not a winebibber, and he ought not to be fastidious in everything, for this is what the profession demands. He ought to have an appearance and approach that is distinguished. In his dress there should not be an abundance of purple, nor should he be too fastidious with frequent cuttings of the hair. Everything ought to be in moderation, for these things are advantageous, so it is said. Be solicitous in your approach to the patient, not with head thrown back [arrogantly] or hesitantly with lowered glance, but with head inclined slightly as the art demands. . . . [27] [to be continued below as treatise L(a), on pulse taking, etc.,].

K(a). [continuation of treatise K, above] He ought to hold his head humbly and evenly; his hair should not be too much smoothed down, nor his beard curled like that of a degenerate youth. He should not use ointment to excess on his hands or the tips of his fingers.[28] He should wear white, or nearly white, garments. He should be lightly clad, and walk evenly without disturbance and not too slowly. Gravity signifies breadth of experience. He should approach the patient with moderate steps, not noisily, gazing calmly at the sick bed. He should endure peacefully the insults of the patient since those suffering from melancholic or frenetic

---

[25] This sentence is also found in a brief St. Gall treatise from MS 751. (edited by Hirschfeld, p. 363).

[26] For details concerning the subjects a young physician ought to study, see above, treatises I and K, and compare with Isidore's *Etymologies,* iv, 13.

[27] St. Gall MS 751 and Escorial MS a IV 6 (edited by Hirschfeld, p. 363) have a somewhat condensed version of the subject matter of the entire paragraph on Medical Etiquette. The same topic is treated in great detail (with suggestions as to the physician's clothing, jewels, and horses) in the *Flos Medicinae Scholae Salerni,* written in the later Middle Ages (De Renzi, I, 513 ff.; V, 102 f.).

[28] The material on dress, hair, etc., may have been derived from Galen's *Commentary on Hippocrates' Epidemics* (Kühn edition, XVII, part II, 149 ff.).

ailments are likely to hurl evil words at physicians; these should be ignored for they are not deliberate but rather a result of the harsh annoyance suffered by the patient.

[Etiquette with regard to Women Patients]

Such [as the following] constituted the sacred medical oath according to the precepts of Hippocrates.[29] Enter a home without injuring or corrupting it. Beware lest your medicines bring death to anyone. Do not allow women to persuade you to give abortives, and do not be a part to any such counsel, but keep yourself immaculate and sacred.[30] Abstain from fornication, from [relations with] maidservants, children, married women, and virgins or widows. Keep secret whatever you hear or see in the course of healing, or otherwise, unless it be something that ought to be reported or judged.

[The Taking of the Pulse]

L(a). [continuation of treatise L above]. When a female lies before you and you are about to take her pulse, look neither at the top of her head nor at the bottom of her feet, but at the hand you are holding. By taking the pulse you determine the inner ailment. Learn how to take the pulse so that you can do it standing or seated. Sit on a stool that is neither too high nor too low, but so adjusted that you can take the pulse. If you are holding the right hand below the wrist with your right hand, let the fingers be uppermost so that your thumb may be in the middle in a position outside [i. e., the outer side of the wrist]. Moreover let two fingers, namely the index and middle finger, be placed together inside on the upper part of the vein [venae].[31] Hold the pulse for a long time so that you may detect the up and down

---

[29] Of the five manuscripts that contain this treatise (St. Gall 751, Copenhagen 1653, Bamberg L III 8, Zurich C 128/32, and Brussels 1342-50) the last mentioned has, in addition to the name Hippocrates, those of Apollo and Aesculapius. The reference to the Hippocratic Oath and "precepts" is noteworthy. Contrast this with the false citations from the Oath in Jerome's letter (above, treatise A), and the vague references to an oath in treatises C and I. It is obvious from the references to the Oath in treatises G, J and K (appearing in manuscripts dating from the ninth to the twelfth centuries) that the Oath was known in the early Middle Ages. It may be that it was known at second hand since it is not found in any of the medical manuscripts of this period. The earliest manuscript version cited by Diels is from the thirteenth century. R. Cantarella's " Una Tradizione Ippocratica nella Scuola Salernitana: Il Giuramento de' Medici" (*Archeion*, 1933, 15, 305 ff.) cites references to the Oath in the thirteenth-century regulations of Frederick II and infers that there was an uninterrupted tradition through the earlier centuries, but presents no definite evidence thereof.

[30] The Zurich mansucript has, immediately after " Sacred," the phrase " a custodian of the faith." The Brussels manuscript is fragmentary.

[31] Here apparently " vena " means artery; " arteria " is used in treatise M, below This somewhat incoherent passage on the position of the fingers, etc., defies complete clarification. In the effort to make sense out of it I followed several helpful suggestions from William Jerome Wilson of the Cleveland Branch of the Army Medical Library. It is my intention eventually to publish an article on the mechanics of pulse taking, with numerous quotations from Medieval texts and with several illustrations from Medieval manuscripts. Usually, it seems, the four fingers were placed on the inner (palm) side of the wrist to register the pulse beat.

F<small>IG</small>. 3

Paris, Bibliothèque Nationale, MS 11219, 9th century, folio 13r.

Text of treatise L(a), "On taking a Woman's Pulse" (continuation of treatise L).

beat by the feeling of the vein. By all means when taking the pulse have your hands warm rather than cold, lest the touch of cold hands upset the warm pulse and make it impossible to determine the true condition.[32] [to be continued below as treatise L(b), concerning sick calls].

The foregoing passage on pulse taking has an almost contemporary parallel in the introduction to a treatise " Concerning the Pulse " (*Peri Sfigmon*) attributed to Soranus. It is found in the tenth-century portion of a manuscript which was written at about the year 900 in the Swiss monastery of Reichenau (it is now at Karlsruhe, MS 120).[33]

M. CONCERNING THE PULSE. Soranus, to his most loved son, greeting. There are many who do not know how long they ought to hold the hand of a patient, and mistakenly think that they have made a true examination. Therefore I urge you, most loved son, to learn early the following method of inspection so that you will never be mistaken. When you visit a patient you should seat yourself in such a position that you may easily see his face, that is, on a stool near the foot of the bed, facing him. In case you are visiting a frenetic patient who would be excited by your facing him, sit near the head whence you can easily see him without being seen. Moreover, if you sit on the bed [do so with a mind to] the conditions of his health, for a slight movement of the person seated there may provoke worse ills, such as a flow of blood or a pernicious reaction or an abundance of sweating or some upset which by lessening in any way the helpfulness of quiet, just that much endangers health by promoting trouble.

Therefore, if this is your first inspection, when you sit down you ought to ask what the bodily affliction is, and how long it has lasted. If it is not your first visit, omit these matters and inquire as to any new ills. Ask if he is sleeping, and

---

[32] A condensed, and apparently garbled, version of the section on pulse taking appears in St. Gall MS 751 and Escorial a IV 6 (edited by Hirschfeld, p. 363). The Paris text and the Karlsruhe treatise (below, treatise M) constitute the most detailed account of the subject that I know of in early Medieval literature. The later Salernitan treatise (below, treatise P) is briefer, and has no additional items. As to the Classical sources for the material, Galen's numerous pulse treatises (Kühn edition, vols. VIII-IX and XIX; especially VIII, 803 ff.) contain no passages exactly like those from the early Middle Ages. It is possible that the Medieval material was taken from the corpus of pulse lore that was transmitted from Classical times to the later Middle Ages under the names of Theophilus, Joannes Philoponos, Meletius, Actuarius and Philaretus (see Temkin's article cited above in note 1, especially p. 54 ff.; also A. Hesse, *Ein Pulstraktat* . . ., Leipzig, 1922).

[33] The text was edited by Rose (*op. cit.*, II, 275 ff.) from A. Torinus' edition in *De Re Medica* (Basel, 1528) and Karlsruhe MS 120. Diels (*op. cit.*, II, 94) cites the Karlsruhe MS and also Chartres MS 62. As a matter of fact the Chartres MS contains only the first few lines of the treatise, after which the text shifts to another pseudo-Soranic treatise which ends with the misleading explicit, *Explicit Peri Sfigmon Ysagogus.* With the exception of the first few lines of *Peri Sfigmon,* this text is the *Ysagogus* or *Horus Ysagoge* mentioned above in note 14; in Thorndike and Kibre's *Incipits* it is listed as *Morus Ysago*.

how often and how much; also if bowels and bladder are functioning normally. After this questioning pause a little, lest the patient has been terrified through timidity or awe at the presence of the physician, or lest he has been upset by his suffering or wakened from sleep. [Give him an opportunity] to compose himself; you might take time for repose by walking about. Then prepare your hand for the pulse taking. Have it moderately warm so that nothing in the hand itself will mislead you; not too warm, not too cold, not sweaty. Such conditions prevail if the hands have been warmed at a fire or heated vessel, or in hot water. It is better to prepare the hands by friction or by placing them next to the chest and under the armpits.

Know which hand to hold; if the patient is lying down, the right hand is better for inspection, or the hand closer to the physician. But it should be on the patient's upper side since the weight of the body from above, pressing on the part underneath, is likely to dominate a normal pulse. Hold the patient's hand with three or four fingers in contact with the artery (*arteria*); with the tips of the fingers press down lightly holding the hand immobile so as to detect the strength, order, and every difference in the movement of the pulse. [treatise continues with a discussion of various types of pulses].

[Sick Calls]

L(a). [continuation of treatise L(a), above]. For those who are ill, you ought to get up early so as to inquire about the preceding night, finding out the order of the causes [of the ailment] and the necessary treatment. At midday pay another visit, not so much to see about the patient's food as to plan for the beginning of a cure. For a third time, visit at about nightfall, staying for an hour in order to make arrangements for him to pass the night [comfortably] so as to be fortified to meet the next day unimpaired. . . . [Treatise ends with an unrelated postscript concerning the study of medicine; apparently it belongs with the succeeding letter: see above, note 19.]

We conclude our series of translations with four treatises, of which the last three are outstandingly practical, being concerned with the bedside manner in particular, and in general with those practices that might be called "tricks of the trade." Although traceable to the age of monastic medicine, these practices seem to have been derived originally from the later Hippocratic treatises, such as *Decorum* and *Precepts*.[34] Apparently it was the late and declining age of Greek medicine that stressed such superficial aspects of medical practice. It is noteworthy that it also was the late, but not declining, age of Medieval medicine that stressed these same factors, which had been known but neglected during the age of monastic medicine. Suffice it to say that this type of late Classical (and also late Medieval) etiquette is distinctly secular in character. In fact,

[34] It seems likely that there were Latin translations of these works as early as the fifth and sixth centuries, and presumably there were copies in the ninth and tenth centuries. I have, however, found no evidence of extant manuscripts in any European collections.

it has a distinctly modern flavor, even though it came out of a declining classicism and was nurtured by a " dark age " of ascetic piety. It is also significant that, when the monastic compilers of these late treatises cited authorities, they were Christian rather than Classical. At the same time there is evident a broader, more detailed and increasingly secular expression of the early medieval ethics and etiquette. The last two treatises (from the twelfth century) exemplify the final transition from monastic to Salernitan domination.

The first of the four treatises is so brief and condensed that it might have constituted a code for medieval physicians. It is a noteworthy synthesis of Christian and Hippocratic ideals, despite the fact that the sole authority invoked is the God of Christianity. The treatise seems to have been popular; it appears in at least eleven manuscripts, dating from as early as the ninth, and as late as the fifteenth, century.[35]

N. [Epistle of Hippocrates. Epistle of Galen].[36]

Meanwhile I warn you, Physician, even as I was warned by my master. You ought always to read, and to shun indolence. Visit with care those whom you accept for treatment, and safeguard them. (Hold fast to the cures that you know. Never become involved knowingly with any who are about to die or who are incurable. Do not take up with the daughter or wife of your patient).[37] Cherish modesty, follow chastity, guard the secrets of the homes [you visit]. If you know anything derogatory concerning a patient, keep quiet about it. Do not detract from other [physicians]; if you praise the character and cures of others you yourself will have a better reputation. (At the outset, accept at least half of the

[35] Paris BN 11219, Brussels 3701-15, Glasgow Hunter V, 3. 2, Zurich C 128/32, Rome Angelica 1502, Rome Vat. Regina 1443, Rome Vat. 2376, and 2417 (according to Diels, op. cit., I, 123), Carpentras 318, Paris BN 15456, and Paris BN 6988A. In the textual analysis of certain manuscripts of this treatise, and also in the translation, I am indebted to my colleague Professor B. L. Ullman for generous assistance.

[36] Although four of the eleven manuscripts have no author caption, the treatise is attributed to Hippocrates in three (Brussels 3701-15, Rome Vat. Regina 1443, and Paris BN 6988A) and to Galen in three (Paris BN 15456, Rome Vat. 2376 and 2417). The attribution to Isidore of Seville by Hirschfeld (p. 361), Sigerist (p. 32) and Thorndike-Kibre (Catalogue of Incipits, under " Interea ") is doubtless due to the fact that in Rome Angelica MS 1502 the treatise is preceeded by " Incipit Liber Ysidori." This caption is incorrect both for this treatise and for those that follow it (see Wlaschky's edition in Kyklos, 1928, 1, 103 ff.). In BN MS 15456 the treatise begins as follows: " I urge you, O Physician, and with exhortation I warn, and with warning I enjoin you even as I was warned. . . ."

[37] Neither of the passages in parentheses occurs in the pre-eleventh-century manuscripts, excepting the second passage (concerning fees), which is in the tenth-century, South-Italian, version from the Glasgow MS. Was this brutally practical factor in medieval medical ethics Salerno's first contribution to the de-spiritualization of " the Art "?

remuneration without hesitation, for he who wishes to buy [your services] is disposed to pay and to beg [for treatment]. Get it while he is suffering, for when the pain ceases, your services also cease).[37] You will win more thanks if you do all these things, and no physician will be greater than you [in reputation]. Read felicitously, be progressive, fare well, and God's grace be with you, in the practice of medicine and [your other] undertakings. Let healing come from God, who alone is the physician. Amen.[38]

Of a more practical trend is the second treatise, which is concerned solely with the bedside manner. It occurs in at least five manuscripts, dating from as early as the tenth, and as late as the fifteenth, century.[39] It is our only treatise on medical ethics and etiquette that appears earliest in a South-Italian manuscript from the Salernitan region.

O. In What Manner You Should Visit a Patient.

You do not visit every patient in the same manner. If you wish to learn all, heed [the following]. As soon as you approach the patient ask him if he has any pain. If he says he has, then ask if the pain is severe and constant. After this take his pulse and see if he has fever. If he is in pain you will find the pulse rapid and fluid. Ask if the pain comes when he is cold; also if he is wakeful, and if his bowels and urine are normal. Inspect both parts and see if there is perchance any serious danger. If the ailment is acute inquire as to the beginning of the illness. If it is chronic you will not recognize it at all, for the beginning of such illness is at a time when the patient begins to feel a lesion when performing accustomed functions, as if he could not perform them. After this ask what former physicians said when they visited him, whether all of them said the same. Inquire concerning the condition of the body, whether it is cold or otherwise, whether the bowels are loose, sleep interrupted, the ailment constant, and if he has ever had such ailments before. Having made these inquiries you will easily recognize the causes of the illness and the cure will not be difficult.[40]

Our third treatise comprises a twelfth-century text from a famous Salernitan manuscript (Breslau 1302),[41] and its fourteenth-century amplification attributed to a certain Archimathaeus (ca. 1100 ?). In De Renzi's edition (*op. cit.*, II, 35) the treatise was lauded for its uniqueness among medieval treatises on the relations of physician and patient.

[38] Carpentras MS 318 has a more pious ending: "Amen, and He lives and reigns and rules through eternity."

[39] Monte Cassino 97, Montpellier 185, Rome Vat. Barberini 160, Carpentras 318, and Paris BN 6988A. The text is found in De Renzi, II, 73; Neuburger, *op. cit.*, II, pt. I, 257; and Sigerist, p. 31 f.

[40] The Carpentras manuscript has a slightly different ending.

[41] Concerning this manuscript, see De Renzi, II, 74 ff.; Sudhoff, " Die Salernitaner Handschrift in Breslau " (*Archiv Gesch. Med.*, 1920, 12, 101 ff.); and Henschel, " Die Salernitanische Handschrift " (*Janus*, 1846, 1, 40 ff.).

Factual evidences, such as the pre-Salernitan treatises already quoted, indicate that it was merely a link, though an important one, in the development of medieval medical ethics and etiquette. It is clear that this treatise in particular, and Salerno in general, mark neither the beginning nor the revival of highmindedness and intelligence in medical practice. They do illustrate the late-medieval shift of emphasis from ideals to practical considerations.

The Salernitan treatise repeats some of the early medieval idealism that stemmed from both Christian and Classical sources; notably the invoking of God's aid and the Hippocratic warning against immorality. But the treatise is more concerned with a hitherto unimportant factor, the materialistic side of medical practice. Even though it treats of the age old topics, it treats them in a spirit of unrestrained ambition and selfcentered individualism. For the most part, professional cleverness overshadows Hippocratic and Christian idealism. This new secular emphasis, often designated nowadays as modern-mindedness, did not originate at Salerno. It evolved out of earlier practices, during the late-medieval era of rapid urbanization. It was widely prevalent in Italy and elsewhere, meeting with the approval of leaders in the profession: Arnold of Villanova, Henry of Mondeville, Guy of Chauliac, Albert of Bologna, Jan Yperman, and John Arderne.[42] This trend might be said to mark the despiritualization of the medieval physician.

Inasmuch as the Salernitan treatise has appeared in English translations that are readily available,[43] we present the subject matter thereof in condensed form with a few quoted excerpts that are of unusual significance.[44]

P. CONCERNING THE PHYSICIAN'S APPROACH TO THE PATIENT.
Therefore, O physician, when you call on a patient, be a helper in God's name. Let the angel who accompanied Tobias [Tobias 3:25. Vulgate] be your spiritual and physical companion. On entering the home try to find out through the messenger [from the household] how sick the patient is and what sort of an ailment he has. This is necessary so that you will not seem to be entirely ignorant of the ailment when you approach him. . . . [Detailed instructions follow: e. g., ask whether

---

[42] Excerpts from the works of these men (quoted in Miss Welborn's article cited above in note 1) show a marked resemblance to the Salernitan treatise (P, below), which in turn resembles treatises L, M, N, and O (above).

[43] Francis Packard, in *The School of Salernum* (New York, 1920) p. 18 ff.; and George Corner, in " The Rise of Medicine at Salerno," (*Annals Medical Hist.*, 1931, 3, 14 f.).

[44] The text is in De Renzi, II, 74 ff.

the patient has confessed to a priest; pretend that the case is serious; thus, whether he survives or dies, your reputation is safe; in the sick room greet those present and pay compliments concerning the household before turning to the patient]. Make him feel secure and quiet his spirit before you take the pulse. Take care lest he lie on his side or have his fingers over-extended or drawn back into his palm. Support his arm with your left [hand] and consider the pulse beat at least to a hundred. Also take note of the different kinds of pulses. . . . [Inspect the urine for color, subtance, and quantity; on leaving tell the patient that he will get well but tell the servants that he is very sick; do not look with lecherous eyes on women of the household; if invited to dine, do not be officious or overly fastidious; during the meal, enquire about the patient; on leaving, show your appreciation; etc., followed by advice concerning diet, cupping, digestion, etc.; on later visits during the patient's convalescence, the physician is advised to be cheerful and to promise the patient a speedy recovery. Finally] with as much as possible of honest promises go in peace, Christ your guide.

The expanded version of the Salernitan treatise appears in a fourteenth-century manuscript (Paris BN MS Lat. 7091). The final paragraph serves as an excellent expression of the increasingly secular and materialistic spirit of late Medieval medical practice. This tendency, which is seldom emphasized by those optimistic modern commentators who sing the praises of Salernitan medicine, was marked by a strong emphasis on the importance of good public relations. The following quotation (with which the treatise ends) seems very modern, and somewhat reprehensible, by reason of the clever psychological approach, with its hint that the physician should assume a hypocritically cheerful attitude in the interests not only of the patient's health, but also of his own purse.[45]

[It is advised that the convalescing patient be encouraged by having congenial friends visit him; boy-friends for young convalescents, old man for senile patients, and for noblemen, friends who will chat concerning dogs, horses, and falcons. The physician himself, when he calls, should enter the room] with a hilarious countenance and a joyful voice saying: " Hey there, what do you say? What sort of fun are you having? " . . . With such words the patient is encouraged. Finally, accept your remuneration graciously, and with a full purse and with joy and delight for one and all (if that be possible), by their leave go in peace.
Explicit. Book of Instruction for the Physician, according to Alquimathaeus [i. e., Archimathaeus].

In all fairness to the Salernitans, it should be noted that they also had treatises expressing the higher ideals of the profession. This is exemplified in our last treatise, taken from a work attributed to Constantine the African who lived and wrote at about 1100. In late Medieval

[45] The text is in De Renzi, V, 348 f.; see also I, 513 and V, 102 for verses from the *Flos Medicinae Scholae Salerni* concerning fees, dress, etc.

manuscripts (of the thirteenth and fourteenth centuries) and in early printed editions (the 1515 Lyons edition of Isaac contains the earliest version), the treatise appears as the prologue to Book I of Constantine's *Liber Pantegni*; Theorica, De Communibus Medico Cognitu Necessariis Locis. I know of no manuscript prior to the thirteenth century, but it is possible that the treatise was compiled by Constantine at about 1100 from Arabic material or from works such as we have noted in the early medieval compilations. At any rate it resembles treatises G and N, quoted above, and appears to be a synthesis of materials long in circulation and originally derived in large measure from Hippocratic sources such as the Oath.

Q. What Sort of Person a Student of Medicine Should Be.[46]

He who wishes to obtain the mantle of medicine ought [so to act] that he is an honor to his master, is praised [by him] and is subject to him just as to his own parents. . . . The master should be honored so that [his disciples] may learn how to handle difficult situations. Whomsoever the master takes for instruction should see to it that he is a worthy disciple. He should teach [only] worthy disciples, without pay or expectation of future emolument; and he should be sure to keep unworthy persons from entering this learned profession. The physician should work for the healing of the sick. He should not heal for the sake of gain, nor give more consideration to the wealthy than to the poor, or to the noble than the ignoble. He should neither teach, nor aquiesce in teaching anyone how to give a harmful potion, lest some ignorant person should hear of it and on his authority mix a death potion. He should not teach anyone to bring about abortion. Moreover, when he visits patients, he should not set his heart on the patient's wife, maidservant, or daughter; they blind the heart of man. He ought to keep to himself confidential information concerning the ailment, for at times the patient makes known to the physician things that he would blush to tell his parents. The physician should flee luxury and avoid worldly pleasures and drunkenness. These things upset the spirit and encourage the vices of the flesh. He should devote himself with assiduous zeal to the healing of the body and should not neglect reading, so that his memory may aid him when books are not at hand. He should never refuse to visit the sick for thus, by experience, he may become more efficient. He should be pious, humble, gentle, likeable, and should seek divine assistance. [In chapter 2 the author discusses " Six Things which it is Well to Know," among them dialectic and " the entire quadrivium." Incidentally it is suggested that the author's book " is useful above all others."].

---

[46] The text in Migne *Patrologia Latina*, vol. 150, 1563, is similar to the sixteenth-century versions.

CONCLUSIONS

In summarizing the possible sources of the above examples of medical ethics and etiquette, we note that many of them bear a marked resemblance to the dicta in certain Hippocratic writings.[47] Neither in Greek nor in medieval times, however, did these dicta constitute an enforced code of conduct; they were merely a set of ideals which the high minded physician was urged to follow. Jones' remarks in the introduction to his translation of the Hippocratic *Law*, to the effect that Greek physicians were subject to neither legal penalties nor a universal guild organization, could be applied equally to medical practice in the Early Middle Ages. The only hint of legal controls is found in the above mentioned Visigothic Spanish laws concerning women patients (treatise B) and in the form letter for the instruction of the governmentally supervised physicians in Ostrogothic Italy (treatise C).

Our second conclusion is that both Greek and Medieval physicians were subjected to two somewhat divergent influences, one of which was idealistic, the other practical; in other words, ethics and etiquette. So far as ethics are concerned, the early Medieval writers seem to have combined Hippocratic and Christian ideals without any apparent feeling of conflict or inconsistency. They repeated much of the ideology of the Hippocratic Oath, notably the moral injunctions against giving poisons or abortives, and against violating the patient's confidence or the virtue of his womenfolk.[48] The Medieval exhortation that the physician keep himself " immaculate and sacred " (treatise K[a]), may be a reflection of the " pure and holy " clause of the Hippocratic Oath. Furthermore, the array of virtues recommended for members of the medieval medical profession (especially in treatises F, G. H and K) reads much like the standard set for Greek physicians in the Hippocratic works concerning the *Physician* (Chapter I) and *Decorum* (Chapter V; also III, VII and

[47] See W. H. S. Jones, " Greek Medical Etiquette (*Royal Soc. Med., Proc.*, 1922-23, 16, Hist. pp. 11-17) ; *The Doctor's Oath* (Cambridge University, 1924) ; and the introductory essays in his *Hippocrates*, II, pp. xxxiii ff. and 257 ff., also I, 295 where he describes travesties of medical ethics such as the practice of abortion (described in *Nature of the Child*, which was a startling contrast to the anti-abortion pledge of the Oath. See also Edelstein *The Hippocratic Oath*, p. 63.

[48] These ideals, plus those from the *Decorum* and *Precepts* concerning fee collecting, were widely prevalent in Ancient and Medieval times. Exigencies of space prevent our citation of the extensive modern literature on Hippocratic ideals among Medieval Jewish physicians, the Arabs, and in China, etc.

XII).[49] In like fashion the Medieval analogy concerning seed planting and medical education (treatise J) is similar to chapter III of the Hippocratic *Law*. The importance of starting medical education early in life is found in both Ancient and Medieval works (treatises H and K, and note 24). One factor not found in Hippocratic writings is the Medieval emphasis on a broad background of liberal-arts education (treatises I, K, L, and Q).

Turning to the realm of everyday medical etiquette, one finds even more noteworthy parallels between the Hippocratic and the Medieval writings; for example, (1) admonitions for the physician to avoid the use of wine to excess (compare treatises F, L, and Q with Hippocratic *Decorum,* chap. XV), (2) to avoid excessive use of ointments (compare treatise K[a] with *Precepts,* chap. X and *Physician,* chap. I) and (3) to avoid ostentation in dress and manners (compare treatises G, L and K[a] with *Precepts,* chap. X and *Decorum,* chap. II-III, VII); also (4) the bedside manner, especially the exercise of patience with difficult patients (compare treatise K[a] with *Decorum,* chap. XII), (5) the withholding of information from the patient (compare treatises C and P with *Decorum,* chap. XVI), and (6) restraint in pressing for payment of fees (compare treatises N and P with *Decorum,* chap. II and *Precepts,* chap. IV).[50] Finally, (7) in both literatures there is evidence of the contrast between the high ideals of physicians for their own profession (compare treatises A, C ff. with *Decorum,* chaps. V-VI, XVIII) and its low moral repute among the general public (compare treatises B, J and K[a] with *Art,* chaps. I, IV-V; *Law,* chap. I; and *Decorum,* chaps. II, VII). It seems that the inefficiency and waywardness of medical practitioners has been condemned by lay critics in all ages.[51]

Perhaps the chief surprise that comes to the student of early Medieval medical manuscripts is the rarity of instances of that pious other-worldly spirit which is supposed to have hung like a cloud over the Middle Ages. To be sure this spirit is the dominant element in two of our seventeen treatises (D and E), and in two others (A and N) it is combined with an approximately equal amount of classical or contemporary pragmatism.

[49] The Hippocratic works cited here and in the succeeding sentences are found in Jones, *Hippocrates,* vol. II, except for *Precepts,* which is in vol. I.

[50] With regard to fees, medieval writers, especially in the later centuries, recommended more drastic measures than those found in Greek writings. See the articles by Welborn and Sigerist, cited above in note 1; also Diepgen's chapter (IV) on the subject.

[51] This can be seen in the works of Pliny the Elder, Seneca, Sidonius, John of Salisbury, Petrarch, and Molière.

In most of the treatises, however (to be specific, in thirteen out of seventeen), it is almost completely eclipsed by the viewpoints of secular medicine.

Our explanation of this paradox is the obvious fact that " everybody who talks about Heaven " is not intent on it at all times. Medieval *religious* literature to the contrary notwithstanding, during the Middle Ages most people lived in *this* world. The public utterances of the monastic writers who monopolized early Medieval literature were likely to be piously religious when concerned with ideals; though in writing of *medical* ideals they often used Hippocratic substitutes. Practical activities, medical or otherwise, were discussed in a more earthly manner. Thus it is that, whereas the treatises on medical *ethics* often manifest a highly Christian ideology, those on *etiquette* are more secular. When one passes from the era of our survey to the later Medieval centuries, he finds still less of otherworldliness and more of those characteristics which seem to be widely prevalent among medical men of all civilized ages.

It might be enlightening for modern folk to think of the early Middle Ages in somewhat the same perspective in which we think of our primitive and rather pious pioneer ancestors of frontier days. The otherworldly utterances of their preachers reflect only one aspect of their civilization. Their medical practices, like other aspects of their everyday lives, were highly practical and secular. So it was in the early Middle Ages. The progressive, secular trend that is exemplified in the Salernitan treatises evolved out of the monastic-Hippocratic environment of the preceding centuries,[52] long before Salerno's rise to prominence in the twelfth century. This trend is to be attributed, not to an Italian Renaissance of Hippocratic classicism, but to the Christian " Hippokratismus " which persisted through the disintegration of the Western Empire and the early Middle Ages, then expanded as the gradual secularization of Medieval life, under the influence of industry, commerce, and other phases of urban civilization, turned men's minds more and more to this-worldly affairs.

---

[52] A noteworthy point in the transmission of Hippocratic ethics and etiquette to the monastic West is the lack of Galenic influence. Galen's commentaries on various Hippocratic works existed in early Medieval Latin versions, but (as has been indicated above in several footnotes) the Medieval texts on ethics and etiquette seldom show as close relationships to Galenic works as they do to late Hippocratic treatises such as the *Oath, Decorum,* etc.

APPENDIX

THE HIPPOCRATIC OATH (Fourth-Century B. C.).[53]

I swear by Apollo Physician and Asclepius and Hygieia and Panaceia and all the gods and godesses, making them my witnesses, that I will fulfil according to my ability and judgment this oath and this covenant:

To hold him who has taught me this art as equal to my parents and to live my life in partnership with him, and if he is in need of money to give him a share of mine, and to regard his offspring as equal to my brothers in male lineage and to teach them this art—if they desire to learn it—without fee and covenant; to give a share of precepts and oral instruction and all other learning to my sons and to the sons of him who has instructed me and to pupils who have signed the covenant and have taken an oath according to the medical law, but to no one else.

I will apply dietetic measures for the benefit of the sick according to my ability and judgment; I will keep them from harm and injustice.

I will neither give a deadly drug to anybody if asked for it, nor will I make a suggestion to this effect. Similarly I will not give to a woman an abortive remedy. In purity and holiness I will guard my life and my art.

I will not use the knife, not even on sufferers from stone, but will withdraw in favor of such men as are engaged in this work.

Whatever houses I may visit, I will come for the benefit of the sick, remaining free of all intentional injustice, of all mischief and in particular of sexual relations with both female and male persons, be they free or slaves.

What I may see or hear in the course of the treatment or even outside of the treatment in regard to the life of men, which on no account one must spread abroad, I will keep to myself holding such things shameful to be spoken about.

If I fulfil this oath and do not violate it, may it be granted to me to enjoy life and art, being honored with fame among all men for all time to come; if I transgress it and swear falsely, may the opposite of all this be my lot.

[53] The following translation is reprinted from Ludwig Edelstein, *The Hippocratic Oath*, Baltimore, 1943, p. 3.

THE LONG TRADITION: A STUDY IN FOURTEENTH-CENTURY MEDI-CAL DEONTOLOGY

*

MARY CATHERINE WELBORN

I swear by Apollo Physician, by Asclepius, by Hygeia, by Panacea and by all the gods and goddesses, making them my witnesses, that I will carry out, according to my ability and judgment, this oath and this indenture. To hold my teacher in this art equal to my own parents; to make him partner in my livelihood;—I will use treatment to help the sick according to my ability and judgment, but never with a view to injury and wrong-doing. Neither will I administer a poison to anybody when asked to do so, nor will I suggest such a course.—But I will keep pure and holy both my life and my art.—Into whatsoever houses I enter, I will enter to help the sick, and I will abstain from all intentional wrong-doing and harm, especially from abusing the bodies of man or woman, bond or free. And whatsoever I shall see or hear in the course of my profession, as well as outside my profession in my intercourse with men, if it be what should not be published abroad, I will never divulge, holding such things to be holy secrets. Now if I carry out this oath, and break it not, may I gain for ever reputation among all men for my life and for my art; but if I transgress it and forswear myself, may the opposite befall me.—HIPPOCRATIC OATH.[1]

THE medieval physician, although he lacked skill and knowledge in the art and practice of medicine, in his humanity toward his patients and his desire to do the utmost to help them, was equal to the best of our medical men today. These high ideals were held not by a few of these early doctors only but were the code of the profession. Now laws are made, usually at the instigation of the physicians themselves, and are enforced by the courts to curb as far as possible unethical practices, although many vitally important

[1] For a discussion of this oath see W. H. S. Jones, *The Doctor's Oath* (Cambridge, 1924).

204

problems are still left to the judgment of the individual physician. But in the Middle Ages there were merely rules and
regulations made either by physicians who passed them on
to their university and private students, or by groups of
doctors in universities or guilds,[2] sometimes with and sometimes without the sanction of the city or state governments.[3]
The main sources for the ethical ideas of the ancient and
medieval periods are those chapters devoted primarily to
medical deontology which are so often found in the general
writings of physicians and surgeons, especially in the later
Middle Ages.

By examining some of the principal works of representative
doctors of the fourteenth century, we can come to certain
definite conclusions concerning the rise and development of
contemporary medical ethics and, what is more precious, to
a better understanding of the fourteenth-century doctor, who
has been so reviled by famous writers like Petrarch[4] and by
other humanists. The deontological chapters reveal the true
nature of the physician and show us the real man—a vital,
intelligent human being who, despite his woeful lack of
scientific knowledge, in many cases was honestly trying to do
his best both for the sake of humanity and for the love of his
art. It is true that many quacks and charlatans existed in
that century, as well as in our own, who neither preached nor
practiced in an ethical manner, but we have no right to condemn in a wholesale way, as did Petrarch, all doctors on
account of the errors of some of their profession. Modern

[2] David Riesman, *The Story of Medicine in the Middle Ages* (New York, 1935),
pp. 226–32.

[3] Frederick II issued in 1241 a statute, *De medicis*, to regulate the manners and
fees of medical men (see J. L. A. Huillard-Bréholles, *Historia diplomatica Friderici
Secundi* [Paris, 1854], IV, Part I, 235).

[4] Petrarch, *Contra medicum*, *Opera* (Basel, 1581), pp. 1087–1131. For a discussion of Petrarch's remarks see A. W. E. T. Henschel, "Petrarcas Urtheil über die
Medicin und die Aerzte seiner Zeit," *Janus*, I (1846), 183–223. For the remarks of
one of his predecessors see John of Salisbury, *Polycraticus*, Book II, chap xxix;
Migne, *Patrologia Latina*, CXCIX, 475–76.

critics have been too prone to ignore these ethical sections of the medical works and to spend all their time criticizing the information, or lack of it, displayed in other parts of these writings, thus giving us a more or less one-sided picture of the medieval doctor.

The medical works of the fourteenth century present an especially interesting basis for the study of the development of ethical ideas because they are the first since classical times to contain lengthy and detailed chapters on this subject.[5] These doctors were no longer so inhibited from expressing their own ideas as were the scholastic writers of an earlier century. They were constantly receiving more and better translations of Greek and Arabic medical works, which were the main sources of these ideas, and thus their writings best reveal to us the historical development of the medical code of ethics.

Too often have editors of fourteenth-century medical works claimed that the men of this century had higher ethical principles than the doctors of the centuries immediately preceding. They try to make us think that this is true because of the innate superiority of these men over those of earlier times. But an examination of many of the works of this age and of preceding ones, by placing fourteenth-century writings in their true perspective, shows us why the men of this particular century have a more highly developed professional code; it shows us that their main principles were taken more or less directly from classical writings beginning primarily with the Hippocratic corpus.[6] For even when medicine was

[5] E.g., the *De subtilioribus cautelis medicorum* of Arnold of Villanova, although it was written as late as the latter part of the thirteenth century or the very beginning of the fourteenth (Arnold died in 1311) could not have been one of the chief sources on this subject for the fourteenth-century writers, since it deals more with prognosis than with deontology. See also the writings of Bartholomeus Anglicus, the *De corpore humano* of Giles of Corbeil, and many others.

[6] Georg Weiss, "Die ethischen Anschauungen im Corpus Hippocraticum," *Archiv für Geschichte der Medizin*, IV (1911), 235–62.

yet in its infancy, physicians and surgeons, by their written and spoken words, began to formulate ethical precepts for their fellow-craftsmen, which were repeated by generation after generation of doctors, usually in the introductions to their writings.

A summary of the most important remarks made by these fourteenth-century doctors, as far as possible in their own words, will be used to prove the claims mentioned above. They deal with the qualifications a man must have before he can become a good physician or surgeon, his appearance, his general culture, his relation to and general treatment of his patients, his proper attitude toward other doctors, and, of great importance indeed, his fees.

According to Jan Yperman,[7] the

doctor must be well-shapen and of a healthy and strong constitution. His outward appearance must be good, for as al-Rāzī says, an ungainly appearance is not likely to go with a good heart, and ibn Sīnā says that a fine face will probably hide a fair character. The surgeon must have shapely hands, taper fingers, and he must be strong. His fingers should not tremble and he must have keen eyesight.[8]

John of Arderne[9] adds a little to this: "The leech should also have clean hands and well-shapen nails cleansed from all blackness and filth."[10] Almost identical descriptions are to be found in the *Cyrurgia* of Guy de Chauliac,[11] and in the one by Henri de Mondeville[12]; both authors stating that they

---

[7] A Flemish surgeon who died about 1330 in Ypres.

[8] *De cyryrgie*, Book I, chap iv; ed. E. C. van Leersum (Leiden, 1912), pp. 12 ff.

[9] An important English surgeon who lived in the last part of the fourteenth century.

[10] *Treatises of Fistula in Ano , . . . by John Arderne, from an Early Fifteenth-Century Manuscript Translation*, ed. D'Arcy Power ("Early English Text Society," Original Series, No. 139 [London, 1910]), p. 6.

[11] *La Grande chirurgie* (1363), ed. E. Nicaise (Paris, 1890). Guy was a French surgeon (died *ca.* 1368), the personal physician of Popes Clement VI, Innocent VI, and Urban V.

[12] A French surgeon who taught in Montpellier and Paris; died *ca.* 1325. His chief work, under the title *Chirurgie de maître Henri de Mondeville*, has been translated into modern French by E. Nicaise (Paris, 1893).

have copied their remarks from ʿAlī ibn Ridwān's[13] commentary on Galen's *Ars parva*.

It was not enough to be fine-looking and cleanly, but the doctor must also be very careful of his dress and deportment; otherwise he would bring contumely upon himself and his profession.

In clothes and other apparel he should be honest, and not liken himself in apparel and bearing to minstrels, but in clothing and bearing he should show the manner of clerks.[14] For why?; it seemeth any discreet man clad in clerk's garb may occupy the boards of gentlemen. And be he courteous at the lord's table, and be he not displeasing in words or deeds to the guests sitting near by, hear he many things but let him speak but few. . . . . And when he shall speak, let the words be short, and as far as possible, fair and reasonable and without swearing. Beware that there never be found double words in his mouth, for if he be found true in his words few or none shall doubt his deeds. . . . . Be he not temerarious or boastful in his sayings or in his deeds. And above all this it shall profit him that he always be found sober; for drunkenness destroyeth all virtue and bringeth it to nought. Also let a leech neither laugh nor play too much. . . . . Let him be content in strange places with the meats and drinks found there, using measure in all things. . . . . Scorn he no man for it is said, "He that scorneth other men shall not go away unscorned." . . . . And as far as he can without harm, flee the fellowship of knaves and dishonest persons.[15]

Jan Yperman says about the same things, then adds:

He ought to devote himself entirely to the patients; in the latter's house he may not broach any other subject than that which concerns the treatment; neither may he chat with the mistress of the house, the daughter or the maidservant, nor look at them with leering eyes. For people are soon suspicious, and by such things he is apt to incur enmity while the doctor had better keep on friendly terms with them.[16]

[13] Flourished in Cairo in the middle of the eleventh century. His commentary was translated by Gerard of Cremona. George Sarton, *Introduction to the History of Science* (Baltimore, 1927), I, 729.

[14] Cf. the remark of Hippocrates, "You must also avoid adopting, in order to gain a patient, luxurious headgear and elaborate perfume. For excess of strangeness will win you ill-repute but a little will be considered in good taste, ... Yet I do not forbid your trying to please, for it is not unworthy of a physician's dignity" ("Precepts," in *Hippocrates*, ed. W. H. S. Jones [London, 1923], I, 327).

[15] John of Arderne, *op. cit.*, pp. 4–7, *passim*.

[16] *Op. cit.*, chap. iv.

Also he warns against making fun of anyone because one can never tell who can stand jokes. John of Arderne impresses upon his readers that the doctor

should never unwarily reveal the confidences of his patients, neither those of men or of women, nor set one person against another. For if a person sees that the physician keeps another man's counsel he will trust him more.[17]

Alberti de Zancarii,[18] who summarizes these same ideas in the Introduction to his *De cautelis medicorum habendis* and tells us that he is basing his paragraph on the writings of Hippocrates, adds in conclusion, "The physician should not be too trusting towards people, nor too credulous, nor too austere, so that he will not lose their respect by being too gullible nor make them avoid him by being too severe."[19]

The doctors themselves knew that their reputations were not all they should be, and in all the deontological chapters they warn against those persons who would make infamous proposals to doctors because from "time immemorial it has been an article of faith with the common people that every surgeon is a thief, a murderer or a swindler."[20] No wonder that so many of their books have stressed the idea that they must do everything in their power to be of good repute in all things. That they have succeeded in making their profession one of the most honored in all countries goes without saying.

Unfortunately these chapters on ethical matters do not go into detail on the subject of a doctor's education, but they all warn their readers against illiterate practitioners who wish to treat the art of medicine as a rude handicraft. Most of a fourteenth-century doctor's knowledge had to come from books and university lectures, although they could inspect

[17] *Op. cit.*, p. 8.

[18] A Bolognese physician who flourished in the first half of the fourteenth century.

[19] Manuel Morris, *Die Schrift des Albertus de Zancariis aus Bologna* (Leipzig, 1914), p. 12.

[20] Mondeville, *op. cit.*, p. 104.

cases in a few hospitals such as St. Bartholomew's in London and could accompany older practitioners on their professional visits. Hence the translations of Greek and Arabic works as well as the writings of contemporaries and immediate predecessors were of utmost importance to doctors young and old, although Mondeville gives the timely warning that "too much faith in books chokes natural talent."[21] That he must have a fairly broad education is evident from several different sources.

He must not only have knowledge of medicine, but he must also know the books of nature, which is called philosophy. Grammar, logic, rhetoric and ethics are the four sciences which are necessary to examine things judiciously. With the help of logic things can be tested reasonably; grammar gives us the meaning of the words in Latin, rhetoric teaches us to talk properly, as we hear from the philologers, who however have not acquired this art from books, but by practice. The doctor must also know ethics, as this science teaches good morals.[22]

Guy de Chauliac was even more explicit in his warning:

It should be as Galen said in the first of the *Therapeutics*, that if the doctors have not learned geometry, astronomy, dialectics, nor any other good discipline, soon the leather workers, carpenters, and farriers will quit their own occupations and become doctors.[23]

Cases were not always accepted by reputable physicians in classical and medieval times. According to Mondeville,

a surgeon ought to be fairly bold. He ought not to quarrel before the laity, and although he should operate wisely and prudently, he should never undertake any dangerous operation unless he is sure that it is the only way to avoid a greater danger. . . . . He ought to promise a cure to every sick person, but he should refuse as far as possible all dangerous cases, and he should never accept desperately sick ones.[24]

The reasons for such remarks have often been misinterpreted by our own writers and editors, who claim that it was only

[21] *Ibid.*, p. 103.

[22] Jan Yperman, Book I, chap. iv; cf. Isidore of Seville, *Liber etymologiarum*, Book IV, chap. xiii.

[23] *Op. cit.*, p. 18.   [24] *Op. cit.*, p. 106.

because these earlier doctors had a selfish and cowardly desire to escape all blame and criticism. A careful analysis of these fourteenth-century works and a study of their sources show that this fear is not merely a personal one but is professional as well—the laity were already too prone to distrust the medics, and, if the latter promised cures when they knew the case to be a hopeless one, this distrust would be increased. Hippocrates gives us the real key to this problem:

> First I will define what I conceive medicine to be. In general terms, it is to do away with the sufferings of the sick, to lessen the violence of their diseases, and to refuse to treat those who are overmastered by their diseases, realizing that in such cases medicine is powerless. . . . . For if a man demand from an art a power over what does not belong to the art, or from nature a power over what does not belong to nature, his ignorance is more allied to madness than to lack of knowledge.[25]

A surgeon should also be careful to

estimate the strength of a patient before he operates. If a patient dies of the operation and not of mere weakness the surgeon is held excused so long as the friends think the wound looks healthy, but if the wound looks badly the surgeon is credited with the death even though the patient has simply died of weakness.[26]

If a doctor has accepted a case that he later realizes is undoubtedly going to prove fatal, there are two alternatives: he may refuse to continue the treatment or "if the relatives still insist on continuing the treatment, do not neglect to inform them in good time of the impending calamity, for if the end would be fatal you shall not be blamed and shall retain their friendship."[27]

Of equal importance with medical care in effecting cures was the state of mind of the patient. Each writer has his own ideas on the methods to be employed to bring about the correct mental condition, but all agree that few diseases can be overcome if the patient is in the wrong frame of mind. First

[25] "The Art," *loc. cit.*, II, 193, 203.

[26] Mondeville, *op. cit.*, p. 109.   [27] *Ibid.*

of all one can begin improving the mental state of the patient "by music of viols and ten-stringed psaltery, or by forged letters describing the death of his enemies, or if he is a churchman by telling him that he has been elected to a bishopric."[28]

Always warn the patient that the cure will take a long time, in fact make it twice as long as you really think it will be so that the patient will not be in despair. Then if the patient recovers sooner and

considers or wonders or asks why he was told the time of curing would be longer, say that it was because the patient was strong hearted, and suffered well sharp things, and that he was of good complexion, and had able flesh to heal; and feign other causes pleasing to the patient, for patients are made proud and delighted by such words.[29]

John of Arderne's advice is often very religious and in places quite scholastic in tone, although he admits the necessity of merry tales:

And another sayeth, "He may never be in rest of body that is out of rest of soul; I will suffer less things that I suffer not more grievous." It beseemth a great hearted man that he suffer sharp things, he forsooth that is weak of heart is not on the road to recovery, for why? for truly in all my life I have seen but few laboring in this vice healed in any sickness; therefore let wise men beware that they have nothing to do with such. . . . . If patients complain that their medicines are bitter or sharp then the leech shall say to the patient, "It is read in the last lesson of Matins of the Nativity of Our Lord that Our Lord Jesus Christ came into this world for the health of mankind to the manner of a good leech and wise." And when he cometh to the sick man show him medicine, some light and some hard; and let him say to the sick man, "If thou wilt be made whole this and this thou shalt take." . . . . The physician should comfort the patient in admonishing him that in anguish he be of great heart. For a great heart maketh a man hardy and strong to suffer sharp things and grievous. . . . . Also it is advisable that a leech tell good tales and honest that will make the patients laugh, as well of the Bible as of other tragedies; and any other things which may make or induce a light heart in the patient or the sick man.[30]

Connected with the problem of the proper conduct of the physician in regard to their patients is the obedience of the

[28] *Ibid.*, p. 100.

[29] John of Arderne, *op. cit.*, p. 6.   [30] *Ibid.*, pp. 7 and 8.

patient and what the doctor should do to obtain it. According to Mondeville,

> the method by which the surgeon can compel the obedience of his patients, is to explain to them the dangers of disobedience. He may exaggerate these if the patient has a bold and hardy spirit, or he may temper and soften the warnings, or keep silent altogether if the patient is faint hearted or good natured. . . . . The surgeon also should promise that if the patient can endure his illness and will obey the surgeon for a short time he will soon be cured and will escape all of the dangers which have been pointed out to him; thus the cure can be brought about more easily and more quickly. . . . . If the patient is defiant, seldom will the result be successful; as Galen says "as many patients who have confidence in a doctor, that number will recover." Therefore the surgeon must see to it that either by his own efforts or by those of some one else, the patient has confidence in him. . . . . And if he knows that the patient has no faith in his ability, he must not accept the case.[31]

There will be no cure if the surgeon does not believe "that the patient has confidence in him and will obey him, otherwise the surgeon cannot visit him with the proper solicitude." Also a doctor should not accept a case if

> the patient imagines that neither confidence, obedience, nor the surgical operation will be of any benefit, unless the doctor states in advance the danger to be feared [from this lack of confidence]; or that he is persuaded to accept it by supplications, a large fee, and unless the nurses and friends of the patient consider the doctor shall be entirely and absolutely exonerated from all the accidents which might happen.[32]

The patient must be warned against consulting more than one doctor at a time because, if he calls in a crowd of them, there will be endless disagreements and different suggestions, and in the meantime the patient will suffer from lack of care. However, the doctor or the patient may call in two or three for a consultation, but it is better if one doctor who seems to know the most about the case should continue the treatment alone.[33]

The doctors are warned against professional jealousy; if a doctor is asked about a colleague, he "should neither set him

---

[31] *Op. cit.*, p. 145.   [32] *Ibid.*   [33] *Ibid.*, pp. 174 ff.

at nought nor praise him overmuch but should courteously answer: 'I have very little knowledge of him but I have learned nothing but of his goodness and honesty,' and thus shall the honor be increased for each one."

The physician or surgeon must be wary when his advice is asked by another doctor:

> It is better if he have good excuses that he may refuse their demands. . . . . He may feign an injury, or illness, or some other likely excuse. But if he accepts their demands let him make a covenant for his work and make it beforehand. . . . . Clearly advise the other leech that he will give no definite answer in any case until he has seen the sickness and the symptoms of the patient. After he has visited the sick person and if he thinks that the latter will recover, nevertheless he should warn the patient of the perils to come if the treatment is not carried out as he himself ordered.[34]

Another obligation put upon the attending doctor is to see that his patient has proper and careful nursing.

> If the assistants [attendants or relatives] are not careful and conscientious, and are not obedient to the doctor in every possible way they will set at nought the work of the surgeon. For example, if the assistants have not made ready all necessities at the appointed time so that the surgeon cannot have a fire, dressings, bandages, or wine, he will have to change the order of treatment. Also if they are chatterboxes and if by chance they tell the patient bad news concerning his condition, ... they will cause the patient to have an access of choler and high fever and the surgeon will have to change his treatment and it may mean death for the patient. Also if the assistants quarrel among themselves, or mutter or scowl, they are liable to excite the irritation and fear of the sick one. In cases like this the surgeon should take every precaution.[35]

Not only will the attendants sometimes cause trouble for the doctor but often the wives or husbands will make difficulties.

> It often happens that the wife or the husband is angry at the patient; more often it is the wife than the husband, because to-day in France it is more often the wife who commands and the husband who obeys, and everything that the surgeon orders for the care of her husband the wife considers to be entirely useless, although that which he orders for the wife, the husband thinks will be of great benefit. . . . . If he [the doctor] fears

[34] John of Arderne, *op. cit.*, p. 5.   [35] Mondeville, *op. cit.*, pp. 172 ff.

troublesome raconteurs, he must not let any outsiders in to talk with the patient. If he fears the noise made by neighboring artisans, such as iron-smiths, carpenters and others, bad air, noisome smells, smoke from the coal which the Parisian smiths commonly use, or anything else coming from outside which might be injurious to the patient, he must eliminate them as far as possible, before they have caused any damage.

But taking care of the sick was not the only duty of a true physician for he must also advise his people how to prevent ill health

because the treatment which stops the onset of a new disease is more useful to a patient than all other treatments. But this is, as one can see, useless and harmful to the surgeon because he thus stops the appearance of a disease whose treatment would be advantageous to himself. Thus he should give this advice to only five classes of people; 1. to those who are really poor, for the love of God, ... 2. to his friends from whom he does not wish to receive a fixed revenue or a definite sum of money, ... 3. to those whom he knows to be grateful after a complete recovery, ... 4. to those who repay poorly, such as our seigniors and their relatives, chamberlains, justices, and bailiffs, avocates, and all those to whom he does not dare refuse counsel, ... 5. to those who pay completely in advance.[36]

But Mondeville also says that from all of these the doctors should expect to receive gifts, so they will not lose out entirely. In order to prevent disease, the doctor should advise his patients to eat, drink, and live abstemiously. John of Mirfeld,[37] an English physician of the first half of the fourteenth century, said that people should not only follow a proper diet to maintain good health but that they should also have plenty of exercise, preferably out of doors. He advised prelates "to have a rope in their rooms suspended from the ceiling, knotted at the end, on which they could exercise by swinging or raising themselves." He also told them "to carry weights in their hands while walking about their homes if they could not take enough outdoor exercise."

In regard to the problem of determining the fees for each case and the manner of collecting them, one must admit that

[36] *Ibid.*, p. 110.

[37] *Floriarium Bartholomei*, BM MS Royal 7, fol. 11.

the fourteenth-century attitude on this ever delicate subject, although a little more considerate than that of the two preceding centuries, was not up to the standard set by the Hippocratic ideal.[38] Medieval physicians were seldom shy in admitting in their works that they often charged high fees and became very wealthy from their practice. As John of Arderne says:

> And if he sees that the patient is busily following the cure, then after inquiring about the state of his health, ask boldly for more or less [in fees]; but be he ever wary of scarce asking, for over scarce asking setteth at nought both the market and the thing.[39]

That they were often avaricious is evident from many sources, sometimes even from the frank confessions of the doctors themselves. John of Mirfeld relates a charming story to warn his students concerning this grave fault. He tells about the doctor whose patient had owed him thirteen pounds for three years. When the doctor was dying, and his priest urged him to accept the Eucharist, all the poor man could say was "thirteen pounds in three years."[40]

Henry of Mondeville must have had an especially difficult time in collecting fees or have been a very grasping person, for he devotes many paragraphs to the subject of charging for services and making patients pay.

> The surgeon must take into account three things when a patient comes to him. First his own standing in the profession, then the condition of the patient, and the seriousness of the illness. . . . . The main objective of the sick is to get rid of their diseases, but when once they are cured, they will most likely forget to pay. But the object of the doctor is to obtain his money, and he ought never to be satisfied with a mere promise to pay, nor with a pledge, but he should either take the money in advance or demand a bond for it. . . . . The doctor ought not to have too much faith in appearances. Rich people have a bad habit of appearing before him in old clothes, or if they do happen to be well-dressed they make up all sorts of excuses for demanding lower fees. They claim that charity is a flower when they find some one else who will help the poor, and thus think that a surgeon

[38] Hippocrates, "Precepts," *loc. cit.*, I, 327.

[39] *Op. cit.*, p. 5. [40] *Floriarium Bartholomei*, BM MS Royal 7, fol. 20.

should help the unfortunate; they however would never be bound by this rule. . . . . I tell these people, then pay me for yourself and for three paupers and I will help them as well as you. But they never answer me, and I have never found a person in any position, whether clerk or layman, who was rich enough, or honest enough to pay what he had promised until I made him do so.[41]

These fourteenth-century medical ideals can best be summed up in the words of one of their own doctors:

I say that the doctor should be well mannered, bold in many ways, fearful of dangers, that he should abhor the false cures or practices. He should be affable to the sick, kindhearted to his colleagues, wise in his prognostications. He should be chaste, sober, compassionate and merciful: he should not be covetous, grasping in money matters, and then he will receive a salary commensurate with his labors, the financial ability of his patients, the success of the treatment, and his own dignity.[42]

41 *Op. cit.*, pp. 111, 188, 199, 200, 201.

42 Guy de Chauliac, *op. cit.*, p. 19.

THE HIPPOCRATIC OATH IN ELIZABETHAN ENGLAND *

SANFORD V. LARKEY

Of all medical writings there is probably none so well known as the Hippocratic Oath, and in all ages it has been a guide to the physician in his relations to his patient and to society. Even in our own times it is held up as embodying the essential ethical principles of the medical profession, although some of its provisions are obviously not applicable to modern conditions, representing as they do the very specific obligations of a guild-like system. It is of interest that in Elizabethan England these very passages are omitted by one writer, John Securis, when discussing the Oath in relation to the current problems of medical practice.

For in sixteenth century England the Hippocratic Oath was, as in all periods, a model to the physician, and of all the Hippocratic writings was the most frequently printed in English. Their appreciation of the Oath and of Hippocrates may be seen in the preface to one of the versions:

> " The othe of Hippocratus which he gave unto his desiples and scollers, which professing Phisicke and Chirurgerie, is very worthie to be observed and kept faithfullie, of everie true and honest Artest, although he himselfe were but a heathen man, and without the true knowledge of the living

* Read before the Johns Hopkins Medical History Club, the Institute of the History of Medicine, Baltimore, Maryland, December 2, 1935.

God, yet for his noble and excellent skil in Phisicke and Chirurgerie, he ought not to be forgotten of us his posteritie, but to be had in an honorable remembrance for ever." [1]

The only other work of Hippocrates known to have been printed in English earlier was a rearrangement of the *Aphorisms*.[2] Although the ideas of Hippocrates and Galen were known in English through the writings of others, the only other works that I know of as printed in English were the *Prognostic*[3] and the *Discourse on Humane Nature*.[4] Of course the *Works* were available in Latin editions as early as 1525.[5]

There were four English versions of the Oath in the Sixteenth Century, the earliest known appearing in John Securis' *A Detection and Querimonie of the daily enormities and abuses committed in physick,* London, 1566. Securis gives part of the Latin text by Janus Cornarius and an English translation. The chief interest in this version lies in the way Securis relates it to the questions of his own day, for, as the title of his book tells us, he is attacking the abuses of medicine. His work will be considered later.

The next version was in Thomas Newton's *The Olde mans Dietarie*, 1586, while there were two more in surgical books in 1588 and 1597. These are in John Read's translation of Arcaeus' *A most excellent method of curing woundes* and Peter Lowe's *The whole course of chirurgerie.* Thus it will be seen that the Oath reached a wide circle of medical readers. These four versions differ markedly from each other, and it is clear that they are independent translations, each one exhibiting certain individual variations that make them of especial interest in themselves. These changes either give a different interpretation to certain passages of the Oath, as we

[1] From John Read's translation of Arcaeus, *A most excellent and compendious method of curing woundes*, London, 1588. Misprints corrected.
[2] In H. Lloyd's translation of John XXI, *The treasury of healthe,* London [1550?].
[3] Peter Lowe in his *The whole course of chirurgerie,* London, 1597, included not only the Oath of Hippocrates (see fig. 7, 8) but also *the Presages of divine Hippocrates.*
[4] This was one of five treatises in *The key to unknowne knowledge,* London, 1599, from the translation of John de Bourges.
[5] *Hippocratis Coi Medicorum Omnium longe Principis, octoginta Volumina.* [Colophon] Romae ex aedibus Francisci Minitii, 1525.

220

know it in modern translations, or add further injunctions, which, while not in the original, are in keeping with the tradition of the Hippocratic physician.[6]   The reader is referred to the reproductions for all of the variant passages.

The first difference that is of importance is a phrase defining the relation of the student to the master who taught him the art.   You will remember that Francis Adams translates this passage:

> " to reckon him who taught me this Art equally dear to me as my parents, to share my substance with him, and relieve his necessities if required; "[7]

This appears to be repetitious, and the English writers avoid this by giving a broader meaning.   Thus Newton says:

> " That I shall yeeld and give unto my Maister, of whom I have bene taught, and by whom I have bene trayned in this Art, no lesse reverence and duetie, then to myne own natural Father that begat me.   That I shalbe conversant in life with him: And that I shall to the uttermost of my power and abilitie, minister unto him all such things as I shall understand he hath need of." [8]

This may more nearly represent the meaning of the original Greek, καὶ βίου κοινώσεσθαι.

Nowhere in the original versions of the Oath is there any mention of treatment of the poor, but Newton modifies the passage on teaching the art to the sons of his teacher, without fee or covenant, to read:

> " That I shal not be squeimish to bestow my skill in this Arte upon the poore and needie, freely, without either fee or other covenant certainly agreed upon."

There is authority for such a statement in the *Precepts* of Hippocrates, which says:

---

[6] These are reproduced in figs. 1-8.
[7] Francis Adams, *The Genuine Works of Hippocrates,* London, 1849.
[8] In this and in the following quotations the original spelling and punctuation have been retained, except for lengthening of contractions, and modernizing of certain typographical features (s; v and u; i and j).

" I urge you not to be too unkind, but to consider carefully your patient's superabundance or means. Sometimes give your services for nothing, calling to mind a previous bene-faction or present satisfaction. And if there be an oppor-tunity of serving one who is a stranger, in financial straits, give full assistance to all such. For where there is love of man, there is also love of the art." [9]

There is also a similar admonition in one of the Arabic versions:

" A doctor must be prepossessing and charitable, soft-speak-ing, accessible and keen on caring for the poor and indigent sick. He must ask them neither salary nor recompense." [10]

Such an attitude is certainly one of the ideals of medicine, and really belongs in an ethical document.

In discussing the rules for treatment of the sick, both Newton and Lowe again interpolate a rather striking thought on prolonging the patient's illness. We all know that this is a charge that is sometimes unfairly made against the doctor, and it evidently was made in those days. Newton says:

" That I shal not deferre, ne linger my cure longer then I neede, keeping my Patient thereby the longerwhile in grief and paine: and that I shall not offer any wrongfull dealing to any maner of person."

There is one Latin manuscript that expresses the same idea.[11]

Peter Lowe is very precise in regard to the giving of poison. He swears:

" That I shall minister no poyson, neither councell nor teach poyson, nor the composing thereof, to any."

There is one injunction that appears only in Lowe, but it is a most interesting one, and certainly a good bit of advice to the young medical student:

[9] W. H. S. Jones, *Hippocrates with an English translation*, The Loeb Classical Library, London and New York, 1923, Vol. I, p. 319.

[10] From Al-Ghāfigī, *Isis*, XXII, 1934, p. 223.

[11] See the Latin text in W. H. S. Jones, *The Doctor's Oath*, Cambridge, 1924, p. 35.

> " I shall patiently sustaine the injuries, reproaches, and loath-
> somenesse of sick men, and all other base raylings: and
> that I shall eschew as much as I may, all venerious lascivious-
> nesse."

Again we find such a thought in an Arabic paraphrase,[12] and also in
an early Latin manuscript.[13] The Arabic text is:

> " He should be patient of insults, because many mad and
> melancholic persons meet us with such, wherein we should
> bear with them, knowing that such conduct does not proceed
> from them but is really caused by a disease external to their
> proper nature."

Lowe, continuing, then makes a curious mis-reading of the section
dealing with secrecy, combining part of the previous sentence with
the first of the next to achieve this idea:

> " Moreover I protest, be it man, woman, or servant, who is
> my patient, to cure them of all things that I may see or heare
> either in mind or manners."

Otherwise the secrecy clause is practically the same in all.

The imprecation on violating the Oath is so expressed by Read
that it applies even to his patients!

> " God graunt that as I truelie observe and keepe this my
> oath, I may have prosperous successe in my Arte and living.
> And according to the performance heereof, each man may
> sounde my perpetuall praise. But if I transgresse and breake
> the same, I wish to God that in all my cures and other affaires
> I may have evill successe, and that everie one may discom-
> mend mee to the worldes ende."

The variations found in these English translations can in most
cases be traced back to some earlier version, but they are not all
found in any single text, so it is impossible to assign the sources of
our English writers.

[12] From Ibn abi Usaybia as quoted by Jones, *The Doctor's Oath*, p. 59.
[13] Ernst Hirschfeld, *Deontologische Texte des frühen Mittelalters*, Archiv für
Geschichte der Medizin, Bd. 20, Heft 4, Leipzig, Johann Ambrosius Barth, 1928,
p. 368.

That the Oath was of more than literary interest and was considered in an almost legal sense is seen in its application by John Securis. As I have said, he omits the portions that deal with the relation of the student to his master, with teaching, and with the penalties for violation of the Oath, but emphasizes the rest of the Oath, the more practical aspects.

" Nowe therfore, before I speake of the abuses and enormities of phisike, I wil shew and declare first, what is the part office and condition of a good Phisition. Thus doyng I wyl first alledge of *Hippocratis Iusiurandum,* that is, the oth that Hipocrates wold that every phisition shuld take before he practise any phisike. I wil not recite the hole chapter, but the chiefest parte first in latin, than in english. Caeterum quod ad aegros attinet sanandos, dietam ipsis constituam pro facultate, et iuditio meo commodam, omneque detrimentum et iniuriam ab eis prohibebo. Neque vero ullius preces apud me adeo validae fuerint, ut cuipiam venenum sum propinaturus, neque etiam ad hanc rem consilium dabo. Similiter autem neque mulieri talum vulvae [text has vulnae] subdititium ad corrumpendum conceptum vel foetum dabo. Porro praeterea, sancte vitam et artem meam conservabo. Nec vero calculo laborantes secabo, sed viris chirurgiae operariis, eius rei faciendae locum dabo. In quascunque autem domos ingrediar, ob utilitatem aegrotantium intrabo, ab omnique iniuria voluntaria inferenda, et corruptione cum alia, tum praesertim operum venereorum abstinebo, sive muliebria, sive virilia, liberorumve hominum aut servorum corpora mihi contigerint curanda. Quaecunque vero inter curandum videro aut audivero, imo etiam ad medicandum non adhibitus in communi hominum vita cognovero, ea siquidem efferre non contulerit, tacebo, et tanquam arcana apud me continebo. The englishe is this: And as concernyng the curyng of the sycke, I will ordeyn and devise for them as good a diete as shall lye in my power and judgement. And I will take hede that thei fal in no domage nor hurte. Nor yet any mans praiers shall so much prevail with me, that I geve poyson to any man, neither will I counsaile any man so to do. Likewise I will geve no maner of medicine to any woman with chylde to destroy her childe. Moreover I will use my life and science godly. I will not cut those that have the stone, but I will commit that thyng onely to the Surgions. In what house so ever I shall come in, my commyng shalbe for the pacients commoditie and profite. And I wil refraine willingly from doying any hurt or wronge, and from falshode, and chiefly from venereous actes, what kynd of bodies soever it shal chance me to have in cure: whether it be of men or women, of fre or bond servants. And whatsoever I shal see or heare among my cures (yea although I be not sought nor called to any) whatsoever I shall know among the people, if it be not lauful to be uttered, I shal kepe close, and kepe it as a secrete unto my selfe: " [14]

The purpose of his book was to improve the standards of medicine and particularly to curb the activities of the quacks, who were a menace then as they are today. He poses a question that we still find puzzling: " Why will the public countenance such obvious charlatans? " He says:

" Verily I muche mervaile at one thynge that many which be of the higher sort, reputing them selves to be of no small gravitie and wisedom will sometymes geve credite to suche lewde persons, counterfayting the phisitions. In dede I suppose that they be partly deceived by the vain persuasions and faire flattering speche of suche fellowes. Their communication is so faire, swete, gentill, plesant and amiable: and their promise and waranting so earnest and great, that they will go nye to deceave the wisest man that is, yf he have not the more grace, and be very ware of them." [15]

But he also criticizes the medical men themselves for their behaviour, citing as rules of conduct not only the provisions of the Oath, but other ethical writings of Hippocrates, Galen, and of his own master,

[14] Sig. A$_2$^{R}-A$_3$^{V}. The quotations from Securis are taken, by permission, from a copy of the 1566 edition, in the Huntington Library, San Marino, California.
[15] Sig. C$_2$^{V}-C$_3$^{R}.

Jacobus Sylvius. He quotes the *Precepts* of Hippocrates in regard to consultations. One of his criticisms is still valid.

" Some there be also (leste I wene that other men should learne their cunning) that wil rather scrible then write a recept, and will make such dashes and strange abbreviations in theyr billes, that theyr writinge semeth rather to be arabicke, or like the writinges of the Cabalistes, then Latin. I feare me that they that write so, are ashamed of their owne occupation, and feare leaste that if they shoulde write playne, their errours and faultes should be espied. He that is a playne man will deale playnelye, will speake playnely, and write playnely." [16]

He speaks feelingly of the greed of some physicians:

" Item, some phisitions ther be, that be so greedy and of so an unsaciable desier, that they care and passe not in what daunger they caste them selves in, what shame and damage they sustain, so that thei may have many cures, wher somtimes one would suffice them well enough and be more perchaunce then they can well bring to passe. They be so covetous that they wold have all, and do al them selfe, and they have envy many tymes at other honest men having cures, when they have none. Thys doinge verelye they bringe them selves in greate contempte, and dothe as it were abate and blemishe the honorable science of phisicke, which requireth rather to be sought earnestly with greate sute, with humilitie, reverence and prayinge, then to be offered, and as it were objected undiscretely to every man, and in every place, lyke a blinde harpers songe or a Pedlars packe. The common proverbe saith, that offered service stynketh. And I have harde oftentymes saye, that phisicke unles it be earnestly sought and well payde for, it will never prosper nor woorke well with the pacientes, I meane not by this but that the Phisition muste be alwayes liberall and mercifull to the poore, on whom his living dependeth not but on the rich." [17]

[16] Sig. C$_6$^{v}.   [17] Sig. C$_8$^{R}-C$_n$^{R}.

There had been earlier efforts to regulate the practice of medicine, and the founding of the College of Physicians in 1518, under the influence of the great Humanist, Thomas Linacre, had done a great deal to better conditions in London, the College having the duty of examining and licensing those to practise physic within seven miles of London. Although this privilege was extended to all of England by a statute of Henry the Eighth in 1523, it appears that it was not being properly enforced in Elizabeth's reign. Securis is most concerned with the relaxing of educational requirements, charging that many who presumed to be physicians based their knowledge solely on what they read in works available in English. He inveighs against such unlearned persons with typical Elizabethan vigor:

> " Then were it a great foly for us to bestow so much labor and study all our lyfe tyme in the scholes and universities, to breake oure braynes in readynge so many authours, to be at the lectures of so many learned menne, yea and the greatest follye of all were, to procede in any degree in the Universities with our great coste and charges, when a syr John lacke latin a pedler, a weaver, and oftentymes a presumptuous woman, shall take uppon them (yea and are permytted) to mynyster Medicine to all menne, in every place, and at all tymes. O tempora, O mores, O Deum immortalem." [18]

To remedy these faults he proposes a law of seven articles, governing the activities of physicians, surgeons, apothecaries, and midwives, and providing punishment for unlicensed practitioners:

Seven Articles concerning the ministration and use of Phisike.

The fyrst.

It were very mete, expedient and necessary that no phisition shoulde practice phisicke in any dioces, unles he were fyrste allowed by some universitie: or at the leaste having sufficient learninge in the saide science, he were allowed and licensed by the byshop or his chaunceloure in that dioces wherin he dwelleth.

[18] Sig. B$_2$^{v}.

The second.

It were good and necessarye that no Surgion shoulde practyse his surgery, unles he coulde reade and write, and had knowledge and experience in the simples belonginge to his art. And that he presume not to let bloud or undertake any hard cure, without the physitions counsell, if he may conveniently have it.

The thyrd.

That no Poticarie should minister of his owne heade, or ordeyne any purgation or other composition of Phisicke for any man: or that he shoulde prepare and make any purgation or notable confection, withoute the Phisitions advyse and counsell, unles that the Phisition hadde fyrst sene and vewed the Ingredientes, wherof the compositions are made, and speciallye the purgations.

The fourthe.

It is not decent nor profitable for the common weale, that any ignorant lewde or ill suspected person, be he man or woman, shoulde be suffered to make, sell or minister medecines to any bodie, but that suche kind of persons (beyng duely examined and convycted by the learned Phisitions of the dioces) should have condigne punishment appoynted them by the Byshop or his chauncelour.

The fyfthe.

That no Physition do take upon him the name of anye degree of Schole, as bachelour, maister of Arte, or Doctor: or cause and permit any writer or printer so to terme him, unles he can approve it to be so in dede by any universitie.

The syxte.

That no midwife should disdayne to come aske counsell of the Phisition, as often as any woman beyng in laboure of childe, is in danger. It were good also that the midwives

wer first sworne to the byshoppe, before they take uppon them their office.

The seventh.

It were also good and expediente that (as the use of London is, graunted by an acte of Parliament) that the Phisitions in every other dioces one or two, or more, shold have licence of the byshop, to searche and vewe the poticaries shoppe, once a yere at the leaste, and see whether their stuffe and medecines be good and lawfull or not.

These Articles above rehearsed I thought good here to allege, (although under correction of my superiors) because that some occasion may be geven to refourme the enormities and abuses in the science of Phisicke. And here let no man think, that I meane to speake any thing in any point against the privileges and liberties graunted by an act of Parliament to the company or corporation of the Phisitions of London, for I mynde not, nor may not medle with their privileges.[19]

In all of the efforts to improve the conditions of medical practice and the position of the doctor, the Hippocratic Oath was an important influence and served as a basis of such endeavours. The practical regulations proposed by Securis, in line with the legal enactments of the time, were an effort to realize the ideal doctor of physic as portrayed in the Oath, while the English versions of the Oath, with their interesting variations, would tend to the same goal, the greater integrity and dignity of the medical profession.

---

[19] Sig. B$_6$^{v}-B$_8$^{v}.

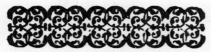

Hippocrates his Oath.

 Take Apollo the Phiſi-
tion, and Æſculapius, and
Hygias and Panaceas, the
ſonnes of Æſculapius, and
all the Gods and Goddeſ-
ſes to witneſſe: That I (ſo much as in me
ſhal lye, and ſo farre as my iudgement and
ſkill ſhall ſtretch) will obſerue & performe
all the things contained in this Oath and
in this Booke. viz.

That I ſhall peeld and giue vnto my
Maiſter, of whom I haue bene taught, and
by whō I haue bene trayned in this Art,
no leſſe reuerence and ductie, thē to myne
own natural Father that begat me. That
I ſhalbe conuerſant in life with him: And
that I ſhall to the vttermoſt of my power
and abilitie, miniſter vnto him all ſuch
things as I ſhall vnderſtand he hath need
of.

That I ſhall make no leſſe accompte of
his Children, thē of myne own Brethren,
D 3   and

FIG. 1-4. The Hippocratic Oath as it appeared
in Thomas Newton's *The Olde mans
Dietarie*, London, 1586.

(Reproduced by permission of the
Huntington Library)

Hippocrates his Oath.

and so to repute and take them.

That I shal not be squeimish to bestow my skill in this Arte vpon the poore and needie, freely, without either fee or other couenant certainly agreed vpon.

That I shal freely, faithfully, and truely deliuer all my Precepts and Secretes vnto myne owne and also to my Maisters Children, and to other such Scholers as haue addicted, vowed, bound, and sworne themselues to the Studies and Lawes of Phisicke, and not to any others.

In curing of the Sicke, I shall vse to the vttermost of my power, knowledge, and iudgement, such things as bee good, wholesome, souereigne & profitable: That I shal not deferre, ne linger my cure lenger then I neede , keeping my Patient thereby the longer while in grief & paine: and that I shall not offer any wrongfull dealing to any maner of person.

That I shall not (although I be there-vnto required) giue deadly poyson to any person: neither counsell the same to any other: nor giue it to any woman being with childe, to kill the Infant in her wombe.

That I shall preserue and keepe both my

FIG. 2

Hippocrates his Oath.

my life and myne Arte , free and cleare
from iust obloquie and slaunder, and from
all such occasions as may iustly disparage
and emblemish the same.

That I shall not presume to cut any
persons diseased with the Stone , but re-
ferre that action to others skilful therein.

That , vnto what house soeuer I shall
goe for the practise of myne Arte, I shall
onely respect and carefully employe my
selfe to relieue and recure the partie diseased, my Patient, vnto whom & for whom
I purposely goe.

That I shall auoyde, eschewe and renounce all wrong, all lewdnesse, all filthi-
nesse, al wanton daliaunce and venereous
actions, whether they bee womens bodies
that I haue in cure, or mens bodies: and
whether they be the bodies of Free, or of
Bondmen.

That whatsoeuer during the tyme of
any cure I shall either see or heare , or o-
therwise (beside my cure) shall knowe in
any many life , vnderstanding that thing
to be such as requireth secrecie and silēce,
I shal not vtter nor bewray to any maner
of person, but shal herein faithfully keepe
his

FIG. 3

232

Hippocrates his Oath.

his counsell.

To these Articles cõprised in this my present Oath, I protest myne obedience & assent : the which if I inuiolably & faithfully obserue and keepe , my prayer and wish is , that all things aswell in my life as in myne Arte and profession, may haue prosperous successe and happie ende; with perpetuall fame, renowne and glorie : as contrariwise , if I treacherously transgresse , or wilfully herein forsweare my selfe, let all things fall out vnto mee contrarie.

FINIS.

Fɪɢ. 4

The othe of Hippocratus

which he gaue vnto his desiples and scollers, which pro-
fessing Phisicke and Chirurgerie, is very worthie to
be obserued and kept faithfullie, of euerie true
and honest Artests, although he himselfe
were but a heathen man ; and without
the true knowledge of the liuing God,
yet for his noble and excellent skil
in Phisicke and Chirurgerie, he
ought not to be forgotten
of vs his posteritie, but
to be had in an hono-
rable remembrāce
for euer.

 Sweare by Appollo the Phisitian , by
Æsculapius , by Higea , and Panacea : yea
and I take to witnes all the Gods and Goddesses : that to my power I will vprightlie
obserue this my othe : I will accompte my
Maister which taught me this arte , my fa-
ther: in his case hee shall commaund my life, and whatsoeuer hee needeth I will giue it him . As for his Children
I will hold his sonnes as my brethren, and if they desire the
knowledge of this arte, I will teach it them without stipent
or couenant. I will instruct my sonnes, & my maisters sonns,
yea & such as by hand wrighting are my scholers & sworne
and adicted to Phisicke, the precepts, rules, and whatsoeuer
else belongeth to the knowledge of the saide profession , or
touching the cure of diseases. I will appoint them a diet , to
my power : and in my iudgement commodius . And I
will defend them from hurt and iniury , neither shall the requests and petitions of any man, be they neuer so earnest,
so much preuaile with me to giue poyson to any person to
drinke , neither will I giue my counsell or consent there-
tos

FIG. 5-6. The Hippocratic Oath from John Read's translation of
Arcaeus' *A most excellent method of curing woundes*,
London, 1588.

(Reproduced from a copy of the 1612 edition
in the Welch Medical Library)

...in like manner I will refuſe the miniſtration of any ſup-
poſitorie, to the hurting or corrupting of the childe, in the
time of my life. And in my profeſſion, I will ſhew my ſelfe
pure, chaſt, and holy. I will neuer cut any perſon that hath
the ſtone, but will giue place to ſtone-cutters, in the cure
thereof, what houſe ſoeuer I come into, it ſhall be to the patient his profite. I will offer no iniurie voluntarelie to anie
man. I will eſchew all wickedneſſe to my power, eſpeciallye
the vice of Venerie, whether it bee my chaunce to deale
with men or women, freeman or bondſeruaunt, whatſoeuer
in any cure I ſhall either ſee, heare, or know, or in any other
matter, yea though I bee not called to the cure my ſelfe. I
will keepe it ſecret and vnreuealed, ſo that ſilence therein be
expediēt. God graunt that as I truelie obſerue & keepe this
my oath, I may haue proſperous ſucceſſe in my Arte
and liuing. And according to the performance heere-
of, each man may ſounde my perpetuall praiſe.
But if I tranſgreſſe and breake the ſame, I
wiſh to God that in all my cures and
other affaires I may haue euill ſucceſſe, and that euerie one may
diſcommend mee to the
worldes ende.
(∴)

FIG. 6

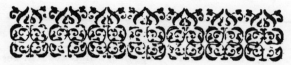

❡ The proteſtation and oath of diuine *Hippocrates.*

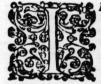Hippocrates doe vow, promiſe and proteſt to the great God *Appollo* and his two Daughters *Higine* and *Panadee,* and alſo to all the gods and goddeſſes, to obſerue the contents of this oath, or tables wherein this oath is carued, written or ingraued, ſo farre as I can poſſible, and ſo farre as my wit or vnderſtanding ſhall bee able to direct me, viz. that I yeild my ſelfe tributarie and debtor to the Maiſter and Doctor who hath inſtructed me and ſhewed mee this ſcience and doctrine, euen as much or rather more then to my Father who hath begotten me, and that I ſhall liue and communicate with him and follow him in all neceſſities, which I ſhall know him to haue ſo farre as my power ſhall permit, and my gods ſhall extend. Alſo that I ſhall loue and cheriſh his children as my brothers, and his progenie as mine owne. Further, that I ſhall teach, ſhew and demonſtrate the ſayde ſcyence (gratis) without rewarde or couenant, and that I ſhall giue all the Cannons rules and precepts, freely, truely, and faithfully to my Maiſter his children, as to myne owne, without hiding or concealing any thing, and to all other Schollers who ſhall make the ſame oath or proteſtation, and to no others. Alſo that in practiſing and vſing my ſcience towardes the ſicke, I ſhall vſe onely things neceſſary, ſo farre as I am able, and as my ſpirit and good vnderſtanding ſhall giue vnto mee, and that I ſhall cure the ſicke as ſpeedy as I may, without dilating or prolonging the Malady. And that I ſhall not doe any thing againſt equitie, for hatred, anger, enuie, or malice, to any perſon whatſoeuer : Moreo-

Tributarie to his Maiſter.

Loue his Maiſters children.

A 3   uer

FIG. 7-8. The Hippocratic Oath from Peter Lowe's *The whole course of chirurgerie,* London, 1597.

(Reproduced from a copy of the 1612 edition in the Welch Medical Library)

The Oath of Hippocrates.

uer, that I shall minitter no poyfon, neither councell nor
teach poyfon, nor the compofing thereof, to any : Alfo,
that I fhall not giue, nor caufe to be giuen, nor confent that
any thing be applied to a woman breeding, or bigge with
child, to deftroy, or make her voyd her fruite. But I proteft to keepe my Life and Science purely, fincerely and in-
violably, without deceipt, fraude, or guile. And that I
fhall not cutte, nor incife any perfon hauing the ftone, but
fhall leaue the fame to thofe that are expert in it : and furthermore, I fhall not enter into the Patients houfe, but
with purpofe to heale him: & that I fhall patiently fuftaine
the iniuries, reproaches, and loathfomneffe of fick men, and
all other bafe raylings: and that I fhall efchew as much as I
may, all venerious lafciuioufneffe. Moreouer I proteft,
be it man, woman, or feruant, who is my patient, to cure
them of all things that I may fee or heare either in mind
or manners, and I fhall not bewray that which fhould be
concealed and hidden, but keepe inuiolable, with filence,
neither reueale any creature, vnder paine of death. And
therefore I befeech our Gods, that obferuing this Proteftation, promife and vow intirely and inuiolably, that all
things in my life, in my Art and Science, may fucceed
fecurely, healthfully, and profperoufly to me, and in the
end eternall glory. And to him that fhall violate, tranfgreffe
or become periured, that the contrary may happen vnto
him, viz. miferie, calamitie, and continuall maladies.

Not to mini-
fter poyfon.

To giue no-
thing to wo-
men, to caufe
abortment.

To beare
with the fick.

Heere Hippo-
crates fhew-
eth, that the
place of blef-
fed is eternall,
and the paine
of the wicked
infinite.

The end of the Proteftation.

The

FIG. 8

SAMUEL SORBIÈRE AND HIS *ADVICE TO A YOUNG PHYSICIAN*

FRANK LESTER PLEADWELL

I.

SAMUEL SORBIÈRE (1615-1670); PHYSICIAN, PRIEST, AND PHILOSOPHER

In December, 1922, in an assortment of autographs acquired by purchase in New York, I found a Latin letter by Samuel Sorbière, or de Sorbière, as he sometimes called himself (see fig. 1). A translation of this letter into English follows:

Samuel Sorbière, to the Most Illustrious and Most Learned Doctor Justus Rickward, Doctor of Medicine. Felicitations!

Most Distinguished and Most Kind Rickward,

On my way back from Rotterdam on Sunday, whilst I thought over the great courtesy with which you received me, so insignificant a man, one to whom you owed nothing, and who had long been a mere victim of fate, suddenly, I grew somewhat ashamed of my silence, in that I seemed not sufficiently to have responded to signs of so great a benevolence, and feared lest you might think poorly of me, and hold me altogether unworthy of so many offices of kindness. Yet I have never been guilty of being an ungrateful soul; and as often as kindnesses have been done me, I have never failed openly to attest both what they were, and to whom I owed them; nor have I failed also to try to repay in the same or better measure, if possible. But I know what happened, and why my words came more reluctantly than usual. There is no reason for me to wonder why I had no answer ready to words of unaccustomed goodness. For some years now I have been living among men ignorant of kindness, so empty that they give sound of hollowness. There are no trusty friends about me, no men of true worth, such that their words are not only on the lips, but come from the inmost marrow of the soul. What wonder then, that I was dumfounded, stricken at the unaccustomed brightness of such goodness. Such is my usual way of behaving, Most Illustrious Rickward, and I know that this has happened before; once especially when I experienced the ineffable kindness of the illustrious Grotius, that godlike man. So that I would not have you doubt that your kindness went deep into my heart; and that I would have you be to me in the future what you have been in the past.

---

[1] An abridged version of this paper was read at the twenty-second annual meeting of The American Association of the History of Medicine, at Lexington, Kentucky, May 23, 1949.

My private affairs take me to France, my uncle Samuel Petit [2] having died last December, and literary people demand that I should no longer put off the appointed journey; for many learned men eagerly await the translation and erudite commentaries on Flavius Josephus which he spent nine years preparing, until, before his time, yet broken by immense labors, he gave his deserving soul to God. There are many whose mouths are watering for his writings, among others the Jesuits. If these [writings] got into their hands what outrage would come to the fame of the venerable dead, what peril to our family, and what harm to truth! This, God forbid! But you, kind Rickward, be always greatly solicitous that I may achieve my purpose speedily, both by advising your other friends of it in word and letter; and then, since you have much influence with the great and good Dr. Swartecron, [3] by urging him to the same end. I hope that you will do this willingly, since by no other act can you more clearly prove how anxious you are to help me, and how fond you are of your obedient servant. Farewell, and greet Dr. Swartecron in my name.

Written at The Hague, the ninth of May, 1644.

If you have occasion to write to me, address the envelope to M. Renaud [4] on Pooten Street, near M. the Count William. [5]

To Monsieur Rickwaerd, Doctor of Medicine, Princes' Street, right across from the small church, at Rotterdam.

It is pertinent to inquire, who was this Sorbière who wrote so feelingly to his friend Rickward some three hundred years ago?

Samuel Sorbière was born September 17, 1615, in the town of St. Ambroise, in the diocese of Uzes, France. He was the child of Estienne Sorbière and Louise Petit, a sister of Samuel Petit, a clergyman of Nîmes, of some notoriety also in the republic of letters. His father, his uncle, and all his family were Protestants, as was Sorbière himself for a good many years. His parents died when he was quite young, and he was adopted by his uncle Petit, also his godfather, who took him into his home and assumed charge of his education. In 1639 Sorbière went to Paris for theological studies, but finding these alien to his tastes, shortly turned to the study of medicine, in which he made rapid progress. He appears to have left Paris for Leyden in 1642, either to complete his medical studies, or to enter upon the practice of his profession. In *Sor-*

[2] Samuel Petit (1594-1643) was a native of Nimes, and by profession a Protestant clergyman and professor of Greek at the College of Arts in that city. The manuscript of his Commentaries on Flavius Josephus is stated by François Graverol to have been purchased by the Earl of Clarendon during his exile at Montpellier, and is now in the Bodleian Library. [MS. 4141-2]

[3] The Dr. Swartecron of Sorbière's letter has not been identified.

[4] David Renaud, a fellow countryman of Sorbière's, and his father-in law to be. Lange Pooten is an important street at The Hague.

[5] Count William was probably the grandson of William the Silent, and eventually to become the father of William III of England.

Viro clarissimo doctissimoque
D. Iusto Rickwardo Doctori medico
samuel Sorberius οι̃ πρἀττειν.

Praestantissime & amicissime Rickwarde.

cum Roterodamo die Dominica rodirem, & mecum re-
putarem quantâ excepisses comitate. me tantulum ho-
minem, de te nihil meritum, aduersa diu aegre obluctan-
tem fortuna, subiit sane suppudere silentii cum scilicet
non satis mihi uiderer ab tam prolixa beneuolentiâ.
significationem respondisse, & uererer ne sequiorem
de me suspicionem haberes, indignumque prorsus existima-
res cui tot humanitatis summae officia obtulisses
Non is tamen sum qui ingrati animi morbo unquam
laborarim : nec enim quoties beneficia in me collata.
fuere cessaui palam profiteri quid & cui deberem,
atque adeo eniti ut αὐτῳ̃ τω̃ μέρω κ̀ λω̕ονι, si quâ
possem, rependerem . sed uideo quid factum sit, atque
unde uox mihi praeter moram faucibus haeserit. Verbis

FIG. 1.

Facsimile reproduction of page one of Sorbière's letter to Justus Rickward, M. D.,
May 9, 1644. (From the author's collection)

beriana, a posthumous work of Sorbière's, published in 1694, comprising a mixture of bon mots, bits of history, and remarks on divers subjects, preceded by a biographical sketch by François Graverol, in a passage referring to Claude Saumaise, Sorbière is quoted as saying, " I have had the good fortune of conversing during two years quite familiarly with the late M. de Saumaise, of whom I was a neighbor in Leyden, where I practiced medicine." In the same work there is also mention of his having resided for a short time in Amsterdam, in a furnished room in the home of one La Barre, near the Bourse. Sorbière returned to France in 1645, but in the following year he was back in Holland and married Judith Renaud, daughter of the Renaud referred to in the letter to Dr. Rickward. Renaud was a former fellow-townsman from St. Ambroise. He now resumed practice in Leyden. How much practice he did is difficult to ascertain, but he was an inveterate writer in many fields including medicine. Sorbière seems to have been something of a rolling stone, and by 1649 or 1650 he was again in France, at Orange, where he was appointed principal of the College. In 1653 his wife died. One child, a son, Henri de Sorbière, was born to the couple. Soon after his wife's death he was received into the Roman faith. " I have heard," Guy Patin wrote in 1653, "that our old friend M. Sorbière, master of the college at Orange, has proved a turncoat, and has become a Roman Catholic. . . . Of such kind are the miracles which can be witnessed today—miracles, I say, of the political and economical, rather than the metaphysic order. He is a widower and a clever fellow, but, sharp as he is, I wonder whether with that new shirt of his, he will succeed in making his fortune at Rome, for the place swarms with hungry and thirsty people."

Shortly after his conversion, early in 1654, Sorbière went to Paris, and following the prevailing custom, published a discourse on the event, which he dedicated to Cardinal Mazarin. He became an abbé and wore the appropriate dress with the " petit collet " of an abbé. The frontispiece of this paper shows him in this dress. After Sorbière had been granted a pension of 400 livres, Mazarin promised him an additional 300 livres, but did not live up to his promise. From Louis XIV he received the rather empty title of Historiographer Royal. Subsequent holders of this office were to be Boileau, Racine, and Voltaire. Sorbière's economic state not improving, he decided to go to Rome, where he made himself known to Pope Alexander VII, by writing him a Latin letter critical of the Protestants. When he met the Pope the latter said to him, " Is it not true that you are the nephew of Samuel Petit? ", an indication that his relation to that scholar gave him more standing than his own erudition. He gained little or nothing financially from his Roman visit, and soon returned to Paris. It was now that he published an attack against Jean Riolan, Junior, the anatomist, who had questioned Jean Pecquet's discovery of the thoracic duct and the *receptaculum chyli,* just as Riolan had attacked Harvey's demonstration of the circulation.

Pope Alexander VII died on May 22, 1667, and Sorbière made his second visit to Rome in time to see Cardinal Rospigliosi elected Pope with the title of Clement IX. He had been a correspondent of the new Pope, and no doubt went to Rome to ingratiate himself further; but ill-success crowned his efforts, and he complained, not disagreeably, " that he had more need for a cartload of bread, than a basin of confitures." While in Rome he addressed a letter to Hubert de Montmor, in which he drew up a portrait of the new Pope, with a panegyric in his honor. It was at the home of M. de Montmor in Paris that a group of physicians was in the habit of meeting to discuss, not medical subjects alone, but also those in the realm of chemistry, physics, and natural phenomena. This group was the nucleus that later formed the Academy of Physicians, eventually, in 1666, to become the Academy of Sciences. Hubert de Montmor was president of the society, and for a period Sorbière was secretary. About this time Sorbière reported to the society an instance of the transfusion of the blood of an animal into the vessels of a man. This may well have been the transfusion performed by Jean Baptiste Denys, physician to Louis XIV, on June 15, 1667.

Let us now return to Sorbière's letter to Rickward. Rickward is a surname of English origin, sometimes spelled " Ryckward," or " Rickword," and by Sorbière himself " Rickwaerd." In his various works he mentions Rickward only once. In his famous *Voyage to England* which appeared in the Spring of 1664, he voices his regret over not being able to see several friends in Holland, since he goes direct from England to France, and one of these friends is Rickward, who by this time must have been in practice in Holland for twenty years. Rickward's name does not occur in the compilation of *English-Speaking Students of Medicine at the University of Leyden* (R. W. Innes Smith, 1932), nor in Munk's *Roll,* nor in the *Register of Medical Licenses* granted by ecclesiastical authority, 1511-1830.

It is quite apparent from Sorbière's letter that he is far from happy in Holland, and could claim but few friends of the caliber of Dr. Rickward. The repression of feeling, and inability to express a proper degree of gratitude toward his friend which marred his recent visit, for which he is profusely apologetic, must have arisen from a state of affairs existing in

Holland at this time. The country had long been the scene of strife between the different religious sects. From about the year 1603 the peace of the church and the tranquillity of the state had been rent by bitter controversy over religious questions. The followers of Arminius battled with the followers of Calvin. Hugo Grotius, the great jurisconsult, mentioned by Sorbière, was a supporter of the Arminians. Prince Maurice, the ruling authority, was opposed to Grotius and his associates and, in 1618, they were brought to trial. Grotius was condemned to life imprisonment, confined to the Castle of Louvestein, but in 1621, through the skilful connivance of his wife, he was smuggled out of the castle in a chest, and escaped to live in France for the balance of his career, except for one short visit to Holland in 1631. It is probable that Sorbière made his acquaintance either in Paris, or in Senlis.

Sorbière's concern for the safety of his uncle's work on Josephus, and his fears that the Jesuits obtain premature knowledge of it, or even possession of it, and thus imperil its truthful publication, is set forth feelingly in the letter, but how far this alarm was justified, it is now impossible to say. Both the church and the state exercised a rigid control of publications, as Sorbière himself was soon to learn when Louis XIV suppressed his *Voyage to England*. It was in the year 1663 that Sorbière undertook a journey which was to make him famous throughout Europe, both in the literary and the diplomatic world. About the 10th of June, 1663, he arrived in London and remained in England for three months. We know but little of the details of his doings on this visit. Except for a short stay in Oxford, he spent his time in London or its environs. He wrote in high praise of the English landscape. In London he lodged in the Common Garden, because it was near Salisbury House where his friend Thomas Hobbes lived with his patron, the Earl of Devonshire. Hobbes was in exile from 1640 to 1651, and lived in Paris where Sorbière made his acquaintance. The latter was entrusted with Hobbes' *De Cive,* and saw it through the Elzevir Press at Amsterdam. Sorbière made a translation into French of the work. During the London visit Sorbière was presented to King Charles II, was elected a Fellow of the Royal Society, together with Christian Huygens, visited Hatfield House, where he greatly admired the Park, and at Oxford was shown about by Thomas Lockey, librarian of the Bodleian. He returned to France in early October, and wrote an account of his journey. A few weeks later, by decree of the Council of State, Louis XIV ordered the suppression of the book and condemned the author to banishment in Nantes. The cause of this summary exile was variously explained, but the majority attributed it to a complaint about the book received from the English government. There were political reasons why the French at the time were anxious not to give England any cause for complaint; hence the thoroughness with which Sorbière was punished. However, by October 6, 1664, Cominges, French ambassador to England, wrote to Louis XIV that Charles II considered the author of the work sufficiently disciplined, and recommended him to the royal clemency. Politically the issue died very soon, but for many years the work was still referred to in England as an insolent satire. Much of this perpetuation of feeling was no doubt traceable to the reply to Sorbière which the Rev. Thomas Sprat saw fit to publish in 1665. Of this book Ambassador Jusserand says: " It is a wild, rambling pamphlet, written *ab irato*, the lapse of time having in no way cooled the anger of the author. Sprat is blinded by his passion; his answers in several cases defeat his own intentions, so much that more actual praise of the English nation will be found in Sorbière's book than in Sprat's wild reply." The French edition of Sorbière's *Voyage*, owing to its destruction and suppression, has become a rare book; but copies travelled to Holland and to England, and the work was widely read. Pepys in his *Diary* mentions getting Batty, his man, to read it to him.

Sorbière's interest in philosophy, as well as his contributions in this field, are worthy of notice. He had many friends among contemporary philosophers. Thomas Hobbes, Hugo Grotius, and Christian Huygens have already been noticed. In addition he knew, or corresponded with, Pierre Gassendi, René Descartes, Marin Mersenne, Jean Chapelain, Valentin Conrart, Claude Saumaise, Gilles Ménage, and Guy Patin; strictly speaking not all philosophers, but all scholars of note in Sorbière's lifetime. In the first collected edition of the works of Gassendi, the biography of the philosopher there appearing is from the pen of Sorbière. In 1642, when Descartes was living at Endgeest, near Leyden, he was visited by Sorbière and the account of that meeting has been drawn upon by numerous writers on Descartes. It appeared under " Descartes " in the 14th edition of the *Encyclopaedia Britannica*.

Respecting Sorbière's attitude to Descartes and his system of philosophy, Professor Balz remarks, " As a follower of Gassendi, as physician, man of letters and man of the world, he stood in a complicated situation. Whether from lack of courage or lack of ability, he could neither repudiate Descartes nor follow him. He illustrates the inability of the age either to assimilate the spirit of Cartesian teaching or to escape its influence . . . Sorbière possessed a genuine passion for what we may call physical science. In this he was evidently sincere, whatever may be true for the rest. Science, a universal science of nature, is the very ideal of intellectual effort. The future lies with the physics of Gassendi, however, rather than with that of Descartes; this is evidently his firm conviction. But he is a compromising and none too courageous spirit."

Graverol mentions that of the ancient physicians, Sorbière esteemed chiefly Galen, of whose methods he was a great admirer, although he found him not without faults. The same authority also says that there was never a man who better knew his Rabelais, whose memory he revered. Among his other favorites were Pierre Charron and Montaigne, whom he preferred to Jean Louis Balzac. In *Sorberiana* there are many references to those whom he calls the " great men of medicine "; but many of the names now seem unfamiliar. He says, " I have given Fernel the praise that is due him " . . . " I value highly the narratives and observations of Forestus, Zacutus, Amatus, and Platerus. I esteem the works of Vesalius, Spigelius, and Veslingius."

There are several references to William Harvey in his works. While Sorbière appears most willing to yield to Harvey a considerable measure of praise for his accomplishments, in the final analysis he fails to express himself frankly, either in opposition to or in support of Harvey's contentions on the circulation of the blood. This attitude was no doubt in part due to his sense of loyalty to Gassendi, Patin, and the other French opponents of Harvey's views.

Samuel Sorbière died on April 9, 1670, after an illness lasting three months. The terminal disease was a double pleurisy. He left a number of works in manuscript to his son, one of which, *Sorberiana,* achieved publication in 1694. Another was his *Avis à un jeune Médecin,* which was printed in 1672.

On August 8, 1938, while in the library of the British Museum, it occurred to me to look over the items in the catalogue under Sorbière, and note any new ones or any not before familiar to me. It was then that I found a copy of his *Avis,* 1672. The library press mark was 1038. e. 27. Its description and collation was as follows:

Small 16mo book, bound (rebound) in full leather, with covers loose and tied on with a string. The water-mark in the paper (endleaf) was the familiar bunch of grapes of that period. Collation: Title (2-¾" x 5-⅝"); verso stamp " Museum Britannicum," otherwise blank; " Au Lecteur," pp. ii-v; 7-138; " In Orbitum Samuelis Sorberii Odi," pp.[4]; Approbation, Permission, Consentement, pp. [11].

The French title reads as follows: (see fig. 2):

AVIS / A VN IEVNE / MEDECIN, / SVR / LA MANIERE DONT /
il se doit comporter en la pra / tique de la Medecine; vû la / negligence que
le Public a / pour elle, & les plaintes que / l'on fait des Medecins. / Par feu
Mr DE SORBIÈRE. / [Printer's device] / A Lyon, / Chez Antoine Offray, à
la descente du / Pont de Saône, du côté du Change. / [Rule] M. DC. LXXII.
/ Auec Approbation & Permission. /

A complete verbatim transcript of the text of this small book was made
by the writer in the course of two days, and from the French version thus
obtained a translation into English has been made. This translation
follows.

This work will be recognized as one of those left in manuscript by
Sorbière when he died in 1670, and published two years later by his son,
Henri de Sorbière. There were many obscurities of the French and Latin
texts, which cannot justly be assigned to a scholar of the standing of
Sorbière himself. One is led inevitably to the conclusion that the son, as
editor, was responsible for them, although the printer's carelessness, and
a much worn and broken font of type, may have contributed. This is
evidently one of the works referred to by François Graverol as " of no
great importance."

However, its interest to the medical historian, and its rarity, are perhaps
reasons enough for presenting the translation. It provides a picture of
the medical practice of an average physician of three hundred years ago,
with observations and comments by a man of superior intellect and intelligence. As to its rarity, not one of the fifteen medical-historical libraries
of this country, Great Britain, and Canada, possesses a copy of the book.
For ten years the writer has had a standing order for the *Avis* in the
hands of several booksellers in Europe, and no copy has been reported.

The identity of the " young physician " has been a matter of speculation,
but has not been solved. Could it have been the Justus Rickward of
Sorbière's letter of May 9, 1644?

Much of the advice given to his friend the " young physician " could
apply with equal cogency to present-day practice, but some of it seems a
mere pretext for bringing certain aspects of the medicine of the period
into derision, perhaps deservedly. Sorbière is well in advance of the
thought of his time in his condemnation of excessive bleeding, over
purgation, over dosage, and polypharmacy. Now and then there are
portions of his narrative which are sharply cynical or satirical. In
physiology and pathology his concepts are often purely Galenical and
obsolete, but in other instances he might well be reasoning on the basis of

knowledge available a century later than his own. However, in comparing his acumen about medicine in all its aspects with that of Jean Fernel, who lived a century earlier, one must admit that Sorbière is outranked by Fernel, for whose ideas he once expressed great scorn. Sir Charles Sherrington, in his remarkable book on Fernel's philosophy, remarks that Fernel's orientation to nature and religion was far more reasonable than that of many who came later, and among these we must include Sorbière, although he did assert that Reason and Faith are not opposed. As Professor Balz remarks, " because of Gassendist teachings, because of a faltering spirit, or because of inability to comprehend, Sorbière ignored the Cartesian position as to the necessary linkage of theology, metaphysics, and knowledge of nature."

II.

ADVICE TO A YOUNG PHYSICIAN RESPECTING THE WAY IN WHICH HE IS TO CONDUCT HIMSELF IN THE PRACTICE OF MEDICINE, IN VIEW OF THE INDIFFERENCE OF THE PUBLIC TO THE SUBJECT, AND CONSIDERING THE COMPLAINTS THAT ARE MADE ABOUT PHYSICIANS.

BY THE LATE M. DE SORBIÈRE

TO THE READER.

The sciences, which are at basis quite genuine and simple, become very often grounds for a thousand errors and a thousand abuses, arising from the slender knowledge which the public has of them, or from wrong usage. Medicine, whose origin is wholly worthy, is not exempt from these two shortcomings; it is neither known nor practiced according to the precepts of its founders. It is this state of affairs which has stimulated a learned man of this century to make known to one whom he admires, who is beginning the practice of medicine, the present-day failings of practice; and also to make him aware how far in these times this science functions through craft.

This small and liberal bit of writing has emerged from the cabinet of the late Monsieur de Sorbière. Everyone knows how his various works thus far published have won him the regard of all great men, both in this kingdom and in foreign lands; and as an indication of this it will suffice for us to state that the capital of the world has been witness of the favors, the esteem, and the liberality with which he was honored by Clement IX.

I. THE MOTIVE FOR THIS DISCOURSE.

Sir, since you have done me the honor to profess confidence in me, as you know that I am your admirer, and because you assume that my years have given me more experience than you as yet possess, I feel under an obligation to tell you two or three things which appear necessary in order to correct the bad impression I may have given you of your profession. Now and then you have heard me discuss the subject of medicine a little to its detriment. My desire to procure some advancement for it forces me often to just indignation towards those physicians who do not have at heart sufficiently the interests of that science.

AVIS
A VN IEVNE
MEDECIN,
S V R
LA MANIERE DONT
il se doit comporter en la pratique de la Medecine ; vû la negligence que le Public a pour elle , & les plaintes que l'on fait des Medecins.

Par feu M^r DE SORBIERE.

A LYON,
Chez Antoine Offray , à la descente du Pont de Saône, du côté du Change.

M. DC. LXXII.
Auec Approbation & Permission.

Fig. 2.

Facsimile reproduction (somewhat reduced) of the title-page of the only copy of *Avis à un Jeune Médecin*, 1672, which has been located. (Courtesy of the British Museum.)

II. HOW THE INDIFFERENCE OF THE PUBLIC WORKS A WRONG TO MEDICINE.

For my part, in my writings, I have tried to stress the importance of a public solicitude towards medicine. I have described the inconveniences which arise from the neglect with which the public has treated it. I have inveighed against the quacks, who have usurped the practice of it; and I have been moved to pity for those honorable men who have been obliged themselves to become quacks in order to make a living, or to have employment somewhat in the line of their profession. But you should not be disheartened over this condition. The fault does not rest wholly with the physician; they who are to blame the most oblige physicians to behave as they do. It is true that since those whose duty it is to regulate others, and who alone can remedy the shortcomings of medicine, do not reflect adequately upon the subject, we have no right to be shocked about it; all the more so since they are the sufferers from the irregularities and the dissensions in medicine which come to pass.

III. THAT IT IS NOT FOR ANY ONE INDIVIDUAL TO FIND THE REMEDY.

It is not for you, Sir, who comes before the public possessing intelligence and a knowledge of fine literature, who wishes to advance still further in the sciences, who loves particularly the study of natural history, and who wishes to avoid alienation from your chosen profession; it is not for you, I repeat, who should have some concern for your own interests, to correct the abuses which are found established in civil society. It is for society, which should take a greater share even than you in the health of its citizens, to institute additional measures, and issue a mandate that the science of medicine advance and progress from day to day more efficiently than it has hitherto done, and with more success in the alleviation of disease. You must not lay claim to practice medicine quite differently from others; and all that you should do is to conform to a style as soon as you can, or to a special habit of procedure, with good grace and the approval [of your confreres], each one of whom tried to do the same in order to achieve the promptest establishment of success. You must of course have in mind the cure of the sick, if you can attain to that, but you must also devote yourself to the advancement of your private affairs, and profit from the sale of commodities by which the public benefits.

IV. THAT BAD HABITS ARE NOT EASILY BROKEN OFF.

I have little doubt that before the invention of bread men were long content with acorns; and that even when wheat was sown and flour made, people might be found who had difficulty in deciding to abandon their earlier diet. Each nation has its customs and its deep-rooted absurdities from which it has no desire to swerve. I might recall many examples found among ourselves and in the most ordinary courtesies, presenting perhaps nothing more absurd than uncovering the head in all meetings, or in drinking each others health; thus suffering inconvenience without serving any other purpose. But I should have too much to do if I told you all that I have noticed under this heading, and it will suffice to mention what I heard from an old Scotchman. He assured me that the mountaineers of his country, who are still in a semisavage state, have not agreed to stop entirely the grinding of grain in a mortar, although they find the provision grist-mills very convenient. How true it is that one has much trouble to break off an old habit!

V. WHAT SHOULD BE THE BEHAVIOR OF A RESPECTABLE PHYSICAN?

Too frank and candid a manner, such as I am about to describe, might not be so successful in a young physician, whose practice as yet would not warrant such an attitude. For can you imagine him, Sir, having this conversation with a patient:—" Although I am disposed to be of service to you, and will undertake your cure as an end to be hoped for, and with God's help achieve success, in order to safeguard your interests, I must tell you that medicine is a very imperfect science, that it is quite full of guesswork, that it scarcely understands its subject matter, nor is it familiar with the things employed to maintain it; that the more enlightened only feel their way in it groping amidst a thick gloom; and that after having considered seriously all the matters which may be useful, collected all one's thoughts, examined all one's experiences, it will indeed be a wise physician who can promise relief to a poor patient." Furthermore, that he will hazard nothing new or very unusual in his case, and that if he is not cured, at least he will do all possible to make him no worse; that he will have his cure uppermost in his mind, and for the honor that will come to him and from the basis of affection which he has for him, will redouble his attentions to his person, and will think of him as much when away from as in his presence, proposing to study his case incessantly, and consult in his library the masters of medicine, and what they have to say about such a case; and finally, that [the patient] having done him the honor to confide in him about so important a matter, he will acquit himself of the duty so well, that if he returns to health as soon as he might wish, he begs him to continue to be the recipient of his friendship, and confirm anew that he yields this friendship to him.

VI. THAT HE WILL BE ILL-RECEIVED BY THE UNLEARNED.

Sir, how do you think that an ignorant person would receive such a speech, who, despite everything, would have to admit that it was the language of an honest man? He would conclude that his physician possessed neither education nor experience; that he had never looked into an anatomy, nor prescribed a remedy; for people usually think that if a doctor knows enough to mention the liver, the spleen, and the hypochondriac region, he knows exactly all the workings of our economy; and because he prescribes some wretched purgatives, they are persuaded that these drugs, in obedience to his behest, go to selected places in the diseased organs to draw out the humors that afflict them. In truth, Sir, I fear that the young physician might not have occasion to make a second visit to his patient, and that the latter would seek out another attendant who was more positive.

Although I sometimes inveigh against physicians, nevertheless I have no more than a slight appreciation of the deficiencies of medicine, and I flatter myself not infrequently with the thought that a science so essential to the welfare of life should make more certain that it is regarded with esteem. However, it is not likely that the public, which has made allowances for so many other things, is much concerned with this one. Moreover, such a reasonable view is predisposed to by common sense, above all when the help of medicine is needed. Nevertheless, it is very true that even the most skilful of physicians knows almost nothing about internal medicine, and if what he prescribes as a remedy occasionally yields a good effect, it is mere chance, since physicians practice by a certain routine, similar to that followed by the blind from the *Quinze-Vingts* [6] in going about the streets of Paris; or the blind of the provinces, who, not knowing in which direction to turn, would be in danger of being run down. But it is in the interest of everyone to praise those physicians who are above the common run in the practice of their art; even if they know but little of the substance of medicine, they are better than those who know it not at all. Does one not see how much more is known of the anatomy of the cadaver and of the body than was formerly the case? How many ruined palaces, how many cities levelled or beheld at such a distance that we can grasp nothing of them, but of which one would, nevertheless, like to write the history and relate narratives!

VII. THAT ONE MUST PUT UP WITH THE FOIBLES OF THE IGNORANT.

The people are not of this mind, and since, upon this assumption a patient deceives himself, and in fact wishes to be deceived, the physician runs little danger when making use of an innocent deception in promising him more than he is certain of achieving. The wise conversation of an eminent sceptic is too delicate a viand for the common mind, and it is very needful to guard against making use of it, except with the greatest care. To do so would be comparable to mixing too subtle an essence with grosser matter.

Perhaps it will be of more worth later in this dissertation to show what attitude one should assume in such a situation, mingling always a little assertion with a little of the fortitude of apprehension, and keeping always to a

---

[6] *Quinze-Vingts.* This was the name of a blind asylum in Paris. In *Sorberiana* Sorbière makes use of a similar illustration, saying, " Physicians, in their knowledge of physic, are like the *Quinze-Vingts* . . . who know nothing of the ins and outs of Paris. . . . Physicians do the same about the human body, of which they know the ways by I know not what routine, which conducts them happily where they wish to go, and to places they know nothing about."

certain middle course between hope and despair; for by measures such as these the skilful physician places his reputation in safety, and keeps the mind of his patient at ease. But it is given to few men to practice thus. What I say to you on this subject consists only of the fancies I have formed, like those one has about an orator, a prince, or a republic; and I have known scarcely anyone, nor you perhaps, except the late M. Walaeus and M. Vallot,[7] upon whose careers we might be able to erect such a model.

VIII. THAT ONE SUCCEEDS EQUALLY WELL BY DIFFERENT WAYS.[8]

However, many others have succeeded in reaching their goal by quite different methods, and perseverance is such a fine quality that in bending one's course constantly toward the same point, one arrives at the objective somehow; whereas those who advance, stopping from time to time, or who fall back, or try for a better way, may never arrive. Nothing matters except to follow steadily the same path; for all human prudence would consume itself uselessly in giving rules by which a physician might attain perfection in his art and gain much in reputation, rather than by another method. I have seen some with whom brusqueness has worked well, demanding of those who had the duty of meeting them, "Where is the patient?", and who, in questioning the patient, would speak as arrogantly as a magistrate might to a criminal at the bar. I have known others who have forged to the front through urbanity, good humor, and flattery. Felix's decoction, and earlier, his roadsters with their green saddle-cloths, and the four footmen in similar livery, all have contributed to make the life of this dashing man of Paris pass happily.[9] Another, in trotting about on foot all day, spouting a little Latin, has conducted his business so well that this language has been worth more to him than a hundred thousand crowns. In some circles a long beard and a solemn appearance in their possessors are regarded as evidence of deep learning, and render the physician having them to be much sought after. Piety, and even a

[7] Walaeus, or Jan de Wale (1604-1649), was the celebrated professor of anatomy in the University of Leyden, who by experiment confirmed Harvey's findings on the circulation of the blood. Antoine Vallot (1594-1671) was first physician to Anne of Austria when she was Queen Regent. Suddenly, in 1652, he entered the field of the scholar, became physician to Louis XIV, and published his *Hortus Regius* when administrator of the Jardin des Plantes. In his practice he used antimonial emetics, laudanum, and quinine, contrary to the general run of the faculty. His critics ceased their attacks when Astruc reported the cure of Louis XIV by an emetic wine.

[8] This chapter heading is a paraphrase of the title of Chapter 1 of the *Essays of Montaigne*, which reads: "That Men by Various Ways Arrive at the Same End."

[9] Charles François Felix de Tassy, d. 1705. He was surgeon to Louis XIV, whom he successfully cured by operation of a fistula-in-ano. In consequence of this success the social position of the French surgical class underwent a considerable improvement, and French surgery was rehabilitated.

cowl or a bracelet rosary, such as I have worn at [Rome, 1654 or 1667], have sometimes a similar effect, and yield virtue to the pumpkins, the mellow cheese, the boiled chestnuts, and to the other remedies issuing from such sources. And, on the other hand, there is the physician who has made it the fashion to represent himself a free-thinker, thus confirming what Pietro d'Abano, the Conciliator, alleged against the definition of a physician, *Medicus est vir bonus medendi peritus*,[10] when he said that this art cannot fail to produce vicious persons, because therapeutics is under subjection to astrology and to Venus, which only create the dissolute. With some only the memory of a much-esteemed name serves to make a cunning man out of a madman or a fool; with others an extensive library, a pallid countenance, a wild look, a very odd style of dress, or some such nonsense, have won a great reputation. And we have seen on the Pont Neuf a yellow ruff win over so many patrons from the practice of the tooth-drawers there, that when he was in turn encroached upon by his confreres, he brought suit against them and made them defend their practice; thus much is it true that people allow themselves to be taken in by outward appearances. It is well to be warned about these things, and then each one can help himself wisely.

IX. THAT THE PHYSICIAN HAS MORE NEED FOR POLITICS THAN ANY OTHER PROFESSIONAL.

There is no profession which asks more of a man than medicine. Neither the lawyer nor the clergyman has to win the good graces of those who consult them. The first has only to speak eloquently for his client; the other has only to utter some fine speeches to those he instructs, and, changing his tone when it seems desirable, permits himself to speak in a domineering way to the conscience of his auditor. One has the law on his side, the other has the Holy Scriptures and the Decrees of the Holy Councils.[11] One is the interpreter of his Prince, the other of the Envoy of God; they both speak with authority in imposing places and in ceremonial dress, whereas the physician presents himself in a chamber, dressed like any other man,[12] among women and the unlearned, with whom he is little reverenced. He has for guarantors only Galen and Hippocrates, and he speaks only about uncertain things, with which everyone thinks it is his right to be concerned, because each pretends to some power of reasoning and to some experience; which are the two wings

---

[10] " The doctor is a good man skilled in curing."

[11] The Holy Councils or Sacred Congregations of the Roman Catholic Church. The Envoy of God is the Pope.

[12] Before Sorbière's day the long-robed and short-robed barber fraternity had diminished in number and importance. Portraits of the 15th century still show the physician with the long robe, or a short fur-edged pelisse. Garrison states that when the surgeon was assimilated to the status of a physician he assumed the square cap and long robe of the latter.

of medicine, wings which scarcely lift it, or carry it far. Therefore the physician has more need to be clever than the others. He must be constantly on duty, and he has always to be careful to avoid the snares set for him on all sides. For him, and for those who have the honor to serve Princes, there are only the old guides, who can speak out with authority, making game of mockery, and imposing silence to the endless contradictions met with at every turn in this conjectural science. Others have to be all submission and employ all their wits in seeking to please the patient, as well as his attendants. To be sure, it is sometimes difficult to succeed on a first meeting, so on the second the aim should be to win the confidence of the patient; and since one esteems the things that one understands the least, on these occasions the wise physician always has a few doses of nonsense to bestow.

X. THE PHYSICIAN SHOULD MAKE USE OF DIFFERENT VARIETIES OF NONSENSE.

He should do this with prudence, adroitly serving up those bits which appear to him to be more to the liking of those who listen. Thus, among the people and with the persons who are familiar only with the philosophy of the schools, the Galenic varieties will suffice; provided the physician sets them off with several quotations from his Hippocrates. With others, according to their tastes, he will use Hermes Trismegistus, Paracelsus, and Van Helmont; and he will mention something of the new philosophy, with which, it will be appreciated, the practice of medicine accords perfectly well. Then he will finish where he began, by making a few compliments, and extending his very best wishes for recovery. In taking their leave of a patient, I have known physicians to speak in such a manner, and I noted that it was not badly received: that what he had just touched on in a few words, about the practice of medicine, which he aimed to adhere to, was not infallible; nevertheless, he believed that God would bless their remedies; that such would be granted in answer to the prayers of good people, and that the faithful services rendered to his Divine Majesty, as well as zeal and assiduity in worship, would supplement fully any imperfections of medicine. Then in asking for the name of the apothecary from whom the medicine must come, the physician added that he was happy to have such a man, for he was very certain to have excellent drugs; and concluded with assurances of the happy success of his good intentions.

XI. THE FOUR SECTS OF MEDICINE.

Sir, you may not be averse to the method of mingling in the sick room with a crowd of distressed, boring, and often impertinent persons, and perhaps it would be good also for all the sects of medicine, the Empirics, the Methodists, the Chemiatrists, and the Rationalists, which latter is a mixture of all that is worthy in the first three, to make similar contacts, for they would not find there anything contrary to their maxims. I place the Chemical sect in this list because today it is better regarded than it was when Galen strove against the other two sects in order to establish the Rational, and when Ausonius said, *Triplex forma medendi, quae logos, et methodos, cuique experimentia nomen.*[13]

You know better than I, who have forgotten almost all such things, what these sects were, and the clamor they have made in the schools. I am quite content to refresh my memory a little about them, and that is why I have requested you to accept what I have assembled here in a short review of my ancient studies, and of my own thoughts, for I have always been inclined to indulge in reflections upon what is instructive to me.

XII. THE EMPIRICS.

We must give the Empirics precedence, for neither Serapion, Philinus, Heraclides of Tarentum, Menodotus, Glaucias, nor Apollonius among the Greeks, nor Celsus or Pliny among the Latins, have been the originators of this sect. It is as ancient as man and the other animals; and since their creation until now they have always been retained within it. It serves them even more than our own special tricks serve us, for our distillations, our systems, our arguments, and our experiments do not provide us with remedies more reliable than those suggested to them by instinct. We should have done as they do in seeking out certain remedies for certain maladies; going at once to nature for those that were necessary to them; but we have been unfortunate in failing to search for remedies, or in trying many that were useless or injurious. The serpents choose fennel, the swallows celandine, the weasel rue, the stork marjoram, the wild boar ivy, the elephant wild olive, the partridge laurel, the dog graminaceous plants, the crane rush, and the fowl wall plant. The " signature "[14] of the plants has no association with the above, and there is so little evidence in what is revealed to us about the remedy for the part affected, that what we have that is rational on some plants, lists of which Crollius and others have made, is indeed very little and of small utility. Whatever the conditions, I am not an enemy of the Empirical system. I love its experiments, and I serve it willingly, but I wish that it might be on surer

---

[13] Decimus Magnus Ausonius (310-395 A. D.) was a poet and rhetorician, and held a consulship under the Emperor Gratian, whose tutor he was. The text of Ausonius quoted runs somewhat differently in the modern editions. The passage occurs in *Griphus ternarii numeri* [A riddle of the number three], as follows: *triplex quoque forma medendi, cui logos aut methodos cuique experimentia nomen, et medicina triplex: servare, cavere, mederi.* [Medicine also has a triple form of healing, namely, theory, orderly procedure, and experience; and medicine in aim is triple: preserve health, prevent disease, and heal].

[14] The doctrine of *signatures*, by virtue of which a remedy was applied on account of some fancied resemblance, in color or shape, to the disease, such as turmeric for jaundice, was developed by Paracelsus.

grounds, particularly when it fails to confine itself to topical subjects, and when it ventures to try internal remedies. Let us pass to the other sects.

XIII. THE METHODISTS.

Methodism, which has grown from the Rational sect, as a result of distaste felt for the Empiricists, was the sect to which Themison and Thessalus tended. The Methodists sought to avoid the trouble of experiments, in order not to embarrass their endless rules, among which there was inconsistency. They believed that all maladies are to be attributed to two causes, either obstructions or relaxations of the natural channels. Thus, for a cure it was only required to open or close these by remedies with the requisite qualities. If the Methodists had known about the circulation of the blood, and the irradiation of the nerve force, they would have been well confirmed in their opinion. But I cannot yield my approval of the moderation of their views when they declined to make a more careful investigation of the economy of the human body, as if Herophilus and Erasistratus had labored in vain, or were regarded as too cruel, because they did dissections on the living bodies of criminals given them, in order the better to know the conformation and movement of the organs. This was the only method they had for instruction, from which perhaps at some time, at the price of expending a small number of scoundrels, relief could be extended to numberless innocent and worthy people, who could be cured if the nature of their diseases could be discerned. But even the learned have not yet accepted this view, having up to the present time spared those by false clemency who have spared nothing to gratify their unruly passions, or satisfy their selfish interests.

What Galen sought to accomplish by inveighing against the Methodists is worthy of praise, although he has not been very fortunate in discoveries himself, and has not done much better than they have in binding medicine to broader views. But he opened up the field in his Asiatic style, and he was a man well found in reasoning powers, as well as in experience. His writings contain a quantity of good things for which we are obligated to him. It is a pity that a man of such fine mind did not have the benefit of all the advances which have occurred since his days, nor the aid of the newer discoveries in anatomy, and those in medicinal plants and mineral drugs which the chemists now have among their wares.

XIV. THE CHEMICAL SECT.

The Chemical sect has made up a third division in medicine, and they have become famous by virtue of their wise men, rather than because they wished to discourse on their performances. Their methods comprise no more than analyses and syntheses, brought about by means of heat or by some solvent, about which they do not know very much, either of the action of the process or of the means of regulating it; or not as much as they claim. I have spoken on this subject at length and emphatically in one of my papers, and also on the subject of Glauber, whom I used to see in Amsterdam, so I will not take up again with you what I have already given to the public. It suffices to say that the Chemists are honest artisans who have improved on pharmacy, but who, having been a little more removed than the apothecaries from dissolving and precipitating mixtures, have too soon believed themselves to have reached the final steps in the analyses of substances.

The Peripatetic Philosophers thence derived the four elements. The Chemists resolved the elements into their principles, and in the end believed that salt, sulphur, and mercury were the first principles. But perhaps they are themselves no less deceived than persons who in grammar, being superior only in a knowledge of words to those who divided a language into sentences, believed that they had arrived at the first elements of this science, and boasted of such a discovery. Nevertheless, a word can be divided into syllables, and syllables can be reduced to letters, which would hold much sooner the place of first principles. It is to be presumed also that the Chemists have only gone a step beyond the Peripatetics; and that to go from salt, sulphur, and mercury up to the first principles, there are numerous successions of analyses to pass, which we do not know how to perform, and which we cannot comprehend. This sort of talk, which constitutes the arguments of the Chemists, is so shallow and so frivolous, that I would be ashamed to enter upon it with you. Paracelsus and his fellows of the Chemical sect have done no more than invent high-sounding words, from which they have formed a jargon beneath which they hide the mysteries of their art, and which being interpreted signify nothing by which one may be better served than by the Galenists; although they have made a pretence of taking a stand against these doctors. The Chemists have substituted for the four elements their three principles, with the qualities, the forms, and images of substances, within which knowledge they have included all anatomy, in such a way that to understand medicine well one has only to know the agreement there is between a microcosm and a macrocosm; and in order to practice it, how to join like things together, which is the opposite of the maxim of the others, that contraries are cured by contraries.[15]

XV. THE RATIONALIST SECT.

Although these good people of the Chemical sect are not wholly to be despised, considering the trouble they take, not faltering or failing in their

---

[15] The Galenic doctrine of *contraria contrariis curantur* was violently attacked by Paracelsus and Cardan, who substituted their doctrine of similars. The old Paracelsian doctrine of signatures and similars received a modified revival in Samuel Hahnemann's *similia similibus curantur*.

zeal of working before their furnaces, I would advise you to adhere to the Rationalist sect, as it is called, or the Reasonable, which is that of Galen and Hippocrates, under whose banners you are enrolled. It is undoubtedly the most learned one, and provided that it is not too dogmatic, it will carry you a long way, and more honorably toward the secrets of nature, than will the others. But it is not necessary to do, as I saw some physicians do, at the home of M. de Montmor,[16] who did not take sufficient interest to more than glance at the dissection which the anatomist Pecquet was making to demonstrate the course of the lacteals; nor [is it necessary] to make such a reply as another physician did to this illustrious promotor of the arts and sciences, at whose home we were assembled, when he was trying to show to one of the most famous physicians of Paris the circulation of the blood and the structure of the animal system, which is so beautiful a scheme. " Really," said this elderly doctor, " this seems excellent to me, and I intend to advise some younger man to defend it in the schools, in order to enliven the discussions with such a neat paradox."

Take good care, Sir, to avoid committing such an impropriety; and since the Reasonable sect is founded on reason and experiment, do not think that these are cut and dried, or that there is no longer anything to be discovered, as the older practitioners attempt to persuade themselves. Be positive, I tell you, whenever necessary, and above all do not allow your interest in natural history, or for those things yet to be discovered, to be stifled. And remember what a wise man of Greece had for a motto, " that he became learned in growing old, and that he grew old in learning." You have joined yourself to a philosophy which has a passion for new discoveries, and which has known how to profit from them. Never refuse those which are presented to you, if you have not been fortunate enough to make them yourself, since you would then be able to demonstrate them; and to this practice you must all your life tend. Do not ever, I pray you, get weary of making dissections, of examining remedies, and of reflecting over the causes of disease, founded on the hypotheses you know, and in a mechanical manner, removed from metaphor, allegory, abstraction, and nonsense, although, to entertain you with this last, which I repeat must be employed, it will be well for you to review every day a few pages of your Perdulas,[17] or of the author in whose works you have made your first studies in medicine.

---

[16] Hubert de Montmor was president of the Academy of Physicians in Paris, and dean of the Master of Requests.

[17] *Perdulas.* This may have been some sort of a compendium of medicine. Its derivation is not known.

XVI. THAT IT IS NECESSARY TO GAIN OVER THE SYMPATHIES OF THE PATIENT.

I wish indeed that you might feel a reluctance to follow my counsel, but if it is not less true to declare, *argutiarum omnia plena*, that is to say, *stultorum omnia plena*,[18] why is there sometimes difficulty in joining yourself to the larger number? And so what danger is there in speaking like the others, by contributing something to the scene in which we live, and adjusting ourselves to the methods of practice which are the fashion, and gathering all the advantages one can over the imagination of those with whom we have to deal? For it cannot be doubted that such measures serve to hasten the recovery of the sick, since not only the mind suffers, but it is very often the mind which makes the body suffer; witness the impressions which the caprices of pregnant women transmit to their children, and the cures which have resulted from sensations of joy and of fear when these passions have been excited by chance or design in the imaginations of the very ill. You know the story of the dying cardinal, who in some way was resuscitated following an outburst of laughter which possessed him, when he saw that his servants, who were in his chamber, had brought his monkey with them, and the monkey, at their invitation, had taken the cardinal's red hat and placed it on its head.

XVII. THAT THE IMAGINATION OF THE PATIENT MAY DO MUCH TO BENEFIT HIM.

At this point I might consider more at length those cures which arise from a strong imagination, from charms and talismans, and by bringing forward certain words, or by practicing certain actions which would appear to have no relation to the effects which they produce, and explain to you my ideas on what are called the sympathies and the antipathies of things; and then relate to you in one way or another what I have seen occur sometimes when the " abracadabra "[19] has cured tertian fevers, and tell of others who feel themselves lost unless they do something like taking a pinch of the first herb they find, in a glass of white wine. I have seen the toothache stopped by driving a nail into a letter of the word " Maccabees," written on a board. It is said also that a horse will be pricked in the foot by a nail, if a nail be driven into one of the horse's footprints; and it is believed even today that the first wolf seen causes the voice to disappear; and that bad luck comes to the sheepfold if one meets with a lamb. Vida[20] tells of a peasant whom he had seen at Viterbo, who had the reputation, not only of causing the death of all the

---

[18] " All are full of subtleties " that is to say " all are full of follies."

[19] *Abracadabra.* A cabalistic word written triangularly and worn to cure an ague.

[20] Marco Giralamo Vida (c. 1489-1566), an Italian scholar and Latin poet. He was born in Cremona and died in Alba.

insects, (which might not be a bad accomplishment), but also of all the plants in the garden, by merely gazing at them. There was danger that he might bring about a general desolation of the vegetation in passing through the country.

Nam quocumque aciem horribilem intendisset, ibi omnes
Cernere erat subito afflatos languescere flores.[21]

Several years ago one of our friends led into an assembly of physicians, meeting at the home of M. de Montmor, one of those horses suggestive of a hobgoblin; the horse carried a note in his mane, which note stated that lacking it he would walk lame. We abstracted the note, but nothing happened. In Flanders I have several times seen silver offered to a German soldier in exchange for a charm he had to protect him from musket-balls. He would permit anyone to fire a pistol shot at his arm; something he might not have cared to do without a charm. Eventually they tried it out on a dog which lived on the place. If one believed the popular delusions about these things, then the wounds of the dead would open and bleed in the presence of the murderer; the castrated cocks would die in the presence of a man who holds and presses upon one of his own testicles. But let us leave all these fabulous beliefs with what is called the Powder of Sympathy, and with the pretended communication of the vital forces of the wounded with the particles of vitriol which go to meet each other along the length of the thread, which cannot be seen, but which nothing interrupts. I do not wish to enter upon a discussion of all these superstitious practices, which for the most part are dreams of the Cabalists,[22] and which arise perhaps from a false and unfortunate imitation which the father of lies [23] has introduced to render the omnipotence of God suspect in the work of creation.

XVIII. THAT IT IS NECESSARY TO AROUSE THE PASSIONS, ABOVE ALL, JOY.

To return then to the condescension which one must sometimes extend to the sick, and to the skill with which the wise physician should bring feelings into play, even the violent ones as well as those that are milder, I will cite to you what I have read in past days in your Roderico a Castro,[24] concerning a case of prolapse of the uterus. He states that he had seen this organ restored to its normal position, by producing a red-hot iron and making a pretense of

---

[21] " For wherever he had directed his terrible ray. there it was possible to see the flowers languish beneath the sudden blast."

[22] The Cabalists were the followers of a mystic speculative system of philosophy which flourished from the 10th to the 16th century.

[23] " The father of lies " was Beelzebub, or the Devil.

[24] Rodericus a Castro was a Jewish physician who wrote a treatise on gynecology, published in Hamburg in 1603.

260

applying it to the patient. In a similar instance Horace's physician [25] awoke him from his miserly lethargy by making him open his coffers by the bedside and count his money. Gouty patients have been given wings to flee their chambers upon a fire breaking out. When you desire I will induce one of my friends to tell you how he was cured of a sciatica, which had kept him confined to his bed, by an access of anger which made him forget his helpless condition, and permitted him to grab a stick and chase after one of his servants who had been insolent to him. One has seen people of consequence, rich and miserly, who found themselves improved by having their caskets brought before them, from which they spread out their jewels; just as among well-to-do children, to whom when ill, golden chains and other trinkets are given. It is because joy is the greatest remedy there is for good health, or better expressed, it is joy and what arouses it which contribute to the perfect organization of our body. The body must be looked upon as a machine with an infinity of channels. The grosser humors are returned through certain channels, some of the more subtle materials being delivered to the muscles. One must imagine that the vital forces penetrate the body, restore the membranes, breathe through the pores, and sustain animal life by reason of their action. As long as this action is neither too strong nor too feeble, so long will it do no injury to the organs but give them just enough impulse and maintain them in a state of well-being, just as an organ concert is in correct tune when the stops are open and the wind is distributed properly and at a certain rate. I have no doubt at all that with fear and with sadness, and in the more material illnesses, there is some failure in the irradiation of the vital forces, which forces do not flow in an even manner; or they encounter obstacles in their movement. Joy seems to exert such an effect on them that it opens the pores and enables the vital forces to pass to parts where they had not previously penetrated,[26] all of which is quite evident to the eye; and one may notice how the countenance takes on a heightened and more lively color when such a passion is dominant; whereas one sees the vital spirits disappear when sadness and fear are present, the latter acting as if they closed the doors through which these spirits are accustomed to pass.

---

[25] Horace's physician was Antonius Musa. He was also physician to the Emperor Augustus.

[26] This pretentious explanation of the physiology (or pathology) of the body, under the influence of joy or fear, harks back to Asclepiades, or to Galen's commentaries on Asclepiades, whose theory asserted that the tissues of the body are pierced with innumerable invisible pores incessantly traversed by atoms, and the various vital phenomena were produced by passage of these atoms through the pores, disease ensuing when the course of the atoms was changed either by dilatation or contraction of the pores.

XIX. DESIRABLE ACCOMPLISHMENTS IN A PHYSICIAN.

Sir, I am led to reflect that with all the fine intrinsic qualities which you possess, outwardly agreeable, with neatness, and an unpretentious humor, it will not be difficult for you to attract a clientele. I am reminded that Michel de Montaigne said that a clever physician advised him to associate with a convivial person with a high color, good humor and good temper, in order to ward off a marasmus and extricate him from the debility of that condition, into which he was about to fall.[27]

If an ophthalmia is contagious, and if what nurses believe is true, elderly persons take away the color from their children's faces when they kiss them; contrariwise, it might well be that a smiling face, a fine appearance, a pleasing voice, and neatness in a physician would contribute to the well-being of a patient, by drawing the vital spirits to the surface through the joy he inspires. Generally that is what happens when it is said of certain physicians that they are more successful in their practice than are others, and they are more sought after because they are more agreeable and more tactful; and from these facts it follows that they have more success with their patients. I do not mean to say that there are not other physicians whom I know, whose native sagacity, particular aptitude in choosing remedies and in diagnosis are not found equally in all medical circles, and who, like the others, manage excellently in these directions and in prognostics. Be that as it may, knowing this, and finding the other intrinsic qualities in two physicians, I would prefer the one who was in the prime of life, who carried himself well, and who possessed gay spirits, to a sulky and forbidding old man who comes into my room coughing, and who retires from it, leaving me with thoughts of Charon or Rhadamanthus.[28]

I do not say, Sir, that I would prefer to such a one a young man who was a little too condescending, who spoke affectedly too much, and who deafened me with his idle talk. I want neither the chatterer, who makes his patient apprehensive of a second illness, nor the taciturn one who has no elegance of discourse whatever; nor him who finds only mirth in mishaps; nor him who always knits his brow; nor him who wears too fine apparel; nor him who comes wearing dirty linen, and who sets all the dogs of the house to barking; nor him who with perfumes of musk and ambergris makes the ladies faint when he approaches; nor him who chews tobacco, or who exhales some more villainous odor. I would desire my physician to have a sweet

---

[27] It was Montaigne himself whom the physician Simon Thomas recommended to visit one of his patients possessing the convivial qualities described.

[28] Charon, son of Erebos, conveyed in his boat the shades of the dead across the rivers of the lower world. He is represented as an aged man with a dirty beard and a mean dress. Rhadamanthus was the son of Zeus and Europa. After his death he became one of the judges of the lower world.

breath, and I would not disapprove if he always had a cachou in his mouth. I should take pleasure in seeing him with a well-composed countenance, a little pensive, suggesting anxiety over my illness, study me quite leisurely, speak to me amiably, propose remedies with honest assurance, and finally tell me diverting stories. I do not require of a physician that he never converse about anything except medicine, and I am very glad that without losing sight of that subject, he make some digressions into the news of the day, or about ancient history, or about such other matters which he knows I am interested in; and I desire greatly that he unfold with good grace some pleasant story to make me laugh. But if all that is to my liking, it is perhaps not to that of others, and I do not object at all if you proceed differently with those patients who always want the physician to be serious, austere, and gloomy. The greater number in an ignorant world would lose the respect they have for the sciences if they understood them, and for virtue if they should see it spritely. It is on account of this perhaps, that Heraclitus affected obscurity in these matters.

Clarus ob obscuram linguam magis inter inaneis manes,
Quam de graneis inter Graios, qui vera requirunt.[29]

And with a similar intention, Zeno in his time, cultivated a long beard.

XX. THE UNCERTAINTIES OF THE VIEWS ON THE VEINS AND THE PULSE.

In order to accommodate oneself to the credulity of ignorant people, who are curious to know the conditions and the results of an illness, it has been necessary to make a pretence of learning by an inspection of the urine, far more than it can reveal, or more than is yet to be discovered by an inspection of this fluid; for it is nothing but a serous fluid impregnated with salts filtered from the kidney and going to the bladder, which may indicate the condition of these parts, and very obscurely show the contents of the mass of the blood, whence they have been separated from the circuit it has made from the arteries to the emulgent veins in following the great course of the circulation. Nevertheless, one wishes that from it one could guess the state of all the rest of the body, and could learn from it all that was to happen to the body. This method of observing the urine has given rise to a thousand jests, made at the expense of those physicians who have endeavored to express judgment from a method so uncertain.

One wishes also that more things might be deduced from the arterial pulsations than at present can be inferred; whether they come from the

---

[29] " Distinguished for his obscure tongue, a shade among the shades, rather than for his serious studies among the Greeks, who seek the truth." Heraclitus was a Greek philosopher of c. 540-475 B. C. Zeno was the stoic philosopher, born 488 B. C.

impulse of the blood when the arteries are filled, or are made by a dilatation of these vessels, which have a sort of elasticity. I fear that what is known about this subject may not be very far advanced, and that all this enumeration of the various sorts of pulse, more than thirty, and from which an infinity of others is fashioned, may be created to no purpose and be devoid of evidence; for I defy two physicians who shall have felt at different times the pulse of the same person, to give it the same name, or to make the same description of it. I am sure that each will name it according to his fancy, or according to the diverse names brought forward in his memory. There are almost never two individuals, either sick or well, in whom exactly similar pulsations will occur, and each has his own pulse so far, even as to rate, that I have seen it happen that one observer counted eighteen or nineteen, while the other reported the pulse-rate twelve or thirteen, although seemingly both of them had carried out the examination equally well. There is not at all any fixed standard for this movement, and so the very short time used in feeling the artery is not, in my opinion, either of great value or of great utility. But nevertheless, it is a procedure one must practice, and I do not despair that in time we may be able to derive advantage from it, more than at present; besides, nothing should be neglected in a matter so obscure and for an end so noble and important. For is it not a species of resurrection which medicine undertakes in the cure of the sick?

XXI. ON THE NOBILITY OF MEDICINE.

I speak freely about the nobleness of our art, seeing that it was Pliny,[30] who in some places has treated medicine quite harshly, but who in another passage has said of medicine, *Unam artium, quae imperatoribus quoque imperat.*[31] Before Pliny the *Holy Writing* [*Ecriture Sainte*] had commanded that it be honored, and declared that the King will make gifts to it, that medicine will be exalted by him, and praised in the sight of the great men of all his court.[32] And then there was your Hippocrates, who when the King of Persia sent for him to attend his Premier, Abteritaino, refused to go, saying that he cared more for wisdom than he did for a treasure of gold; but he exposed himself willingly to cross the seas with others called to succor one of the wisest men of the world, Democritus. According to Pliny, Erasistratus, grandson of Aristotle, received from Ptolomeus a recompense of one hundred

---

[30] Pliny the Elder, born 23 A. D. He perished in the eruption of Vesuvius in 79 A. D.

[31] " One art which gives orders, even to emperors."

[32] This refers to the *Words of Wisdom* by Jesus, son of Sirach (Sira), who lived in the first half of the second century B. C. Garrison, in his *History of Medicine* gives the whole quotation, as follows: " Honor a physician according to thy need of him, with the honors due unto him: for verily the Lord hath created him: for from the Most High cometh healing; and from the King he shall receive a gift. The skill of the physician shall lift up his head: and in the sight of great men he shall be admired."

talents, which in our money, according to Bude [Budée of Halberstadt], would be sixty thousand crowns, for having cured his father, King Antiochus. Crinas of Marseilles left means to build the walls of the city, besides other buildings which he caused to be erected at prodigious expense. Louis XI gave up 6000 crowns every month to his physician, Jacques Cottier. A king of India offered as a pledge to Garcias ab Horto the sum of forty thousand crowns. Pierre Texera reports that the Grand Mogul offered nearly a hundred thousand crowns to Mizarene. Philip II gave his physician Valesius six thousand crowns for an illness of seven days.

XXII. THAT THE PHYSICIAN IS NOT ORDINARILY WELL RECOMPENSED.

Despite all the above, it is only too true that the physician is usually very poorly compensated; and moreover, this is one of the reasons why medicine is very badly practiced; for physicians must run about after several patients at the same time in order to make the liberality of the few recoup them for the ingratitude of the many; whereas, it might be preferable for them to engage themselves to a small number of sick, two or three perhaps, as being calculated quite enough to occupy a physician who might wish to observe accurately all the symptoms which arise, and all the effects produced by the remedies ordered for them. It might even be desirable for all measures to be administered by his own hands, since physicians are very badly served, and very ill-informed about what passes in a situation where they have every right to rule. I have often remarked that they do not dare even to put questions about matters needful for them to know, and that they are contented to ask in a wholesale manner if the patient has slept, and what food he has taken, with nothing said, however, about the things we call non-natural, such as rest, excretion, or failure of excretion, state of the mind, temperature of the air, and an infinity of conditions about which the physician should be informed, and from ignorance of which one makes dangerous mistakes. For it cannot be doubted that bleedings and purgations ordered at the wrong time, and carried out after certain other evacuations, or after certain practices, have often cost the lives of those who would have been well advised if they had done nothing except sleep, take a little sustaining nourishment, or a small amount of some cordial to restore promptly their well-being, or to calm their agitation. Thus the wish that physicians should not be so inquisitive, the dislike of variety in remedies, contempt for the simpler ones, fear of the expense of the more elaborate ones, disobeying the physician, doubt of his zeal or his competency, and calling several into consultation at the same time: all this, I assert, has caused much disorder in the practice of medicine and admirably clears the physicians of blame. I wish to say only two or three words on some of these matters.

XXIII. CONSULTATIONS.

Consultations are the most ill-conceived affairs in the world, unless one resolves when attending one of them to lose the friendship of the physician whose advice is not followed. For it is certain, from the way men are constituted, and in view of the liking they have for their own views, that if the advice of the first physician, ordinarily opposed by the consultant, is not followed, the former will do all that he can not to cooperate, or at least he will not be annoyed if things go badly, or that regret exists for not allowing him to carry on. The remedy that might be brought to bear, for your own interest, if you possessed between you sufficiently good intelligence, would be never to contradict the attending physician, and to confirm all his actions, continuing all that he has undertaken before passing on to measures which he (the consultant) might propose, both thus yielding their reciprocal approval and approbation. Perhaps this consideration will not be without benefit to the patient, in view of the uncertainty of remedies, any one of which is scarcely worth more than another; at least it will tranquillize the by-standers who have heard the discussion, and will always be excellent policy for the physician. But the ambition and vanity of wishing to appear more knowing than another is often of more consequence to some than are these considerations, and at the expense of the patient.

XXIV. ON THE DISAGREEMENT BETWEEN PHYSICIANS AND APOTHECARIES, WHICH HAS DONE AWAY WITH THE SPECIFIC REMEDIES.

I wish to state also that the variance of views which has arisen between physicians and apothecaries has done great harm to medicine, because physicians now confine themselves to one or two remedies only, senna, syrup of pale roses and that of peach flowers, opium, and emetic wine; these, with bleeding and injections being all that the greater number employ in all varieties of illness, whereas the cordials and specifics have become almost unheard of in present-day practice, to such an extent that all that is done for internal maladies consists only in the withdrawal of blood from the veins by phlebotomy and the emptying of the lower bowel by purgatives. In this practice one can easily fall into excesses. It is perhaps not always necessary to clean out the bowel to such an extent, for some pool must remain in this part, and some humors in the mesentery to serve as a leaven for the agitations which should occur in these parts. And further, the blood stream should not be dried up or depleted, in order that there remain enough force to drive the blood through the smallest vessels and by obstructions in them, as in the manner sometimes observed when rain-water is held back in the street, and afterwards made to flow more forcibly to carry away by pressure the mud which fills it, by thinning it out in the stream with a rake. It appears that our sour-tempered thinkers aim to achieve this effect in the veins by these antidotes [purgatives and bleeding], which suppress some poisons by a sort of incrustation, or by some alteration in shape [of the vessels], by some property which belongs to them. But there is no occasion for me to explain this matter further, since I have testified elsewhere to the apprehension I feel about frequent blood-letting, which has suppressed the crises of illnesses where it has been employed. I am almost certain that it shortens gradually the lives of those who are subjected to it, and emphatically that it is only practiced with impunity by the merest chance in the world; for one cannot hold to any standard in phlebotomy, either as to quantity or to time, or to the place where it is to be done. Up to the present time no rules have been established on the subject, so that it is dependent upon the caprice of him who orders it.

The temerity of apothecaries who dabble in the dispensing of remedies without the orders of a physician has been open to censure, and it was right to curb it. But really the revenge that has come from the practice has been cruel, and the public who has been sent to the market-place, to the apothecary shops, enticed there by some economy, has renounced thoughtlessly the help that could come to them from the cordials and specifics, which are undoubtedly prepared more easily by the apothecaries, from which procedure physicians have come to abstain almost entirely. Either they dare no more to hazard anything themselves, or they do not care to take the trouble to prepare remedies, or because they are not all equally adroit in putting up these preparations; in addition to which they are so jealous of those prepared by others, that a man of quality whom I will not name, but who is well known to you for his highmindedness and curiosity, told me a short story in days gone by, the principals in which I will name to you whenever you wish. One of his neighbors having been seized with an apoplexy, his family sent to ask for a small quantity of an elixir, which being strongly alcoholic has often revived for some time persons who were in deep lethargy to whom it was given. At the least it served to prepare them for death (and that indeed is the chief thing for the good of the soul), by putting them into a condition to think of salvation, and enable them to make arrangements in their domestic affairs. He gave them rather liberally of his remedy, and they were on the point of taking it to the sick man, when the physician, who arrived unexpectedly, opposed its administration, saying that the patient was his, and that he wished to see first what course the malady would take. The course that it took was that the patient died in a few hours from then, and in a miserable state, devoid of all consciousness, from which neither bleeding nor emetics could ever recall him. This story reminds me of another in my experience, and I will share it with you, to avoid finishing with one which is so distressing. A gentleman of my acquaintance finding that his brother was on the point of death, at all events given up by his physicians, and deprived of all sensibility, decided to give him undiluted wine, then spirits of wine in liberal amount, which having restored him forthwith, those who were present had nothing more urgent to suggest than exhort the sick man to think of God; whereupon the young man, whose mind was troubled and whose temper was naturally fiery, only responded with great extravagance of expression. His brother was very angry with him, and wondered for a time if he was inflamed with a new frenzy; but finally noting the effects of his remedy in restoring the powers of the patient, resolved to give him a second dose, believing that the disorder could not develop further, and that it might be able to effect a new performance of nature that would put matters back again where they belonged. The enterprise succeeded happily, and the dying gentleman is still full of life, despite the prognosis of his physician, through the use of this crude and military restorative.

XXV. CONCLUSION, OPPOSING THE NEGLIGENCE OF THE PUBLIC.

And in all these considerations, Sir, the little attention paid by the public to an art to which one must necessarily have recourse, and which is concerned not less with life than with good health, excuses the attitude assumed by physicians, when they withdraw, each to his own side, caring only for the advancement of their own affairs in the way best calculated to achieve this, or by the more beaten track. They are no more to be blamed in this practice then, since the public is willing that the subject remain where it is, still in the infancy state. No one is any longer astonished over their being at variance over this question; being in considerable numbers and so poorly paid, they must have some employment. No one mocks them any more for their fantastic ideas, or for their frivolous talk, since there is no other language to substitute for theirs. No one is any longer insulted by their ignorance, since the public suffers patiently all the evils that it produces, and because it is very difficult to remedy them effectively, although it may not be wholly impossible. Advice would have to be taken on this subject from intelligent and sensible persons, who have no interest in it except on behalf of the public, and the matter well merits the trouble.

XXVI. HOPES FOR THE ADVANCEMENT OF MEDICINE.

The solicitude that one might be able to inspire in princes to take in the subject of medicine, as well as in commerce, and in the reform of chicanery, might perhaps not be unworthy of them, nor very prejudicial to their reputation. For even if it were not necessary to speak of Phoebus [Apollo] in a matter so serious, nor have recourse at this point to Aesculapius and his sons Podalirius and Machaon, it is certain that Mesua, son of Abdela, King of Damascus, and Avicenna, Prince of Cordova, Sabra and Mithridates, are themselves made celebrated in posterity through medicine, and there are some herbs which still preserve the names of Artemisia and Lysimachus. It is not that I

6

might have a fancy to persuade a great king, occupied in administering justice to his people, watching the schemes of his neighbors, and giving orders about other things of this importance, to descend to the details of medicine. But since it suffices for commercial companies to have their directors, so for war purposes he [the king] directs his commissaries; and as he sometimes takes over the care of his arsenals to prevent fraud, it might indeed be sufficient for a judicious prince, whatever the state of his health and that of his people might be, to give a glance of his eye over the art which assumes to maintain health; and that he summon experts to advise him what should be done in this direction. But it is a Utopian dream! Be that as it may, Sir, to return to what concerns you, and to tell you what I think, if I had like you to practice medicine, I would be of a mind to speak in this way to an intelligent patient, and above all on my first visit. The discourse perhaps would be well tolerated by a liberal man, and, at any rate, if I was not obeyed, I would withdraw from the business, something which happens quite often with physicians.

Here is what I would say to the patient:

" Sir, if you have the intention of not doing much with remedies in your illness, or of doing nothing at all, and allowing nature to operate, which cures maladies, as our Hippocrates bears witness, you could not have applied to a person who enters more willingly into your design, and would be more prompt than I am to praise the patience and courage that you exhibit in this firm resolution. If you are of a mind to try several remedies for your relief, I feel myself capable, please God, to point out to you a great number of them, having a few good authors on the subject, which I have read and consult daily. If you or your friends have any remedies which I do not know about yet, and which are to your liking, I will not oppose your procuring them, and I will even try to find reasons, experiences, and authorities which confirm you in the resolution you have taken to employ them; but if you challenge yourself a little on your sufficiency in these matters, and that of your friends, and if you presume to know something of my studies, my experience, and my affection, you will allow me to carry on, if you please, and I can assure you that I will proceed with as much circumspection for you as for myself. Upon which I dare hope, with God's help, for a happy outcome. It is for you, Sir, to tell me which of these three ways you wish me to employ in this conjuncture, and to order those who serve you that I be exactly obeyed."

That is a little how I should deal with him. I say no more to you on the subject, save that I am, Sir,

Your very humble and very obedient servant,

De Sorbière.[33]

---

[33] In the collation of *Avis à un jeune Médecin* previously given it will have been noted that the book ends with an " Ode on the Death of Samuel Sorbière " by Jacob de la Fosse,

Acknowledgements

My first knowledge of Sorbière was derived from *English Essays from a French Pen. A Journey to England in the Year 1663*, by the late Hon. Jules J. Jusserand. London: 1895.

I am further indebted to the Hon. Mr. Jusserand for suggestions of value in preparing the earlier portions of this paper. Fathers Reynolds and Coady of St. Matthews Parish, Washington, D. C., and an un-named associate in Georgetown University were kind enough to assist in the translation of Sorbière's Latin letter. I am indebted to the Rev. H. H. A. Corey of Honolulu for translations of the Latin texts in the *Avis*, 1670, and in other volumes by Sorbière. Professor Albert G. A. Balz, Corcoran Professor of Philosophy at the University of Virginia, was gracious enough to send me a copy of his article on Sorbière in the *Philosophical Review*. I have quoted freely from his paper. Professor Vincent Guillotin, Professor of French Literature at Smith College, has also written on this subject, particularly on the *Voyage to England*, and I have to acknowledge material benefit from a reading of his work on Sorbière.

I am grateful to Dr. Owsei Temkin for several valuable suggestions made to me during the writing of this paper.

---

of the Missionary Congregation in Paris, "in sadness," in May, 1670. I have chosen to omit the translation of the ode since it adds nothing to our knowledge of the career of the subject whose death is deplored.

BERNARD MANDEVILLE, M. D., AND EIGHTEENTH-
CENTURY ETHICS [1]

GEORGE CLARK

It is ninety years since Leslie Stephen, when he was already thirty, left Cambridge to continue his literary career in London; but for a particular reason he seems to many of us much less remote in time than he actually is. He not only planned the *Dictionary of National Biography* and edited twenty-six of its volumes; in nearly 400 lives from his own hand, he set a standard for that kind of work which is still the best standard we have. No one has ever surpassed him in combining facts with judgments in miniature biographies which can be read as literature and yet provide the scholar with all the indications that he needs for further study. This lecture was founded in his memory by his friends, and it will not be inappropriate to their purpose to discuss a writer whom Stephen dealt with in the *Dictionary* and also in an essay which he incorporated in his great *History of English Thought in the Eighteenth Century*.

In one respect this will not be a typical example of the changes which have come over historical biography since Stephen's time. Research has become so active, and the materials accessible to historians have multiplied so immensely, that it is difficult now to bring order into our over-abundant information about even the minor characters of earlier centuries. With Bernard Mandeville it is not so. We know even less about him than the Victorian writers thought they knew. Leslie Stephen wrote that Mandeville was said to have been hired by the distillers to write in favour of spirituous liquors and was probably little respected outside distillery circles. Here he was misled by an unreliable authority, quite excusably, for it was a work of no small labour to prove, as has been proved, that there is no ground for this whatever, and that Mandeville consistently wrote not in favour of gin-drinking but against it. The disreputable Mandeville of the old tradition has not been entirely rehabilitated, but we are left in astonishing ignorance about the real man. He was born in Holland, to a good position among the prosperous professional class. His great-grandfather Michael de Mandeville was a physician and a head-

[1] The Leslie Stephen Lecture delivered in the Senate House, Cambridge, on 30 April 1965.

master, perhaps the son of a Protestant refugee from France. His father also was a respected physician, and his maternal grandfather, after whom he was named Bernard, served as a captain in the Dutch navy during the first English war. The education of the young Bernard is unusually well recorded; but from his arrival in England we have to be content with disconnected scraps. We know names and dates about his wife and his two children, a boy and a girl, but scarcely anything more. We know which London parishes he lived in at different dates, but not his addresses or whether he owned a house or lived in lodgings. There are hardly a dozen people of whom we can be sure that he ever spoke to them. Everybody knows his description of Addison as "a parson in a tye-wig," but we never hear of him in connexion with Steele or Locke or Garth, let alone Swift or Arbuthnot. The first Lord Macclesfield gave him hospitality, and it is a fair guess that the naturalised Dutch merchant Sir Matthew Dekker regaled him with a slice of pineapple. An obscure wouldbe philosopher, William Lyons, took the young Benjamin Franklin to a pale-ale house off Cheapside where Mandeville ruled genially over a club.[2] That is almost all that we know about Mandeville as a social being.

There are almost certainly other facts lying hidden in archives which are open to enquirers, and perhaps there are many more in one private muniment room which is not open; but it will be a rare chance if anyone ever discovers whether he ever went back to Holland, whether he went to church, or why he dropped the particle "de" before his surname.[3] We have an indistinct picture of a man who did not belong to the fashionable literary circles, but probably identified himself completely in his private life, as he certainly did in his writings, with the life of his adopted country.

He took his degree as a doctor of medicine at Leyden, and less than two years later (in 1693) he was engaged in medical practice in London. This requires no special explanation: Holland was better supplied with doctors than England, and there were already other Dutch physicians in London. Our first intimation that Mandeville had joined them comes from a summons to appear before the president and censors of the College of Physicians. He was to answer the allegation that he was practising without the licence of the College, which the law required him to obtain.

[2] This seems to have been the Horn Tavern, which long afterwards was sufficiently respectable for the monthly meetings of the Society of Collegiate Physicians to be held there from January 1770 to February 1771: see the Minute Book of the Society, Royal College of Physicians MS 287.

[3] Sometimes from 1704, always from 1715.

He did not apply for a licence, but he was more fortunate than another of his countrymen, who was summoned on the same day (17 November 1693) and forbidden to practise.[4] Mandeville went on with his practice undisturbed for many years. Even this does not require much explanation. It was well known, and openly stated in current books of reference, that "there are divers Physicians that have good Practice in London, altho' they never had any Licence, which is connived at by the College."[5]

Mandeville seems never to have become rich or prominent as a physician, and this he explained by writing: "I am naturally slow, and could no more attend a dozen Patients in a Day, and think of them as I should do, than I could fly."[6] He did indeed hold up to contempt those leaders of the profession who collaborated with apothecaries, sometimes even prescribing without seeing their patients. In this he was on the same side as the College of Physicians, which expelled John Radcliffe from its fellowship in 1689, though it reinstated him in the same year. Mandeville wrote on the thorny subject of the relations between physicians and apothecaries with a restrained and balanced appreciation of both points of view; but his summing up, though it is expressed politely, comes down in favour of the men of learning: an apothecary is as well qualified to be trusted as the most able physician if he is well versed in anatomy, and in the economy and history of disease, if he has had twenty or twenty-five years' experience, and if he has seen the practice of able physicians. Mandeville was an avowed admirer of " the great Sydenham." He upheld the ideals of the " practical physicians " against the exponents of systems. He wrote scathingly about the lack of clinical teaching in the medical faculties of Oxford and Cambridge.[7] An undated letter shows him in consultation with Sir Hans Sloane, who, probably when it was written or not long afterwards, was president of the College of Physicians. The contents of this letter are impressive. Mandeville writes with the self-possession of a professional equal. Without the least fuss or circumlocution he admits that his prognosis has been wrong: " A fortnight ago I pronounced him dying; I have often thought of it since, and am not yet certain, whether I ought to accuse *Artis vanitatem an meam*; however I shall make no more prognosticks but continue to be diligent in observing

[4] See the present writer's *History of the Royal College of Physicians*, vol. II (Oxford: Clarendon Press, 1966), p. 450.

[5] J. Chamberlayne, *Angliae Notitia*, issued at intervals from 1682.

[6] *Treatise* (ed. of 1730), p. 351. He puts the words in the mouth of one of the speakers in the dialogue, but in the Preface he writes that "except for some loose sallies" this person represents himself.

[7] *Treatise* (1711), especially pp. 33, 62, 107, 219-220.

and pray God for more knowledge." [8] More than once in his published writings Mandeville showed this creditable willingness to own that he had been wrong.

He wrote one medical book, *A Treatise of the Hypochondriack and Hysterick Passions, Vulgarly called the Hypo in men and Vapours in women* (1711). It is a good book, full of keen observation and sound advice. There are judicious remarks on more than a dozen recent writers, such as Highmore, Willis, Robert Pitt, Baglivi, Sylvius and Tulp. Much of the book is based on the silent experience of painstaking practitioners, especially Mandeville and his father. But it is not in the strict sense a medical treatise. This indeed is suggested by the latter part of the title, which was dropped from the second edition. The book was intended for the use not of doctors but of patients.[9] It consists of a series of dialogues in which a sympathetic physician interrogates, explains, and prescribes. They are written in excellent coloquial English, without any taint of professional pedantry. They deepen the impression of Dr. Mandeville's estimable and benevolent character. Here and there, it is true, there are sentences which seem to conflict with this. The preface scouts as a romantic pretence the idea that physicians write books for any higher purpose than that of advertising themselves. The writings of doctors are not so different from Quack Bills: the common good and benefit of mankind are stalking horses. For a moment we see why Leslie Stephen called Mandeville " the shrewdest of cynics;" but only for a moment.

We hardly see it at all in the only other book which Mandeville published with his full name on the title-page. *An Enquiry into the Causes of the Frequent Executions at Tyburn and a Proposal for some Regulations concerning Felons in Prison, and the good Effects to be Expected from them, to which is added a Discourse on Transportation, and a Method to render that Punishment more Effectual* (1725). This was a pioneering programme for social reform, in part very wise and in part patently impracticable.[10] It gives vivid and horrible descriptions of Newgate and

[8] The letter is reproduced in facsimile as the frontispiece to the standard edition of *The Fable of the Bees* by F. B. Kaye (Oxford: Clarendon Press, 1924). The two indexes in this edition, the editor's and Mandeville's own, are so good that I have not thought it necessary to give page-references for quotations from the Fable.

[9] It was not, however, until the fourth edition that the Latin quotations were translated into English. The Royal College of Physicians has the editions of 1711 and 1730, but both were acquired after its library was catalogued in 1757.

[10] The proposed improvement in transportation, for instance, was, instead of sending criminals to the colonies, to exchange them for Englishmen captured and enslaved by the Barbary corsairs.

Tyburn and the processional route between them. Most of it was first published in the form of articles in the *London Journal*. It contains a cogent argument, written some months before the arrest of Jonathan Wild the Great, against the use of professional thief-catchers and receivers as Crown witnesses. The physician appears in a short justification of the dissection of the corpses of executed criminals for the purposes of anatomical science and teaching. The Dutchman contributes information about the Rasphuis prison in Amsterdam. What Mandeville praises in this institution is not that it treats its inmates with understanding but that it is well-ordered and severe. He writes not as a humanitarian but, without pity, as a hater of crime and vice; not as a cynic but as a man who is not afraid to look steadily at the worst of human nature.

Two other books were avowed as his, not with his full name but with the initials B. M. The first is a collection of verses, some of them in continuation of a mock-heroic poem *Typhon* (1704), which is thus also covered by the avowal. The book takes its title from the *Wishes to a Godson* (1712), the tone of which is undeniably low. In the second, in prose, there are many similarities of style with the other books, along with several medical allusions and several passages about Holland, some of them recondite, all of which together must have made it easy to identify the author. This book has a strange preface, apparently sincere but ironically overdrawn, in which the writer claims to have consciously run into danger in performing a good work " to promote the Interest and Temporal Felicity of the Nation he lives in." It is called *Free Thoughts on Religion, the Church and National Happiness* (1720). Here we come closer to the imputed cynicism.

" My aim," Mandeville writes, " is to make Men penetrate into their own Consciences, and by searching without Flattery into the true Motives of their Actions, learn to know themselves." Much of this book is taken, as Mandeville fully acknowledges, from the great dictionary of Bayle, who was teaching and writing in Rotterdam when Mandeville was a schoolboy there. That is to say, it is a work of the anti-clerical " libertine " movement of the time. It also has considerable traces of Hobbes, as, for instance, in the matter of the origin of society and in the organic analogy of the state, to which our physician gives a turn of his own. The earlier part of the book, about religion, is chiefly concerned to advocate toleration and the control of churches by states; the latter part, by a transition which was easy in the reign of George I, is straightforward Whig propaganda. There is a contrast between the pugnacious arguments and some circumspect reservations. The writer assures us that, poorly as he thinks of priests and priestcraft, and little as he thinks belief by itself can do to make men morally good, he is neither an atheist nor a deist. He says that men should believe the mysterious as well as the historical truths of the Gospel, thus repudiating the deistic principle, *Christianity not Mysterious.*[11] Most readers have thought that this was a mere precaution, and the references to revealed religion in the book are so perfunctory that they have good reason for thinking so. There are, however, passages where Mandeville seems to accept this view for the subsidiary reason that it enables him to glide over his difficulties. In a long argument about predestination, free will, and the origin of evil he supplements Bayle with a brilliant illustration and more, but he concludes that only revealed religion, the Old and New Testaments, are " capable of cutting the Gordian Knot." [12]

None of the three books I have mentioned so far provoked any controversy; those of Mandeville's writings which did that came out anonymously or under pseudonyms. He began publishing anonymously ten years after he arrived in England, and he began with little books of fables in verse. In 1709 he published a dialogue, *The Virgin Unmasked.* All his literary qualities are full-grown in this short work: it is amusing, full of clever characterisation and acute social criticism. There are good things about girls' boarding schools, duelling, Holland, physicians, human motives, love and reason, or, as we might say, sensibility and sense. There are cynical touches about social climbers and about the moralists who say that virtue is its own reward. The book harvested the success it deserved, but Mandeville did not set everybody talking and writing until he published the " second " edition of his anonymous *Fable of the Bees* in 1723. In 1733, a year before he died, at the age of sixty-two, he published his last important book, *An Enquiry into the Origin of Honour and the Usefulness of Christianity in War.* The title-page states that it is by the author of the *Fable of the Bees,* and it is a continuation of the dialogues from the second part of the Fable. By that time the secret was out; it had been general knowledge for several years who that author was.[18] In the meantime Mandeville had published under the pseudonym " A Layman " an outspoken addendum to the Fable, the nature of which is truly indicated by the title, *A Modest Defense of Public Stews.* That was in 1724, in the period of danger after the Fable was first presented

---

[11] P. 297.

[12] Pp. 90, 105.

[18] J. Byrom, *Private Journals and Literary Remains,* ed. R. Parkinson (Chatham Society) vol. 1 (1854), p. 381, entry for 29 June 1729.

by the grand jury of Middlesex as tending to subvert all religion and civil government, our duty to the Almighty, and our love to our country.

That there was real danger is proved, among other incidents, by the misfortunes of Mandeville's exact contemporary Thomas Woolston, a former fellow of Sidney Sussex College and an earnest, if deviant, theologian, who died in prison. Whether Mandeville's anonymity was due to prudence in the presence of this danger we do not know. He may have assumed it from one of the various literary motives which operated commonly enough at that time. He took no precautions to disguise his style or manner, and these are distinctive.[14] But one of the identifying marks is irony. Mandeville practised not only irony but other indirect forms of expression, such as the fable and the parable, where the moral is conveyed by a story, and the dialogue, where the author can hide behind his characters. Once, in controversy, he uses parody, twisting his opponent's words back against him; and above all he practised paradox. All these forms were in favour with writers of the time, but with Mandeville they became so habitual that it is hard to be sure when, if ever, he is speaking his own mind. He enjoyed playing tricks on his readers. At one point he seems to be gravely plumbing the depths of constitutional law until his real purpose suddenly appears, which is to prove that Lord Macclesfield is greater, not only in degree but in kind, than Sir Robert Walpole.[15]

The defence of one main paradox came to dominate Mandeville's thought. He returned to it again and again, sometimes when he was stimulated by contradiction, but sometimes, apparently, because he could not steer his mind away from it. Sometimes he calls it a " seeming paradox." This is a tautology: it is appearance, seeming, that makes a paradox, but Mandeville wants us to believe that his own paradox is not a seeming but a reality, some kind of fact. First he threw it out light-heartedly in one of his fables, four hundred lines or so, sold for sixpence and printed in a halfpenny sheet. It was entitled *The Grumbling Hive*. He called it a story told in doggerel. Nine years later he made a book of it with the much better title *The Fable of the Bees or Private Vices, Public Benefits*. This gave the original verses with a preface, an " Enquiry into

[14] It seems, for instance, that the anonymous dialogue pamphlet of 1714, *The Mischiefs to be apprehended from a Whig Government*, can safely be attributed to him on internal evidence alone.

[15] The earliest example of this playfulness is in *Some Fables* (1703). In the Preface he says that all the fables except two are taken from La Fontaine; but instead of saying which the two are, he tells the reader "Find 'em and welcome." They are " The Carp " and " The Nightingale and the Owl."

the Origin of Moral Virtue," as long as a very long sermon, and twenty Remarks on particular points, the whole amounting to 284 pages. In 1723 it appeared again with further additions, " An Essay on Charity and Charity-Schools " and " A Search into the Nature of Society," besides some shorter pieces about the presentment by the grand jury. In 1729 came the second part of the *Fable of the Bees*, another substantial volume to elaborate and justify the first, consisting of six pretty long dialogues. Taken as a whole, it must be confessed, these two volumes make a clumsy and formless mass, and even that was not all. Of Mandeville's last two publications one had more about the paradox in its preface, and the other was a short reply to the strictures of Berkeley. But it is all good reading; to the last page it is witty and effective.

The Grumbling Hive is the story of

> A spacious hive well stockt with bees
> That lived in luxury and ease . . .
> Was counted the great nursery
> Of sciences and industry.
> No bees had better government
> More fickleness or less content:
> They were not slaves to tyranny,
> Nor ruled by wild democracy;
> But kings, that could not wrong, because
> Their power was circumscribed by laws.

The parallel with England is prettily turned, with satirical sketches of the criminal classes, the lawyers, physicians, and clergy, and we are assured that

> every part was full of vice,
> Yet the whole mass a paradise.

Then we are told that the grumbling brutes cried out for honesty and Jove " in anger rid the bawling hive of fraud." No sooner did the politicians, the traders, the professional men, and the rest cease to cheat than they all sank into poverty, temperance and thrift, so that prices fell, there was no demand for anything but bare necessities, and by becoming honest, the hive ceased to be great.

The story had two morals. At this first stage Mandeville thought perhaps more of the immediate political lesson for England: the Jacobites and nonjurors and tories set up the cry for honesty. If they had their way they would bring ruin on the country. But he generalised the paradox, and as he went on to amplify and defend it, his attention was taken up more and more with the second, underlying moral:

> So vice is beneficial found
> When 'tis by justice lopt and bound;
> Nay where the people would be great,
> As necessary to the state
> As hunger is to make 'em eat.

This paradox was not new; nor is it far-fetched. In the world of action there are few men who have never consciously accepted in a good cause the help of bad men actuated by bad motives. When Mandeville found that his first prose variations on the theme roused indignation, he protested. He had not said that private vices as such were for the public advantage. The elliptical formula " Private vices public benefits " omitted a verb; " may be " was implied, not " are." One critic maintained that there were five different ways in which the gap could be filled. Still, whatever the verb might be, the apparent contradiction remained. Several eminent writers sharpened their wits on it, and it did serve the useful purpose which paradoxes have often served. Adam Smith wrote that it was Mandeville's great fallacy to represent every passion as wholly vicious which is so in any degree and in any direction. Mandeville says that, at least under certain conditions, normally bad dispositions in men bring about consequences which are socially desirable. Moral badness therefore, for instance selfishness or unreasonableness, has no necessary connection with social badness, which resides in the consequences of the acts of individuals.

This paradox did not arise for those who followed either of the two lines of ethical thought, each with a long history behind it, which were taking shape in Mandeville's time. The utilitarian tendency identified the moral goodness of an act with its social benefits: what made an act good was that it was useful. The various doctrines of the moral sense, on the other hand, required no calculation of consequences either on the part of the moral agent or on the part of the impartial judge of his conduct. They maintained that by a necessary harmony moral action was socially beneficent. Mandeville, insisting that self-love and social were incompatible, had to bring in a third factor to force them into agreement. In the original rhyme he wrote that vice was beneficial when it was lopped and bound by justice or statecraft. When he came to explain himself, he wrote that the legislators, among whom he included all the wise men of every profession who promote the good of society, used their power through education, rewards, and punishments to compel self-loving and self-liking men to act in accordance with its interest. " The moral virtues," he wrote, " are the political offspring which flattery begot upon pride."

To account for the existence of these legislators he plunged back into pre-history: " human wisdom is the child of time." [16] To explain why these legislators did not simplify their task by taking the more direct, if arduous, road of encouraging virtue he had only to point out that, as he had said from the first, this would have brought about a starveling greatness like that of Sparta, not opulence and flourishing arts like those of England or France or Holland in his day.

Mandeville had a very active brain. There is no end to the subjects on which he has something quotable, and often extremely funny, to say— fox-hunters, the training of jockeys, chimney-sweeps' boys, freemasonry, cremation, tipping in private houses, the importance of the week in the development of chronology. He was a fertile phrase-maker. I suggest, perhaps rashly, that he was the inventor of a phrase which has become proverbial, and at any rate is characteristic of him: " facts are stubborn things." [17] Although he had this gift for using words, and although he was well-educated and well-read, he was not, strictly speaking, a scholar. He seems to have known no Greek and practically nothing of Greek literature; the Latin classics merely provided him with a few quotations, usually familiar. He often quoted at second hand without verifying his references. Except for Renau on shipbuilding [18] and Ottius on the Anabaptists,[19] the modern authors he mentions, including even the theologians named in his *Free Thoughts*, are those, mostly French and English, who were widely known to the educated world. He used them, as indeed he used the medical authors in his *Treatise*, for their general sense.

Much has been written about Mandeville's anticipations of later writers, which are many in number and sometimes remarkably close. In economics, for instance, he wrote about the balance of trade and the division of labour, and he used words which look like the formulae of *laisser faire*. Adam Smith read his Fable and wrote about it; but there were a good many other writers who wrote more fully about these subjects and to whom Adam Smith devoted more attention. It is not justifiable to make Mandeville a teacher of Adam Smith. The tracing of anticipations and influences through phrases and turns of thought has the attraction that it seems to deal with units more definite and manage-

[16] *Origin of Honour* (1732), p. 41.

[17] *Ibid.*, p. 162. The earliest reference for the phrase in the *Oxford English Dictionary* is to Malkin's translation of *Gil Blas* (1809) ; but the original only says "les faits parlent."

[18] This book, *De la théorie des vaisseaux*, was published anonymously in 1689; Mandeville probably only knew the English translation by J. Senex, which was published in 1705 and gives the author's name as B. Renau d'Eliçagarny.

[19] Johann Heinrich Ottius, *Annales Anabaptistici* (1672).

able than large ideas. The editor of the *Fable*, the late Professor F. B. Kaye, rendered a valuable service by identifying the sources from which Mandeville drew ideas, information, and verbal expressions: he showed that this anticipator was himself often anticipated and that much of his thought was derivative. It is probable that Mandeville also borrowed other passages which have not yet been identified. We may hope that in a more affluent future computers will relieve us of this kind of work. They may help us to deduct from every book everything that is copied from elsewhere, and to distinguish everything that is carried over into subsequent books; but even so they will only carry out an ancillary process. The history of thought is much more than a history of the trading in and out of separable items which, in their temporary combinations, form the stock of one thinker after another. It is the history of the activities of minds. Literary borrowing is not mere transference from one piece of paper to another; it is the incorporation of a selected part of a completed whole in another whole which is being made. Its significance depends on the relation of these two wholes and on the ground of the selection. Identified borrowings are milestones, but the history of thought is a road, or even a tract of country.

In this history one group of Mandeville's anticipations has its place. He was not, as we have seen, a great scholar, nor was he a great philosopher, but he was a scientist. In this, to be sure, he was not alone among the eighteenth-century moralists. John Locke himself was a trained and experienced scientific worker, intimately associated with Sydenham. The materials have only recently become available in print for estimating how much Locke's medical studies contributed to his thought in general. From Mandeville's mind science was never absent for long. His education included anatomical dissections and the use of the microscope; his daily professional work included clinical observation and thinking about it. When he drew parallels and illustrations from the human body he did not, like most of the moralists, compare an object with a mirror-image; he saw both sides in three dimensions.

The value and the limitations of his scientific outlook are shown by two well-known passages.[20] One is a discussion which begins from the then fashionable attempts to apply mathematics to medicine. A speaker in a dialogue asks what insight or real knowledge we have from anatomy concerning the operation of thinking. The answer is " None at all *a priori*. The most consummate Anatomist knows no more of it than a Butcher's Apprentice." In the following pages there are reminiscences of Descartes,

[20] In the fifth and sixth dialogues of the second part of the *Fable*.

of Locke, of Shaftesbury, and very likely of others; but these pages are somehow disappointing. Even the opening words which I have quoted sound as if they mean more than is really in them. When it is asserted that the anatomist has no *a priori* knowledge of the mind, does this deny any proposition that has ever been accepted? What could such *a priori* knowledge be?

In the following dialogue the same characters appear. The questioner's function is to lob up fallacies in order that Mandeville's representative may refute them. He uses a phrase which strikes sharply on a modern reader's ear, though we must remember that for him its meaning was far less momentous than it is for us. "Holy Writ," he says, "has acquainted us with the miraculous Origin of our Species." Then comes an account of the beginnings and rise of civilisation. It allows for no difference between human nature in the savage and the civilized man. Under the name of Providence it postulates that nothing comes by chance. It puts forward ideas which struck the Darwinian Victorians as astonishingly modern: the prodigality of nature, the struggle for life and its relation to the variety of creatures, animism in early religion, the relevance of vital statistics to social evolution. But the sense of power which all this conveys arises less from these conclusions, remarkable as they are, than from the texture of the argument. Throughout it the well-digested findings of science are an essential component. Mandeville enhances the concrete richness of his own thought by referring to Sir William Temple's idea of primitive man and Milton's picture of the Garden of Eden, two specimens of the narrow pre-scientific approaches to the study of human origins. As he draws on chemistry, zoology, human physiology, and psychology, the scientific spirit works outwards from the multiplicity of observable facts to the limits beyond which Mandeville refuses to speculate. Many readers have been reminded of Lucretius, to whom strangely enough there is no reference in Mandeville's work except one inaccurate quotation in a quite different context.

The evolutionary view of civilisation was consistent with Mandeville's ethics. As against Shaftesbury's doctrine of a moral sense, an innate tendency to choose the good, the beautiful, and the true, Mandeville held that there was no virtue without self-denial; and that the social discipline of education and government must be imposed on "silly, reptile man." [21] He insisted that there were no absolute standards, in morals or religion or aesthetics, any more than in mere fashion; but this relativism, or Pyrrhonism as it was called, was not merely negative or destructive.

[21] This expression comes from *Origin of Honour*, p. x, where it is used in contrast with the goodness of God.

Although he seems always to evade the question wherein moral goodness consists, he draws pictures of its operation in the life of society, and of these the most illuminating and profound are in his sketch of evolution. Yet it is only a sketch, brief and summary, brought in as a subordinate, almost an incidental, element in the defence of his central paradox.

Although most of the abuse that was thrown at Mandeville was completely unjustified, we cannot pretend that the tone of his works is elevating. If I understand Robert Browning's address to Mandeville in *Parleyings with Certain Persons of Importance*, of which I am doubtful, Browning penetrated early to some genial appreciation of human goodness below the crust of sneering, and then in his old age hoped for clearer evidence that Mandeville was an optimist at heart. But this was no more than a hope unfulfilled, and where Browning could not find optimism, there was none to find. Mandeville shocked his readers, and it is impossible to doubt that he intended to do it.

He did it even in medical matters, where we know that he was personally kind and conscientious. He wrote that: " A Miser may go directly to Hell, as the reward of his Avarice and Extortion, at the same Time, that the great Wealth he leaves, and the Hospital he builds, are a considerable Relief to the Poor, and consequently a Publick Benefit." [22] In another passage he illustrated the proposition that there is no virtue so often counterfeited as charity. He does this by dissecting the motives of a mean shopkeeper who drives a trade prejudicial to his country and on all occasions grinds the faces of the poor, but in his old age lays out the greatest part of his immense riches in building or endowing a hospital, finally in his will defrauding those to whom he had obligations. Even in details this outrageous paragraph inevitably calls to mind Thomas Guy, the only man who had built and endowed a hospital in England since the Middle Ages. Since one of these passages was published only five years after the death of Mr. Guy, and the other in the year when the trustees of Guy's Hospital reprinted his will, I conclude that Mandeville either meant to undermine the respect for his name or at least was careless whether he did so or not.

The best example of this recknessness is the *Essay on Charity Schools*. We know now, thanks largely to an excellent book by the late Miss Gwladys Jones of Girton, that the charity school movement was one of the best manifestations of eighteenth-century philanthropy. The essay does include much good sense about education and the differences between the sexes, but it tells us no more about the charity schools than *The Fable*

[22] *Letter to Dion* (1732), p. 39.

of the Bees tells us about entomology. It gives a merciless exposure of all the mixed motives which passed for charity in supporting the schools, and it ends with a downright condemnation of their aims. They were meant to give the children of the poor learning and accomplishments which would unfit them for the hardest and most unpleasant work. That work must be done, and therefore in a flourishing society it was necessary that the poor should be many. They must face the hardships which it was " wisdom to relieve but folly to cure."

Mandeville may well have been one of those men who may with equal justice be described as cynics and as idealists; but it was his own fault that so many of his readers saw only one side of his character. Both in practical matters and in theory he subsided into a habit of stopping short when he had exposed an error. He wrote that it was the business of the body politic (or, as we should say, the state) to supply the defects of the society and to take in hand that which was neglected by private persons. He seemed content to leave all social responsibility to the government. He insisted that the notions of right and wrong are acquired, and so he recognised no need for any ethical theory beyond a psychology of the passions and the will. This was not insistence on the application of scientific reasoning to human affairs, but surrender to a hampering limitation. Just as he saw in a paradox not a puzzle demanding solution but a kind of established truth, so he did not follow the lines of thought which might have led him beyond the new counter-orthodoxy, the constricting circle of the " libertine " ideas. In the symphony of English ethical thought, he limited himself to playing a percussion instrument. He had the full score before him, but, while others developed the theme, he supplied only thumps and taps, skilfully aimed and timed, and occasionally a roll that lasted through three or four bars.

I reveal no secret if I say that a new edition of the *Dictionary of National Biography* is under contemplation. When it is written, the new life of Bernard Mandeville should treat him more gently than the old; but the estimate of his ethical thought should remain substantially the same. In time perhaps some master will write a book to supersede Leslie Stephen's history of eighteenth-century thought. He will bring the development of philosophical ideas into its due relation with our accumulated knowledge of the history of science, and of society in many of its aspects. His task will be like that of the practical physicians of the eighteenth century. The history of ideas is the arena of several competing ready-made systems, as the physician's art was in Mandeville's day, but the practical historian has an independent contribution to make, beginning from the principle that facts are stubborn things.

Historical Introduction
to 1975 Reprint
THOMAS PERCIVAL:
MEDICAL ETHICS OR
MEDICAL JURISPRUDENCE?
Chester R. Burns, M.D., Ph. D.

Not a little has been written about Thomas
Percival and his *Medical Ethics*.[1] Symbolized by
this reprint, Percival's legacy is "alive and well"
and still living in the hearts and minds of health
professionals interested in ethical standards. However, certain features of Percival's legacy have
been neglected. Attention to these features allow a fresh interpretation of Percival's place in
the history of Anglo-American medical ethics.[2]
Before accurate generalizations can be made,
Percival's book must be studied in a detailed
fashion. The book was published in 1803, eleven
years after the initial request by the trustees of
the Manchester Infirmary. It was entitled *Medical Ethics, or a Code of Institutes and Precepts,
Adapted to the Professional Conduct of Physicians and Surgeons*. The four chapters of the
book deal respectively with professional conduct
in hospital practice, professional conduct in pri-

284

vate or general practice, conduct of physicians toward apothecaries, and conduct of physicians in cases requiring a knowledge of the law. Prior to examining the content of these chapters, it is important to review Percival's objectives.

He desired to "frame a general system of Medical Ethics; that the official conduct, and mutual intercourse of the faculty, might be regulated by precise and acknowledged principles of urbanity and rectitude."[3] Percival discovered, though, that he could not offer ideals about interactions between practitioners without placing them within a broader conceptual context. In a letter to his son, Edward, this discovery is expressed in a precise fashion:

> "It is the characteristic of a wise man to act on determinate principles; and of a good man to be assured that they are conformable to rectitude and virtue. The relations in which a physician stands to his patients, to his brethren, and to the public are complicated, and multifarious; involving much knowledge of human nature, and extensive moral duties. The study of professional Ethics, therefore, cannot fail to invigorate and enlarge your understanding, whilst the observance of the duties which they enjoin will soften your manners, expand your affections, and form you to that propriety and dignity of conduct,

which are essential to the character of a Gentleman."[4]

There was, therefore, a cloverleaf of four parts
to Percival's understanding of professional ethics.
One involved the physician's image of himself as
a "gentleman" physician. Another involved relationships between medical practitioners, between the "brethren." A third pertained to the
transactions of a physician with his patients. The
fourth dimension involved the relationships of
practitioners to the public or community. An
examination of some of Percival's precepts will
demonstrate the interrelatedness of these four
components.

"Gentleman" signified a cluster of ideals about
the physician *qua* person. A "gentleman" physician should unite "tenderness with steadiness"
and "condescension with authority." Physicians
and surgeons should be "governed by sound reason, just analogy, or well authenticated facts."
Impartial retrospection was necessary in order
to circumvent self-deception and error. There
should be a "decorous silence" in the operating
room. The surgeon should change his apron between operations. There should be a strict temperance on the part of physicians and surgeons.

The competent physician should receive a "regular academical education," and be punctual. Thus, the following adjectives can be used to characterize Percival's "gentleman" physician: considerate, authorative but humble, reasonable, reflective, self-critical, temperate, educated, punctual. For Percival, though, these ideal characteristics were not meaningful if segregated from interactions with practitioners or patients.

The "gentleman" physician must unite "tenderness with steadiness" and "condescension with authority" in order to elicit gratitude, respect, and trust from his patients.[5] The physician and surgeon must be "governed by sound reason, just analogy, or well authenticated facts" in making a clinical decision about using a new drug or method of surgical treatment.[6] The practitioner will avoid self-deception and error only if he conducts an impartial review of the treatment and response in each of his patients, especially if the patient dies. The "decorous silence" in the operating room must be broken if the patient needs reassurance or instructions.[7] The surgeon should change his apron between operations because the sight of blood might evoke terror in the next patient. Temperance was absolutely essential if the practitioner was expected to perform properly, especially in emergency situations. The practitioner must be punctual in order to prevent unnecessary visits to the patient and repetitive questioning of the patient. A "regular academical education" was not absolutely necessary for the attainment of skill in the practice of physic and surgery, and those who had the skill but lacked the academic distinction, should not be excluded from the fellowship of other practitioners.[8] Percival believed in a fundamental connection between "gentleman" ideals, values about interphysician behavior, and norms about the conduct of physicians with patients. These ideals were not rigidly segregated from each other, as will be demonstrated again by examining the other components.

The second part of Percival's framework involved the relationships of a physician or surgeon with his "brethren." The following exemplify some of Percival's precepts about these intraprofessional relationships. The physician or surgeon should be cautious about damaging the reputation of a colleague by accusing him of improper conduct. Any complaints should be lodged with the staff of the hospital before any private or public accusations are made. If a practitioner is ignorant or negligent, he should discuss this situation with the "gentlemen of the faculty," unless the patient's life is threatened by the ignorance or negligence. If the latter situation occurs, the practitioner should regard interference with the other practitioner's care of that patient as a duty.[9]

Numerous rules involved consultation.[10] An orderly presentation of consultative opinion was desirable, with the succession from junior to senior physician. A distinction between the provinces of physician and surgeon should be sustained, but consulting physicians and surgeons should agree about procedures in all important operations. Consultation, discussion, and cooperation between physicians, surgeons, and apothecaries must be encouraged. In rural areas, Percival noted, apothecaries usually know considerably more about the patient than anyone else. If there was direct and friendly communication between the apothecary and the consulting physician or consulting surgeon, the patient would benefit ultimately. Consultation and discussion were desirable, not only for improving the skills of the practitioner, but for making adequate and judicious decisions about the care of a patient.[11] Permeating all of these rules of intraprofessional decorum was a belief that ethical ideals about relationships between practitioners were intimately connected to values associated with a "gentleman" practitioner and to standards that pertained to the welfare of a patient.

Fifty-seven of the seventy-two precepts contained in the first three chapters of Percival's book dealt explicitly or implicitly with the care of the patient.[12] The following are additional examples.[13] A practitioner should have considerable regard for the feelings, emotions, and prejudices of the sick. Privacy of interrogation was absolutely necessary. The use of quack medicines and the dispensing of secret nostrums should not be prescribed. "Gloomy prognostications" should not be made by a practitioner. Practitioners should discuss the problem of a last will and testament with the relatives of a dying patient. These and other norms reflect Percival's foremost regard for the welfare of patients.

The realm of society-at-large or the public trust was the fourth major component in Percival's conceptualization of medical ethics. A careful study of Percival's book, including the fourth chapter, will reveal the extent to which this component is illustrated with precepts about hospitals, absentee certificates, and legal circumstances.

Percival urged communities to establish more

asylums and hospitals. He specifically mentioned insane asylums and an asylum for women with syphilis.[14] He believed that the hospital staff should keep comprehensive registers. Those registers would include important facts about the care of the hospitalized patients. A study of these registers would enable concerned professionals and citizens to correlate disease patterns with age, sex, occupation, climate and seasons.[15]

As acts "due to the public," physicians and surgeons should prepare any certificates required to justify the inability of public officials, military personnel, jurors, or others from performing their work. Each person's claim should be carefully studied and no false or dubious declarations made by the practitioner.[16]

Percival believed that the laws of a nation or community circumscribed significant moral relationships between practitioners and that nation or community. In England, the law exempted physicians and surgeons from certain civil duties, such as military service or jury duty. In return for these privileges, the law made certain demands on these practitioners.[17] A physician could be required, for example, to make a decision about the mental abilities of a sick person who wanted to prepare a will and testament.[18]

A practitioner could be called to testify in cases of sudden death and he should know the differences between justifiable, excusable and felonious homicide.[19] Medical practitioners, therefore, should attend all judiciary proceedings requiring their professional knowledge.

To reiterate, there were four components in Percival's approach to medical ethics. The personal values of a practitioner were fundamental. In Percival's time, these values were subsumed under the label "gentleman." The second group, norms about the behavior of a practitioner toward his colleagues, involved more than simple courtesy or kindness. Undergirding most of these ideals was the welfare of the patient. Finally, the ethical demands of a community, including those represented by its laws, were morally binding for medical practitioners. Each group of values was logically and practically interconnected. Percival himself did not claim that one part was more important than another.

Other features of Percival's legacy need emphasis. Percival admitted that his book was incomplete. He also knew that it had been written in a piecemeal fashion.

Originally, he had been asked to draft a code of rules that would regulate and govern practice at the Manchester Infirmary. Percival was expected to write a set of rules for a hospital, not a general work on medical ethics. As ecclesiastical institutions, many medieval hospitals had adopted definite systems of admission rules, daily regulations, and penalties for disobeying these rules and regulations. Even the Manchester hospital had adopted such a code of rules and regulations when it was established in 1752. But such rules needed revising, as the conditions of medical practice changed and as hospitals became exclusively concerned with the care of the sick. The hospital was a new stage for the expression of ethical conflicts by British physicians, surgeons, and apothecaries. The oaths of antiquity, the moral maxims of the traditional guilds, and the legally binding statutory responses to these professional hierarchies were no longer satisfactory.

Percival fully appreciated the moral significance of those legal statutes that pertained to medical practice. He knew that a society could create new professional obligations, such as requiring medical testimony at judicial proceedings or the inscription of absentee certificates. He also recognized that some laws could be wrong, such as those that permitted the beating of lunatics.[20] Moreover, he recognized that a practitioner could experience conflicts between legal stipulations and professional ideals. For example, Percival believed that a practitioner's personal judgment about the validity of capital punishment should not interfere with his medical testimony in a particular case.[21]

The importance of legal influences on professional ethics was revealed in Percival's distress about the title of his book. The original manuscript had been privately circulated with the title of "Medical Jurisprudence." Since some of his friends objected to the term "Jurisprudence," it was changed to "Medical Ethics." A significant glimmer of displeasure is evident in Percival's pronouncement that "according to the definition of Justinian, however, Jurisprudence may be understood to include moral injunction as well as positive ordinances."[22] An understanding of Percival's belief in the profound relationship between law and ethics is essential for a complete understanding of Percival's legacy.

Percival was also well-versed in religion and moral philosophy. He was a devout Unitarian, imbued with Christian ideals. He had read the works of several moral philosophers including Paley's *Principles of Moral and Political Philosophy*, Smith's *Theory of Moral Sentiments*,

Hutcheson's *System of Moral Philosophy*, Grove's *Ethics*, and Gisborne's *Enquiry Into the Duties of Men*. Percival also demonstrated remarkable acquaintance with a number of legal works written by such important scholars as Foster, Blackstone, Hawkins, and Burn. Finally, Percival was thoroughly familiar with the traditions of professional ethics in British medicine. With such a remarkable background as a medical practitioner and as a student of religion, moral philosophy, and law, why did Percival not construct a theoretical system of professional ethics for medical practitioners?

Percival demonstrated some ambiguity in his attitude toward speculative systems.[23] He objected to speculation about the nature of God and excessive rational analysis of biblical precepts. On the other hand, he heartedly approved of metaphysical inquiries about nature and human nature. But, speculation that led to dogmatism or simplistic systems was to be rejected. Percival favored experimentation based on observation, the use of principles of correct logic and inductive reasoning, and the judicious use of analogy. Perhaps Percival believed that a speculative system of professional ethics would become dogmatic and counterproductive in a manner similar to the various systems of therapeutics so popular in his day.

Percival also believed that knowledge did not automatically insure virtuous behavior.[24] He believed that a man could be virtuous even though scientifically immature. The wisdom of God and the Gospel had made the possession of goodness a matter of the heart rather than that of the mind. Thus, Percival was not interested in preparing a multivolume treatise on a theory of morals in medicine.

How, then, to declare one's values about the conduct of practitioners? By writing specific rules and using concrete examples, Percival offered the same pattern of ethical education to his fellow doctors as he did to his own children.[25] Individual precepts illustrated with specific examples and framed within the context of religious sentiment, moral theory, and legal prescription, provided Percival with the provocative balance between the specific and the general, the concrete and the abstract.

Percival's *Medical Ethics* was a little more than a pragmatic code and a little less than a systematic treatise. It was a set of maxims that represented four basic dimensions of a medical practitioner's obligations. It was a set of rules that partook of both the practical and the theoretical, a set that allowed margins of freedom for their interpretation in particular professional and social circumstances. Perhaps, this is why the volume was so influential, especially in Great Britain and the United States, and why it deserves to be re-printed again and studied by all persons inter-ested in the nature of professional ethics in medicine.

NOTES AND REFERENCES

1. Forbes, Robert, "Medical ethics in Great Britain," *Wld. Med. J.*, 1954, *1*:297-299; Lester King, *The Medical World of the Eighteenth Century*. Chicago: University of Chicago Press, 1958, pp. 253-260; "Thomas Percival (1740-1840) Codifier of Medical Ethics," *J. Amer. Med. Assn.*, 1965, *194*:1319-1320; H. M. Koelbing, "Die 'Ärztliche Ethik' des Thomas Percival," *Schweizerische Medizinische Wochenschrift*, 1967, *97*:713-716.
2. For additional comments, see Chester R. Burns, "Reciprocity in the Development of Anglo-American Medical Ethics, 1765-1865," *Proceedings of the XXIII International Congress of the History of Medicine*. London: Wellcome Institute of the His-tory of Medicine, 1974, Vol. 1, pp. 813-819.
3. Percival, *Medical Ethics*, p. 1.
4. *Ibid.*, pp. viii-ix.
5. *Ibid.*, p. 9, (I, I). In parentheses, I shall indicate,

first, the number of the chapter and, secondly, the number of the precept. This will make it easier for the reader to locate each in this reprint.

6. *Ibid.*, p. 15, (I, XII).
7. *Ibid.*, p. 21, (I, XXIII).
8. *Ibid.*, pp. 37–38, (II, XI).
9. *Ibid.*, pp. 14; 32–33, (I, X; II, IV).
10. *Ibid.*, pp. 19–22, 33–38, (I, XIX–XXIV; II, V–XII).
11. *Ibid.*, pp. 53–55, (III, II).
12. "Implicitly" means that the precept would be senseless without reference to patient care.
13. Percival, *op. cit.*, pp. 10–14; 44–45, (I, III–VIII; II, XXI).
14. *Ibid.*, p. 24–27, (I, XXVII–XXVIII).
15. *Ibid.*, pp. 15–18, (I, XIV–XV).
16. *Ibid.*, pp. 43–44, (II, XX).
17. *Ibid.*, pp. 61–62, (IV, I).
18. *Ibid.*, pp. 63–66, (IV, II).
19. *Ibid.*, pp. 71–99 (IV, VI–XV).
20. *Ibid.*, pp. 68–69, (IV, IV).
21. *Ibid.*, pp. 108–112, (IV, XIX).
22. *Ibid.*, p. 7.
23. *The Works, Literary, Moral, and Medical of Thomas Percival, M.D.* London, 1807, Vol. II, pp. 175–188.
24. *Ibid.*, pp. 115–123.
25. As early as ·1775, Percival began writing a book of precepts and examples specifically designed to teach principles of morality to his children. Two years later, he added a second installment to these tales, and a third portion was completed in 1800. All of these were published with the title: *A Father's Instructions to His Children: Consisting of Tales,*

Fables, and Reflections: Designed to Promote the Love of Virtue, A Taste for Knowledge, and an Early Acquaintance with the Works of Nature.

*   *   *   *   *   *

Note: It would be ungracious not to acknowledge publicly my thanks to Doctor Chester Burns for his very helpful, detailed, and critical analysis of Percival's *Medical Ethics.* My gratitude to him is deep. He has done well what was beyond my capacity to do. Clearly he shows how much of Percival was a product of the "Age of Enlightenment." I am honored by Doctor Burns' contribution.

Chauncey D. Leake
Holidaze, 1974

Morals are judgments on individual activity: the various ethics are socially derived generalizations induced from individual morality.

C. R. Burns

Galveston, Texas (U.S.A.)

Reciprocity in the development of Anglo-American medical ethics, 1765–1865

From the beginnings of recorded human history, ideals *and* ideas about values have been associated with the personal and professional activities of medical practitioners. The professional values can be classified best under the following four headings: (1) the education of medical practitioners, (2) consultations with other practitioners, (3) transactions between physicians and patients, and (4) relationships between medical practitioners and communities. During the one hundred years encompassed by this study, Anglo-American physicians experienced value changes within all four of these categories of interpersonal relationships. These changes are well illustrated by the ideals of three British physicians: John Gregory (1724–73), Thomas Percival (1740–1804), and Michael Ryan (1800–41).[1]

After joining the Edinburgh faculty as professor of medicine in 1765, Gregory gave several introductory lectures about the qualifications and duties of physicians. He published six of them in 1772. His ideals primarily involved the education of a physician and the nature of medical science. He strongly believed that a formal education in particular subjects constituted the ethical basis for medical practice. Education, science, and ethics were inseparable. Even when dealing with the public, Gregory's scientific emphasis continued. He was less concerned about what physicians should do for the community than about what laymen *qua* scientists could do for medicine. Somewhat randomly he exhorted his students to attend to the professional decorums that underlay interactions of practitioners and transactions between practitioners and patients. A more detailed analysis of these latter two groups of professional ideals was made by Thomas Percival, a Manchester physician who had carefully studied Gregory's book.

After a decade of private practice, Percival was appointed physician to the Manchester Infirmary. As hospitals became more exclusively concerned with the care of the sick during the eighteenth century, they provided a new arena for the struggles of British physicians, surgeons, and apothecaries. After verbal and emotional conflicts persisted among the physicians and surgeons of the Manchester hospital, Percival was asked – in 1792 – to draft a code of rules to regulate and govern practitioners at that hospital.

Since he had no vested interest in the principal London guilds, Percival could view the nexus of traditional relationships as an outsider, so to speak. He realized that the moral statutes of the various colleges of practitioners exerted little significant influence in hospital practice. But, by altering and expanding these statutes, particularly those of the Royal College of Physicians of London, and by using the highest moral sentiments of the age in dealing with the practical problems of hospital practice, Percival cleverly adapted guild regulations to the hospital setting. These rules were accepted by the trustees two years later, and they eventually became the first chapter of a book on medical ethics. After adding three chapters – one about private practice, one about relationships with apothecaries, and one about the legal duties of practitioners, Percival published his *Medical Ethics* in 1803.

There were major differences between the ideals of Gregory and the precepts of Percival. In view of Gregory's thorough discussion, Percival probably thought it superfluous to devote much attention to educational and scientific ideals. Besides, Percival did not believe that an 'academical' education was absolutely necessary for a medical practitioner even though he himself was a scholar and an ardent proponent of the experimental philosophy.

Gregory had offered a few standards about interactions of practitioners and about patient care. In appreciating the centrality of consultation in both private and hospital practice, Percival offered many precepts about transactions between physicians, surgeons, and apothecaries. In contrast to the guild statutes, though, Percival emphasized that all matters of consultative decorum should be judged in terms of better patient care. For example, in rural areas, apothecaries usually knew considerably more about the patient than anyone else. Thus, consultation and cooperation between physician, surgeon, and apothecary were desirable not only for professional improvement, but also for a more judicious decision about the care of the patient. In fact, ideals about the conduct of practitioners towards patients were pre-eminent in Percival's code.

There was a third major difference between Gregory's values and those of Percival. Gregory had urged laymen to devote their attention to basic problems of health and disease, but he had not discussed the social obligations of medical practitioners. Percival not only attended to public health obligations, but he also recognized the ethical significance of legal requirements. In return for exemptions from military service and jury duty, for example, physicians were required to meet certain demands of society, including testimony at judicial proceedings requiring medical evidence. This recognition of the impact of laws on professional ethics was a unique contribution by Percival. When applied to medicine, 'jurisprudence' meant primarily forensic medicine to the majority of British physicians who practised in the eighteenth and nineteenth centuries. 'Jurisprudence' signified moral injunctions to a few, including Percival and Michael Ryan.

A medical graduate of Edinburgh and a member of the College of Physicians in Edinburgh and in London, Ryan was editor of the *London Medical and Surgical Journal* in the 1830s. In 1831, he published a manual of medical jurisprudence, and, five years later, he issued an enlarged edition. The three sections of Ryan's compendium dealt respectively with medical ethics, laws in Britain relating to medicine, and forensic medicine.

Written primarily as a text for students, Ryan wished to prepare a 'concise and comprehensive compendium of the moral and legal duties of a medical man'. In the section on moral duties, Ryan essayed a history of medical ethics – probably the first in the English language. He did not analyse basic problems of professional values, as had Gregory and Percival.

Nevertheless, Ryan is singularly significant because he attempted to correlate medical ethics, health legislation, and forensic medicine. He realized that any society could incorporate its values about professional behaviour into civil statutes and, consequently, impose both moral and legal obligations on professional persons. Moreover, practitioners could not satisfactorily discharge professional obligations without understanding community expectations embodied in laws, and a satisfactory fulfilment of certain community obligations involved a special knowledge of law as well as medicine. Thus, Ryan sustained Percival's emphasis on the moral import of laws as well as his understanding of the forensic responsibilities of practitioners.

Various editions of Gregory's monograph, Percival's code, and Ryan's manual appeared between 1770 and 1850. In using these, British and American physicians began to deal with problems of medical ethics in a more thoughtful and organized fashion.

Physicians in the United States who considered problems of medical ethics were well acquainted with the writings of these three men. Benjamin Rush had read Percival's *Medical Ethics*, but, above all else, Rush had been profoundly influenced by his teacher, Gregory. As a professor in Philadelphia, Rush gave at least seven lectures about particular aspects of medical ethics. For example, in 1789 and again in 1801, Rush lectured about the immorality of scientific falsehoods in medicine. Medicine would be vastly improved if the scientific causes that retarded medical progress were removed. Rush repeated some of the causes that Gregory had listed in 1772, and he added some of his own.[2]

After Gregory's lectures were reprinted at Philadelphia in 1817, his influence became even greater. Hugh Hodge, in an oration to the Philadelphia Medical Society, reiterated Gregory's suggestions about the importance of certain subjects in medical education. Hodge had also studied Percival's book, and an abridgement of the same was published at Philadelphia in 1823. In that same year, the New York State Medical Society adopted its first code of medical ethics. However, it was not the first American code.

A few rules of professional ethics had been included in the by-laws adopted by some of the medical societies established in the United States before 1800. During the first half of the nineteenth century, these norms were frequently separated from the main group of by-laws and incorporated into codes of ethics, etiquette, or police. The first code was adopted by the Boston Medical Association in March of 1808. Known as the *Boston Medical Police*, this code had been prepared by a committee of doctors who claimed that they used the writings of Gregory, Percival, and Rush. Actually, all of the precepts in the *Boston Medical Police* could be found in the second chapter of Percival's *Medical Ethics*, the chapter that discussed such situations in private practice as consultations, arbitration of differences, interferences with another's practice, fees, and seniority among practitioners. Furthermore, the Boston physicians did not explain their reasons for ignoring Percival's precepts about hospital practice, apothecaries, and laws. Although there were few apothecary-practitioners in the United States at this time, there were hospitals, druggists, and medically-related laws. In spite of these exclusions, or, perhaps because of them, the *Boston Medical Police* became *the* model for codes of medical ethics adopted between 1817 and 1842 by at least thirteen societies in eleven states, New York not included.

The New York physicians did not simply imitate the Boston code. They included the forensic obligations so important to Percival. On the other hand, they championed Gregory's ideal about the social arrangement of medical practitioners. Percival had desired that a rigid distinction be maintained between physicians, surgeons, and apothecaries whereas Gregory had challenged British practitioners to learn and practise all branches of medicine. In agreeing with Gregory, the New York physicians expressed the sentiments of other American practitioners who saw no value in supporting the British hierarchy of social distinctions.[3]

The code of the New York State Medical Society exerted obvious influence on those who prepared a code for the Medico-Chirurgical Society of Baltimore in 1832.[4] The committee of Baltimore physicians also used the code of the Connecticut Medical Society (based on the *Boston Medical Police*) and the writings of Percival, Gregory, Rush and Ryan. In that same year, R. E. Griffith of Philadelphia, had issued an American edition of Ryan's *Manual of Medical Jurisprudence*. To the fifth chapter of this edition, Griffith added a synopsis of Rush's list of duties for patients. This synopsis became part of the fifth section of the code adopted in Baltimore and part of the first chapter of the code adopted by the American Medical Association fifteen years later.

Rush had offered his ideals about the obligations of patients in another lecture to students in 1808. According to Rush, patients should select only those physicians who have received a regular medical education. Moreover, patients should select only those doctors who have regular habits of life and are not devoted to company or pleasure at the theatre, turf, or chase. Patients should send for the doctor in the morning but be ready to receive him at any time of the day. They should communicate the history of their complaints fully but not relate the tedious or unimportant details. They should promptly obey the doctor's prescriptions. They should express appropriate gratitude and pay their fees promptly. Thus, the Baltimore doctors added a new dimension to American medical ethics by codifying the ideas of Rush regarding the responsibilities of patients toward their physicians.

With the momentum generated by local and state societies and their codes, it is not surprising that one of the earliest resolutions passed by the delegates to the first national medical convention in the United States involved the creation of a code of medical ethics. The committee who drafted this code reported that 'a great number of codes of ethics adopted by different societies in the United States,' were 'all based on that by Dr. Percival'.[5] In preparing their code, the committee attempted to preserve the words of Percival, although a 'few of the sections were in the words of the late Dr. Rush', and 'one or two sentences' were from other writers. On the afternoon of 6 May 1847, the committee's report was adopted as the first code of medical ethics for the American Medical Association.

Between 1765 and 1847, therefore, interested Americans unquestionably studied and utilized the British heritage bequeathed by Gregory, Percival and Ryan.[6] This heritage was essential to the beginnings of American medical ethics. In fashioning their ideals, American physicians borrowed many, but not all of the values offered by the British doctors. Furthermore, there was a major paradox in the transmission of professional values from Great Britain to the United States. Americans had rejected the British arrangements of medical practitioners and had grouped together in local, state, and national societies. In preparing codes of ethics for these societies, though, the Americans adopted many ideals about professional conduct that Gregory and Percival had offered to improve relationships between members of the British guilds. Nevertheless, with the adoption of the national code in 1847, American values and ideals returned to influence British doctors.[7]

The AMA code was divided into three chapters. The first dealt with the duties of physicians to their patients and, vice-versa, the duties of patients to their physicians. The latter section was exclusively Benjamin Rush. The former included summaries of the comments about patient care scattered throughout Percival. Chapter 2 reviewed the obligations that physicians had toward each other. It included all of the aforementioned precepts about consultations, interferences, and disagreements. Chapter 3 included the obligations of the profession to the public and, conversely, the obligations of the public to the profession. The latter were generalizations based on the requisites of Rush. The former preserved the concerns of Percival and Ryan by obligating American doctors to attend to matters of public health and forensic medicine.[8]

In 1849, a third edition of Percival's *Medical Ethics* was published in London, but the momentum of American influences was strikingly increasing in Great Britain. In an essay that appeared in the *London Medical Gazette*, W. B. Kesteven quoted several clauses from the AMA code.[9] The London publishing firm of John Churchill reprinted the AMA code and some essays on the duties of physicians written by a Boston physician, John Ware.

The most important American author, though, was a private practitioner in Connecticut, Worthington Hooker. In 1849, Hooker published a monograph with the following title: *Physician and the Patient or, a Practical View of the Mutual Duties, Relations, and Interests of the Medical Profession and the Community*. With this book, Hooker became the only American physician to write an extensive interpretation of the AMA code, and he was also the only nineteenth-century American physician to write a comprehensive monograph on the subject of medical ethics.

In 1850, an edition of Hooker's book was published in London. The editor, Edward Bentley, understood the historical significance of Hooker's book. 'It has been the subject of common remark', said Bentley in his preface, 'that no work upon the mutual duties, relations, and interests of the medical profession and the community has hitherto appeared in England, and considering the many able men capable of performing this task and whose opinions and experiences in such matters would carry weight and add importance to this interesting subject, it certainly is a matter of surprise . . .'. It is difficult to say which was more surprising to Bentley: the fact that no British physician between 1803 and 1850 had written a monograph on medical ethics, or the fact that a Norwich, Connecticut, practitioner had written one that so forcefully illustrated the dimension of mutuality or reciprocity in physician-patient relations. Although calling Hooker 'William' instead of Worthington on the title page of his London edition, Bentley could not change the fact that an American doctor had made a significant contribution to Anglo-American medical ethics.

Hooker believed that physicians had profound obligations to develop the highest of professional skills, especially those involved in clinical observation and evaluation. He also expected the public to correct their errors about professional skills and to learn how to distinguish between good and bad practices. Furthermore, physicians must understand and adhere to all of the rules of professional decorum, and the public must also understand these rules and appreciate the consequences of interfering with the activities of competent practitioners. With these and other analyses of the mutual obligations of physician and patient – of the medical profession and the community – Hooker championed the ingenuity of the AMA code and brilliantly depicted a feature of professional ethics that was not emphasized by Gregory, Percival, or Ryan.

The American novelty was widespread codification culminating in the AMA code of 1847. This code was voluntarily adopted by many state societies during the ensuing eight years. In 1855, the AMA resolved that all state and local societies had to adopt the code if they wished to send delegates to its annual convention. But compulsory acceptance did not guarantee higher standards or uniform enforcement. In 1857, one critic of codification observed that professional conflicts and abuses were as evident in England where there were no codes as they were in America with codes. Hooker might have retorted that the goods of professional life were more recognizable in the United States with codes than in Great Britain without codes. No American claimed that codes guaranteed medical righteousness. Codes simply provided physicians with some knowledge of the difference between right and wrong professional conduct. Without some ideals and some means of institutionalizing them, there would be little chance to alter professional evils anywhere.

Spurred by the AMA code, the British Medical Association attempted to develop a code of ethics. Prior to 1858, at least two committees faltered. At the Edinburgh meeting in July of 1858, a thirty-four-member committee was established with Charles Hastings as chairman and T. Herbert Barker and Alexander Henry as secretary. At the meeting in 1859, Barker was granted additional time to prepare his report. It had not materialized by 1865.[10]

The American efforts afforded British doctors a mirror by which they could judge the relevant and less relevant parts of their own professional values. Perhaps the British practitioners understood the problems of enforcement and compromised professional freedom inherent in codes. Whatever the reasons, Great Britain did not have a nationally accepted set of ethical guidelines by 1865.

In summary, the international exchange of professional ideals was not exclusively from Great Britain to the United States between 1765 and 1865. Primarily one-way before 1830, the influences began to shift afterwards. By the middle of the nineteenth century, British practitioners were well aware of developments in the United States, including the adoption of the AMA code in 1847 and the publication of Worthington Hooker's *Physician and Patient* in 1849. After 1850, practitioners in both countries recognized the challenge of a principle of mutual obligations between practitioners and patients and they reciprocally influenced each other as they created and changed their professional values.

References

1   KING, LESTER S., *The Medical World of the 18th Century*, Chicago, 1958, pp. 244–60; FORBES, ROBERT, 'Medical ethics in Great Britain', *Wld med. J.*, 1954, 1, 297–99.
2   RUSH, BENJAMIN, *Sixteen Introductory Lectures*, Philadelphia, 1811, pp. 141–65.
3   *A System of Medical Ethics, Published by the Order of the State Medical Society of New York*, New York, 1823.
4   Medico-Chirurgical Society of Baltimore, *The System of Medical Ethics Adopted by the Society, Being the Report of the Committee on Ethics*, Baltimore, 1832.

5   *Proceedings of the National Medical Conventions, Held in New York, May, 1846, and in Phila-delphia, May, 1847*, Philadelphia, 1847, p. 92.

6   Between 1832 and 1847, the writings of Gregory and Percival had been cited by several other American physicians. In 1834, sections from Percival's books were published in an issue of the *United States Medical and Surgical Journal*. In 1836, Gregory's lectures and Percival's book were recommended to candidates for licensure examination by the Massachusetts Medical Society. Robley Dunglison, in 1837, recommended that medical students carefully study the books on medical ethics written by Gregory and Percival. In an address to a group of Lexington doctors in 1839, Thomas Mitchell referred to Percival.

7   Influences from the United States began to be visible in the 1830s. When Michael Ryan revised his book on medical jurisprudence in 1836, he transformed chapter 5 into a section entitled 'American Medical Ethics'. This chapter was actually a reprint of the talk that had been given to the Philadelphia Medical Society in 1826 by John Godman. Ryan had not prepared a history of 'American medical ethics' nor had he mentioned the synopsis of Rush's essay on the duties of patients that Griffith had added to the Philadelphia edition of Ryan's book. But Ryan had acknowledged the existence of an 'American' medical ethics.

8   Thomas Percival's grandson, James Haywood, visiting Philadelphia in December of 1848, expressed his appreciation to one of the members of the AMA committee for their use of Percival's moral precepts. 'In England', said Haywood, 'I believe that my grandfather's Medical Ethics are generally looked upon as a standard work on that subject, and it is gratifying that you have honored him with a similar confidence on this side of the Atlantic.' Letter to Isaac Hays from James Haywood, 3 December 1848; located in Isaac Hays' Papers, Library American Philosophical Society, Philadelphia, Pennsylvania.

9   KESTEVEN, W. B., 'Thoughts on medical ethics', *Lond. med. Gaz.*, 1849, 9, 408–14.

10 *Br. med. J.*, 1858, pp. 657–58; ibid., 1859, p. 631.

THE WILLIAM OSLER MEDAL ESSAY

CABOT, PEABODY, AND THE CARE OF THE PATIENT

THOMAS FRANKLIN WILLIAMS

The art of caring for sick people, the mark of the true physician, is not easily learned. Its acquisition must depend in large measure upon the inspiration to master it which a good teacher adds to the inclination of his students to learn it.

Two among Boston's physicians and teachers who have helped particularly to keep the care of the whole patient in its just place as the highest, challenging goal for their colleagues and for recent generations of medical students are Richard Cabot and Francis Peabody. These two men served as personal examples of physicians worth following, and in addition, by putting their ideas into practical, lasting new forms—in institutions and in their writings—they have influenced the care of patients far beyond their own place and time.

Richard Clarke Cabot was born in Brookline, Massachusetts, on May 21, 1868, the son of James Elliott and Elizabeth Dwight Cabot. His father was a philosopher, overseer of Harvard College, and friend and biographer of Emerson. Both parents came from old Boston families, secure in social and financial ways. At the same time the family was " distinguished for independent thinking and acting ";[1] we shall find plenty of evidence for these very qualities in Richard.

After preparing for college at the Noble and Greenough School, Richard went on, as one would expect, to Harvard, where he graduated *summa cum laude* in 1889. He majored in philosophy, thinking that he might go into the Unitarian ministry, but by Commencement time he had decided on medicine instead. His reasons for making the change are not clear. His mother writes at the time that she is " startled "; she can, however, " see how his quick sympathies and his interest in humanity lead him to think of it." [2] It may very well be that he was seeking, in medicine, a more obviously practical way of serving his fellow-man.

In another of her letters at this time, Cabot's mother gives a picture of

[1] Washburn, Frederic A., *The Massachusetts General Hospital*, Boston, Houghton Mifflin Company, 1939, pp. 459-460.
[2] *The Letters of Elizabeth Dwight Cabot*, edited and privately printed by Richard C. Cabot.

one of his lifelong qualities of character: his inflexible adherence to the truth as he saw it, his driving will to seek it out. This drive was sometimes inconsiderate of others, and the letter gently but firmly criticizes Richard for, at times, forgetting what his mother calls the " shield of good manners." [2] His mother's strong will and clarity and beauty of expression in writing seem to have been reflected in Richard. He was always close and devoted to her.

Cabot crossed the Charles River to the old buildings of the Harvard Medical School in downtown Boston, graduated there in 1892, and interned for 18 months at the Massachusetts General Hospital. For his paper before the Boylston Medical Society, the student medical society which dates back to 1811, he made a study of " The Medical Bearing of Mind-Care "—the system of healing of Christian Science, 25 years old then. One Boylston historian wrote, " In his characteristic way the author [Cabot] had accumulated a vast amount of knowledge by mailing 150 letters to prominent Christian Scientists, and by personally interviewing many of them." [3]

Dr. Cabot's early fame in medicine was due, according to Dr. Paul White, to "his great ability and industry in pioneer work." [4] This industry was already quite evident in his internship, for during it he published his first paper in clinical research, on " Leucocytosis as an Element in the Prognosis of Pneumonia." [5] The subject of leucocytosis was followed up the next year, 1894-1895, when as a Dalton research fellow at the Massachusetts General Hospital he was apparently the first to note that the white blood cell count rises in pyogenic infections, and that leucocytosis is very good supporting evidence for a diagnosis of appendicitis. In discussing this work the Boston surgeons of that day expressed their gratitude for this aid in making the often-difficult distinction between typhoid fever and appendicitis. [6] The Massachusetts General Hospital's historian, Dr. Frederic Washburn, states that Dr. Cabot introduced clinical hematology to the hospital at that time. [7] These studies of the blood were enlarged into his first book, published in 1896, when Cabot was 28 years old and just four years out of medical school. Called

[3] " Catalogue of Boylston Medical Society," 1923, p. 26.

[4] White, Paul D., " Richard Clarke Cabot," *New England J. Med. 220*: 1049-1052, June 22, 1939.

[5] Cabot, R. C., *Boston M. & S. J. cxxix*: 117, 1893.

[6] Cabot, R. C., " Diagnostic and Prognostic Importance of Leucocytosis," *Boston M. & S. J., cxxx*: 277, 292, 1894.

[7] Washburn, F. A., *op. cit.*, p. 126.

A Guide to the Clinical Examination of the Blood, it was, he said in the Preface, " the first book of its kind in English, so far as I am aware." It quickly became the standard text and went through five editions.

In 1894 Cabot married Ella Lyman, a teacher of ethics and psychology in Boston private schools. She shared his temperament and interests and remained for forty years his constant support and inspiration, and his best critic.

The year 1898 saw Richard Cabot serving a short while in the Spanish-American War aboard the U. S. Army Hospital Ship *Bay State.* In the same year he returned to Boston to plunge into a full schedule: private practice, work as a physician to out-patients at the Massachusetts General Hospital, and research and writing in new fields of medicine. A monograph on *The Serum Diagnosis of Disease,* covering mainly the new Widal reaction for typhoid fever, was published in 1899. By 1901 he had prepared the first edition of his *Physical Diagnosis of Diseases of the Chest.* Within the next four years he expanded it to include the rest of the body, and it has been used all over the world as a textbook of physical diagnosis ever since, appearing in twelve editions up to the time of Dr. Cabot's death in 1939.

Dr. Cabot certainly considered the advancement of medical science in his conception of the best care of the patient. That he did so is evidenced by these contributions to the laboratory science, and by the great volume of his own kind of clinical research, which began at this early date and continued over the next twenty years.

His method of doing clinical research was to gather data from large numbers of cases and to arrive at conclusions statistically. An example may help to show the value and weakness of his method. In a study of 784 cases of fever lasting longer than two weeks (all the cases of this type that he could find in the records of the Massachusetts General Hospital—his usual procedure), Cabot found that 90 per cent were produced by tuberculosis, typhoid fever, or pyogenic sepsis. This conclusion he put into a lecture before the New Hampshire State Medical Society in 1907, entitled " The Three Long-Continued Fevers of New England." In this paper he says, " Simply to know the facts shown in this table is of importance, because of the help it gives us in diagnosis by exclusion. If you have a continued fever, a long fever, you are pretty sure it must be one of three things. Then if you exclude two of these three—as you often can—your diagnosis is made." [8] This is typical of his quite useful but

---

[8] Cabot, R. C., *Boston M. & S. J., clvii*: 281, 1907.

not quite complete way of stating things which bothered some clinical purists.

On Dr. Cabot's side it should quickly be added that just this method of gathering data, especially from autopsy material, led to his most important contribution to medical science, his paper on " The Four Common Types of Heart Disease." [9] In this paper, which appeared in 1914, Dr. Cabot classified heart disease according to its causes, and found that rheumatic, arteriosclerotic, syphilitic, and nephritic or nephrogenic made up 93 per cent of all heart disease in the 600 cases studied. In appraising the value of this work, Dr. Paul White writes:

For the first time, proper emphasis was laid on the etiological diagnosis of heart disease, in contrast to the over-emphasis of structural defects that had been current for over two hundred years. The revolution in point of view was amazing. Where at one time, in fact for generations, textbooks and papers had been preponderantly involved with such subjects as mitral regurgitation, myocarditis, and pericarditis, they now present as a primary interest the causes of heart disease . . .—a landmark in medical history, which places him as the greatest contributor to cardiology in our generation.[10]

Dr. Cabot published many other papers of the same type in varied fields of medicine. He might be called one of the last of the great general clinicians, not limited to any special " field within a field." His interest in research was in finding out " What? "—" What are the facts? "—not in answering the questions, " Why? ", or " How? ". Francis Peabody, we shall see, asked the why and how of things.

In those busy years of the early nineteen hundreds one finds the beginnings of two other of Cabot's most important contributions: the case method of teaching, and hospital social service.

The idea of using summaries of cases to teach medicine systematically originated with Dr. Walter B. Cannon, the Harvard physiologist. In about 1898, while still a medical student, Cannon suggested it to Dr. Cabot and others of his clinical teachers, and in 1900 he published several articles on its use.[11] He stated that he got the idea from the new case teaching of the Harvard Law School. Dr. Cabot took up the use of case summaries more enthusiastically than anyone else. He saw it as a way

---

[9] *J. A. M. A., 63*: 1461-1463, 1914.

[10] White, P. D., *loc. cit.*

[11] Cannon, Walter B., " The Case Method of Teaching Systematic Medicine," *Boston M. & S. J., cxlii*: 31, 1900; " The Case System in Medicine," *Boston M. & S. J., cxlii*: 563, 1900; " The Use of Clinic Records in Teaching Medicine," *Bull. Amer. Acad. Med., V*, 1900.

of teaching students about many diseases in addition to those of the patients actually in the hospital beds at the moment.

In 1902 Cabot published a tiny book of 43 case summaries, called *Exercises in Differential Diagnosis*. On each page was a short summary of a case, ending with the questions, " Diagnosis? Prognosis? Treatment? " He used these for teaching his students, making them commit themselves to the diagnosis first, then discussing the cases with them in his stimulating style. He considered the act of making a decision—committing yourself—the most important part. By 1906 he had enlarged the book to 77 cases, now called *Case Teaching in Medicine*. There was a student's copy containing the same three important, inevitable questions and some additional questions on differential diagnosis, with blank spaces for answers. The teacher's copy had the answers conveniently and, one may say, didactically printed in it. To the student Cabot says, in the Introduction, that the goal in reading the case is to answer the question, " What is the gist of it all? "—a principle that is still taught medical students when they first begin studying case summaries.

Dr. Cabot soon became impressed with the usefulness of having a definite, final answer, in the form of a pathological lesion found at operation or autopsy, to give to the question, " What is the diagnosis? " Furthermore, it added to the value of the teaching session to relate the clinical picture to the pathological one. As early as 1905 he was calling such sessions " clinico-pathological exercises." [12] From here it was an easy step to the large-scale Clinico-Pathological Conference, for which Dr. Cabot deserves full credit as originator.

He tells his own story very well:

As soon as I began to have the opportunities of ward service at the Massachusetts General Hospital, beginning with 1908, I was much impressed by the undesirable separation between the clinical men and the pathologists. One day I discovered in an old volume of bound records a case diagnosed as neurasthenia (or nervous prostration), and looking at the final lines of the record saw that the patient had died and that an autopsy had been performed. Yet the diagnosis of neurasthenia still stood as the only clinical diagnosis, both on the record and in the index. This curious blunder aroused me so much that I went at once to the Pathological Laboratory and looked up the post-mortem record of the case. I found that the patient had died of cancer of the pleura but had had neurasthenic symptoms and vague intercostal pain, which had misled the clinicians. What especially impressed me was that the clinical diagnosis had never been changed, presumably because the clinicians were unaware of the post-mortem result.

---

[12] Cabot, R. C., and E. A. Locke, " The Organization of a Department of Clinical Medicine," *Boston M. & S. J.*, cliii: 461, 1905.

312

Soon after this, at the beginning of the year 1910, I began, on my own initiative, to hold exercises with the house officers and medical visitors to the hospital—a weekly exercise in connection with Dr. James Homer Wright, modeled essentially like the later clinical pathological conferences. . . . The test of the student's diagnostic powers in reviewing the whole clinical record, physical examination, and laboratory findings and committing himself to a diagnosis in writing, is of great value because each student knows that within a few minutes the autopsy record will prove him right or wrong and usually make clear why he was wrong and how he can correct his thinking for the future.[13]

These Clinico-Pathological Conferences grew rapidly in popularity and spread to other medical centers. An English visitor to them, years later, gives a good description:

The clinic was an experience and an inspiration. Cabot read out in detail the history, the results of investigations and the general findings in each case. The audience was a motley gathering of newly qualified internes, colleagues on the staff, and elderly visiting physicians—a Negro, a Chinese, any type and every type. Cabot sat on a table with his legs dangling and asked for suggestions as to diagnoses. Smilingly he extracted comments and criticisms from complete strangers both young and inexperienced and old and hard-bitten and worked up a lively discussion. At the end he summarized with beautiful clarity the various diagnoses made, finishing with his own. Then he summoned the pathologist with his post-mortem notes. As it turned out, in one case Cabot and everybody else was wrong. It is good to remember the spirit in which he took his failure. " That is the third time I have made a wrong guess," he said, and he showed us the steps that had led him astray.[14]

The " CPC," as it has come to be known in teaching hospitals throughout our country, received the praise of Dr. Alan Gregg when he said that it " is the wonder and admiration of many of our foreign visitors, who see in it a candor and fearlessness altogether to the credit of American medicine." [15]

Dr. Cabot himself regularly discussed the medical cases presented until the early 1930's, gradually letting other men take over the discussions. They were printed by the hospital for several years and, after 1923, in the *Boston Medical and Surgical Journal* (now the *New England Journal of Medicine*). Cabot was editor of the write-ups until July, 1935, when Dr. Tracy Mallory took his place. In his own discussions Dr. Cabot relied on his statistics to give him the most probable diagnosis. His temper would occasionally flare up at " CPC's," when the diagnosis would

[13] Cabot, R. C., quoted in Washburn, F. A., *op. cit.*, pp. 115-117.
[14] " Richard Clarke Cabot " (Obituary), *Lancet 1*: 1406, June 17, 1939.
[15] Gregg, Alan, quoted in Washburn, F. A., *op. cit.*, p. 117.

turn out to be some rare, improbable malady, or again when someone else would make the correct diagnosis when it did not seem to him to be the likely one. Such flare-ups were short-lived, however; he would apologize and, as in all his dealings with other people, be extremely willing to admit that he had been wrong. Cabot's disinterestedness in himself, his lack of personal ambition or pride, has been called his greatest quality of personality.[16]

Before leaving Cabot the teacher, we should take note of his lectures and his essays, the ways in which his ideas—the truth as he saw it—were shared with people far and wide. He used a very successful technique for lecturing: he always prepared and followed a careful outline, which was either printed and distributed to the audience or written on a blackboard, so that everyone saw clearly just what point he was making.[17] He gave medical lectures all over the United States in these busy years: in California in 1904, Colorado in 1906, Maryland in 1906.

He was a real master of the constructive and inspirational speech or essay, both much in demand in his day. His essays are still well worth reading today for their beauty, clarity of expression, and logical persuasiveness. In one of his early essays (1903) he wrote about " Truth and Falsehood in Medicine," a subject to which he returned numerous times later. He was quite absolute in his belief in telling the truth at all times; very likely his training in philosophy, in the days when the teachings of Immanuel Kant were in much favor, helped to foster his absolutism. He was, however, often misquoted. Dr. Cabot's central thesis was only that the physician should " make a sincere effort to convey a true impression " to a patient or his family when they ask for it.

A frequent topic of Dr. Cabot's speeches was the hospital out-patient department. He described the situation in the " OPD " pungently: " Out-patient departments are, as a rule, neglected." [18] " I think that if some good newspaper man got a hold and looked into exactly what are the actual results, the good accomplished in our hospital dispensaries, that we medical men and nurses would look pretty cheap." [19] How was the OPD falling

[16] (Perry, Ralph Barton), " Richard Clarke Cabot," *Harvard Alumni Bulletin,* May 19, 1939.

[17] Conversations with Miss Ida M. Cannon and Mrs. Hilbert F. Day, who kindly furnished much information from their long personal and professional association with Dr. Cabot.

[18] Cabot, R. C., " Suggestions for the Reorganization of Hospital Out-Patient Departments, with Special Reference to the Improvement of Treatment," *Maryland M. J.,* 1: 81-91, 1907.

[19] " Social Service Work in Hospitals," *Chicago Medical Recorder,* June, 1911.

down on its job? Mainly, he said, by not being able to get the treatment that the patient needed carried out. This defect Dr. Cabot set about to remedy by establishing Medical Social Service as a necessary part of carrying out *effective* treatment. Many people believe this to be Cabot's greatest accomplishment.

When a hospital undertakes the care of a patient,—Dr. Cabot said,—it ought to do it and not be content with going through the forms of doing it. . . . To order for one patient a diet which he cannot possibly procure; for the next a vacation which he is too poor to take; to forbid the third to worry when the necessary cause for worry remains unchanged; to give the fourth directions for an outdoor life which you are morally certain he won't carry out; to try to teach the fifth . . . how to modify milk for the baby when she understands perhaps half what you say and forgets most of that half—this makes a morning's work not very satisfactory in retrospect to anybody, and hardly more useful than the old-fashioned wholesale drugging.

It was to fill just such needs as we have suggested that there was organized in October, 1905, a small force of social workers to attend to any cases which the out-patient physicians might see fit to send them.[20]

Somewhat similar uses had been made of auxiliary personnel in hospitals before this, and Cabot had learned from them. In London since 1895 the so-called " Lady Almoners," the first paid workers, had helped hospitals check the "abuse of charity," and, as a definitely secondary function, had helped cooperate with government and private social agencies.[21] At the Massachusetts General Hospital the philanthropic " Ladies Visiting Committee" of the hospital had " frequently found need of assistance and quietly given it." [22] And in July, 1905, Dr. Joseph H. Pratt had begun to set up his classes designed to improve the care and treatment of poor tuberculous patients in their own homes. An important part of his plan was the " friendly visitor," as Dr. Pratt called her—a paid woman worker who went into the home regularly, to instruct, advise, and report on conditions and progress. Dr. Cabot, with the idea of social service in his mind for some time,[23] was definitely stimulated by Dr. Pratt's remarkable results to organize his " small force " of workers, to try to make the treatment of the whole OPD effective. This is an example of Dr. Cabot's great ability to recognize the really valuable ideas of his time and to put them into action in lasting form, as in a new institution.

[20] Cabot, R. C., *Maryland M. J., 1*: 81-91, 1907.

[21] Cabot, R. C., " Hospital Dispensary Social Work," *Hospital Social Service, XVIII*: 269, 1928.

[22] Washburn, F. A., *op. cit.*, p. 459.

[23] Conversation with Miss Ida M. Cannon.

The start was unpretentious. One of the first social workers describes it for us: " a little corner of the Out-Patient Department surrounded by screens, with one paid worker and volunteers. Dr. Cabot consulted with and advised the helpers daily, being himself responsible for all financial aid beyond what little might be given by subscription. The work was Dr. Cabot in those days."[24] Cabot said later that, fearful that the paid worker might be accused of loafing if she had nothing to do, and suspecting that she might not, he left her some typing to do. She had typed for about fifteen minutes when a physician appeared with a mother and baby in tow, and, asking the worker to explain infant feeding to the mother, quickly left. From then on there was no time for Dr. Cabot's typing. In 1906, the first full year, 684 patients were seen by the social workers.

Miss Ida M. Cannon, sister of Dr. Walter B. Cannon, became Head Social Worker in 1907 and from then on she shares equal credit with Dr. Cabot for developing this new field, against, at first, much opposition in the hospital.

Dr. Cabot thought and wrote a lot about this new profession that he had helped to create. Probably the best of his writing is in his book, *Social Service and the Art of Healing*, published in 1909. He explores various ideas about social work and concludes that essentially the social worker is an expert—an expert in " the study of character under adversity and of the influences that mold it for good or ill." [25] She must take good care not to be a professional do-gooder, but stick to her specialty just like anyone else. As a professional person she should command expert fees, and have " office hours and private practice as well as public work among the poor." She should be consulted " in all sorts of moral and domestic difficulties, by the parents of difficult children, by the children of difficult parents." [26] " The true business of the social worker," he says, " is psychical diagnosis and treatment." [27]

Since its beginnings 43 years ago, medical social work has come to include hospitalized patients along with out-patients in its care, has developed the case work technique to a high degree, and has added other refinements—even specialists, such as psychiatric social workers. But it has continued to grow substantially along the lines that Richard Cabot set forth.

[24] Lawson, Mary, quoted by P. D. White, *New England J. Med., 220*: 1049-1052, June 22, 1939.

[25] Cabot, R. C., *Social Service and the Art of Healing*, New York, 1909, p. 55.

[26] *Ibid.*, pp. 84-89.

[27] *Ibid.*, p. 65.

Social work also did things for Dr. Cabot. He started out, as he says, merely to practice good medicine by making treatment effective—the goal of any ethical physician. Social service led him to consider the larger problems of man in society, and he spent most of the last half of his life going more and more into social problems and, finally, ethical problems, as we shall see in a little while.

Dr. Cabot had other interests in these, his developing years, besides mere textbook-writing, case teaching, CPC's, reforming the OPD, starting social service, and practicing medicine. It might be expected that he would recognize and be interested in the relation of the mind and emotions to disease, and such is so, for his writings about psychic factors in disease and about psychotherapy are, I believe, remarkable.

As early as 1899 the young clinician had reported a case in which he felt that the ataxic, cerebellar symptoms of a young man, diagnosed as cerebellar tumor by everyone, were shown by a five year follow-up to be due probably to feelings of guilt because of masturbation.[28] Dr. Cabot was one of the earliest American physicians to study and refer to Freud's work, an indication of his wide reading and openness to new ideas. While speaking before the Colorado Medical Society in October, 1906, Cabot quoted with approval an early article on psychoanalysis by Cabot's friend, Dr. James Jackson Putman, Professor of Neurology at Harvard. Dr. Cabot goes on to say, to the Colorado physicians, " Does all this sound to you very fanciful and mystical? Then remember that you are listening to a paraphrase of the words [of Freud], one of the greatest neurologists since Charcot, and further that these conclusions are the result of many remarkable therapeutic successes attained through the use of methods and conceptions here suggested. It is now solid science, and we have been verifying its results at the Massachusetts General Hospital." [29] This was in 1906, three years before Freud came to America on a visit which he calls " the introduction of psychoanalysis into North America." [30]

In this same talk in Colorado Dr. Cabot showed that he understood something of psychosomatic medicine thirty years before it began to be developed as a field, by giving a clear description of emotional factors in exophthalmic goitre as an example.

Dr. Cabot mentions Freud's work in almost every article and lecture of his on therapeutics during these years. At the same time he thought of

[28] Cabot, R. C., " Cerebellar Tumor or Masturbation? " *J. A. M. A. XXXII* : 1027, 1899.
[29] " Mind Cure: Its Service to the Community " *Colorado Medicine, iv*: 5, January 1907.
[30] Freud, S., *History of the Psychoanalytic Movement,* New York, 1914.

psychoanalysis as only one of many psychotherapeutic techniques, other important ones being education, explanation, suggestion, hygiene, rest, and work. He talked of the work of Pierre Janet, another of Charcot's pupils, and of Paul DuBois, a Swiss, as much as he did of Freud. DuBois impressed Cabot with the value of learning to make decisions, and the important role of indecision in producing mental troubles. It may well be that Dr. Cabot's belief in committing oneself on the diagnosis comes from this idea of DuBois.

Finally, Cabot considered religion to be the central, driving force in human beings, and thought that psychotherapy would have to acknowledge and use this force if it were to be as useful and efficient as possible.

All through these busy years we must picture, too, Richard Cabot the choral director, tall and lanky, energetic as always, leading the Massachusetts General Hospital Glee Club on the steps of Bulfinch Building on such occasions as the dedication of the new Out-Patient Building in 1903, or leading Christmas carollers over Beacon Hill and through the wards of the hospital. These things he originated, too. And there is Cabot the philosopher, keeping up his earlier interest by attending Dr. Josiah Royce's famous Harvard Seminary course in logic year after year, and giving lectures in the course in 1903 and 1904, just as if he had nothing else to do.

This pace kept up through 1912-1914. About then Dr. Cabot began to devote more of his time to social problems related to medicine. It seemed to him a logical conclusion of his own experience that, despite all its faults, group medicine, as he had seen it in the teaching hospital, gave better medical care than the private practitioner could give. With his characteristic crusading spirit he spoke and wrote this conclusion. He laid his views first before his own profession, but shortly afterwards he turned to public addresses and magazine articles. Perhaps his most controversial article appeared in the *American Magazine* for May, 1916, entitled " Better Doctoring for Less Money." Here he argued that some system of health insurance, centered around the hospital or group-practice system, was the way to give better medical care for less money—even at the expense of the doctor-patient relationship if that were necessary.

These statements to the general public, with Dr. Cabot's somewhat exaggerated phrases used for newspaper headlines, provoked a strong exchange of letters between him and the Massachusetts Medical Society, published in the *Boston Medical and Surgical Journal* for June, 1916. Despite disagreement with his colleagues, he continued his interest in group practice the rest of his life. He supported the Group Health Association in Washington, D. C., in its early days, and he spoke in favor of group practice, but not in favor of compulsory health insurance, at his last public appearance, at the *New York Herald-Tribune* Forum in October, 1938.

This crusade was turned aside in 1916 by a more urgent cause. Dr. Cabot became convinced that our nation should be fighting the war alongside of Britain and France. With his usual drive to put beliefs into action, he set out on a lecture tour of the Midwest (the center of opposition to our entering the war) to convince people that we should enter it immediately. One story, possibly apocryphal, is that he would play his violin first, to attract the crowd, and then launch into his appeal. When we did enter the war, Cabot served as Chief of Medicine with Base Hospital Number Six, formed at the Massachusetts General Hospital. He was the despair of more militarily-minded people like Dr. Frederic Washburn, the hospital director, because he could never learn to salute or to keep his shoes shined. While in France he helped to set up aid stations for refugees, and he introduced medical social service to France through a series of lectures.

During their service together in France, Dr. Cabot talked often with his friend, Dr. Paul White, about how impatient he was becoming " with the mere healing of wounds and illnesses, and the education to be found in most schools. . . . Morons can be superbly healthy, criminals can be highly educated. It was the spiritual quality of the individual that attracted his attention " now, and " the possibility of its cultivation became to him a challenge." [31] To put such thoughts into action, Dr. Cabot, in 1919, became Professor of Social Ethics and head of the department at Harvard at the same time that he became a full Professor of Clinical Medicine. Throughout the last twenty years of his life he gave more and more of his time to the field of ethics, where, he felt, the key to the care of the whole man really lay.

Believing strongly that we learn most from the lives of great individuals, Dr. Cabot would present his classes in social ethics with his own spellbinding biographies of great men, and would often invite the living great in for a class. One might call this case-teaching, carried from medicine over into social ethics.

Dr. Cabot's many other activities in these later years of his life deserve the attention of a much fuller biography, and can only be listed here. He continued his support of the growing field of social work, serving as President of the National Conference of Social Work in 1931. He was

President of the Massachusetts Anti-Saloon League in 1931-1933 (and a life-long total abstainer himself). At another time he was a member of the Board of Directors of the American Civil Liberties Union. He continued to write beautiful essays on the values of life. Some of his best writing on any subject were the four essays, " Work," " Play," " Love," and " Worship," gathered into the book called *What Men Live By* (1914). Late in life he helped to start the Institute of Pastoral Care at the Massachusetts General Hospital, for the training of ministers in their care of the sick.

One of his last papers, entitled " The Wisdom of the Human body," [32] was delivered by invitation before the Massachusetts Medical Society— evidence of the esteem in which Dr. Cabot and his colleagues held each other, despite their earlier disagreements. In this paper Dr. Cabot gives examples of how his experiences as a physician helped to substantiate his deep religious beliefs. Here again, as in so much of his work, his contribution was to show the inter-relations between fields. He made significant contributions to medicine, sociology, ethics, and religion, but his real genius was in relating one to the other, in the " borderlands " of each of these realms.

The personality of Richard Cabot is best summarized by Dr. Paul White:

In every generation there are restless souls, who cannot be made to fit the common mold. A few of these are valuable in keeping their communities and professions in a ferment by their constant challenge to the existing order of man's thought and action. But when, in addition to possessing these attributes, a rare individual is endowed with the divine fire and makes important contributions to the pioneering programs of humanity, then indeed we recognize a great leader. In the thick of the fray such recognition comes slowly but as the smoke of the battle clears the acclaim is universal.[33]

With such a beautiful characterizing picture of this great and complex man, we leave Richard Cabot and turn to Francis Peabody, no less great, I believe, than Cabot, but one whose life seems to have been one of simplicity and human warmth. He is perhaps an easier person to understand than Richard Cabot.

Francis Weld Peabody was born in Cambridge, Massachusetts, November 24, 1881—thirteen years younger than Cabot—and died of cancer in 1927, at the age of 47. He was the son of the Unitarian minister and

[32] Cabot, R. C., *New England J. Med., 217*: 833-836, 1937.
[33] White, Paul D., *loc. cit.*

Harvard Professor, Francis Greenwood Peabody, and of Cora Weld
Peabody, a gentle, quiet lady who came from the trading and Quaker
families of New Bedford. Francis grew up in the intellectual and
pleasantly religious surroundings of his father's home and of that of
William James, a close neighbor. He went with his family to Europe
twice, for a year each time, learning German as a particularly useful
by-product of those trips. While in Venice in 1899, just before entering
Harvard College, he barely survived an attack of typhoid fever. During
Francis' severe illness the disease killed his brother.

A quiet, unassuming young man, Francis somewhat surprised his family
by graduating *cum laude* from Harvard. By his third year in college he
had decided to go into medicine; he had been thinking of it ever since his
and his brother's typhoid fever. In the Harvard Medical School he was
president of his class, and was vice-president of the Boylston Medical
Society in the same year (1906) that its president, a faculty member, was
Dr. Richard Cabot. Peabody's Boylston paper was on " The Treatment of
Diabetes." The person scheduled to discuss it when it was presented, in
April, 1906, was Dr. Elliot P. Joslin, but he came down with pneumonia
at the time and could not be present. Peabody was already thinking of
the whole patient, for he says in his paper, " We must not forget in
treating Diabetes that we are treating a man and not a disease." [34]

By the end of his third year, in 1906, Francis was considering long-
range plans, and Dr. Reginald Fitz suggested to him that he consider
taking prolonged training for a career in " academic medicine." This was
a new idea in American medicine, for most of our medical school professors
were clinicians who gave a little of their time to teaching, and our medical
research was insignificant compared to that of European countries,
especially Germany.

At this very time a fortunate chance to try out medical research appeared :
Dr. Joseph H. Pratt had just returned to Boston after sound academic
training at Johns Hopkins, under Osler, Welch and Councilman, and in
Germany under some of the great men of that day. Dr. Pratt was preparing to offer for the first time an elective course in clinical research for
fourth-year students. Francis Peabody became his first student in the
course, over the opposition of almost all the clinical teachers in the medical
school except Dr. Fitz—something of a courageous new departure for any
student.

[34] Boylston Medical Society Records, 1899-1908 (bound volume in Harvard Med. Sch.
Library), pp. 307-308.

Dr. Pratt himself describes that year, 1906-1907:

We took a bare room in the newly opened buildings and fitted up a bacteriological laboratory. The problem assigned to Peabody was to isolate typhoid bacilli from the dejections of typhoid patients by the use of new methods. The program I proposed to him would have repelled most students. He had to go from his home in Cambridge each morning to the Massachusetts General Hospital and there gather up the collected feces of typhoid patients and bring them out to the school. . . . Arriving at the school he had to make all the culture media, and to do all the work aided only by an untrained laboratory boy. He completed the research and we published it under our joint authorship, first in German in the *Zentralblatt für Bacteriologie,* and later in English.[35]

Peabody followed up this work on typhoid by developing, during his internship at the Massachusetts General Hospital, a method of growing typhoid bacilli in blood from the earlobe of patients early in the course of the disease. This work he reported before the Section of Medicine of the American Medical Association at its Chicago meeting in June, 1908, near the end of his internship year. Dr. Pratt states that he " can recall no other interne who has reported original work in clinical medicine at a meeting of our national society." [35] Even in this early paper Peabody showed a remarkable interest in the individual patient and in the broader, preventive medicine aspects of his work. " To the individual patient," he said, " early diagnosis in typhoid means better treatment, better nursing, perhaps more adequate domestic arrangements, and often a great saving of strength during the first stages of the disease." [36] And he comments on the importance of early diagnosis in preventing the spread of typhoid, as it had just been shown that it may be spread even before clinical signs appear.

This year of research with Dr. Pratt, Dr. Peabody later said, gave him his first real enthusiasm for medicine—it showed him that medicine is a " growing thing "; he gave Dr. Pratt credit for first showing him " the joy and satisfaction of seeking new truths." [37] Evidently this experience satisfied him about academic medicine, for, immediately after his internship, he turned down an attractive offer to join one of the best clinicians in Boston. Instead, he set out on a training program which in the next

[35] Pratt, Joseph H., " The Personality of the Physician," *New England J. Med., 214:* 364-370, 1936.

[36] Peabody, F. W., " The Bacteriologic Diagnosis of Typhoid Fever," *J. A. M. A., 51:* 978, 1908.

[37] Peabody, F. W., quoted in *Francis Weld Peabody, 1881-1927, a Memoir.* Privately printed (by Francis G. Peabody), Riverside Press, Cambridge, 1933, pp. 18-19. Many of the facts about Peabody's life come from here.

six years made him one of the best-educated internists in America at that time. Two years at Johns Hopkins, in clinical medicine and pathology, were followed by a year in Germany, where Peabody studied organic chemistry with Emil Fischer and with Fresenius. He saw Ehrlich briefly —Ehrlich had discovered " Salvarsan " the year before. Back in the United States, in 1911-1912, he worked as a resident at the new research hospital at the Rockefeller Institute in New York, where he helped prepare a monograph on poliomyelitis which became the standard work for a decade. Finally he returned to Boston to be the first chief resident at the Peter Bent Brigham Hospital, under Dr. Henry A. Christian, from its opening in 1913 to 1915. In planning the research work which they were going to carry out in their new hospital, the two of them and a few others spent several months in Europe, picking up new ideas. Peabody spent a large share of his time with Krogh in Copenhagen; he was one of the first American students to work with that great physiologist.

Thus Francis Peabody obtained the best of foundations in biochemistry and physiology, as well as in clinical medicine. In the next few years he became one of the first to use these growing basic sciences in the study of disease—doing what he called " making clinical applications of the methods of physiology " [38] to diseases of the heart and lungs. In the years 1913 to 1921 Dr. Peabody and people working with him established the importance of the vital capacity as a measure of pulmonary reserve, and showed the mechanism by which the vital capacity is decreased in heart failure and emphysema, and other diseases. This, in a word, was pathological physiology.

Peabody and Cabot were quite different in the kind of research that they did. Cabot, with limited scientific training, and no training outside of Boston, made his valuable discoveries simply by gathering clinical facts —answering the question, " *What* is the state of things? "; Peabody, with thorough, world-wide training, was an early leader in the type of medical research which has been growing so rapidly since his time, which asks, " *Why* or *how* did this state of things come to be? "

Two of Dr. Peabody's papers which are particularly good examples of his clear writing are his Harvey Lecture on " Cardiac Dyspnea," in 1917, and a paper on " Certain Clinical Aspects of Pulmonary Emphysema," in the *Medical Clinics of North America* for 1925. Cabot and Peabody certainly shared the marvelous ability to turn a lucid phrase.

[38] Peabody, F. W., " Recent Advances in the Study of Heart Disease and Their Significance to the General Practitioner of Medicine," *Wisconsin M. J.*, *XV*: 255, 1917.

These active years of research and teaching at the Peter Bent Brigham Hospital were interrupted twice for the performance of public services. In 1914, when only 33, Dr. Peabody was asked to go to China as the only medical member of a three-man commission to study public health and medical education there for the Rockefeller Foundation. Out of this study grew the plans for Peking Union Medical School. Peabody returned to Peking in 1921, with his newly acquired wife, as one of the main speakers at the new school's dedication.

In 1917, when we entered the war, Dr. Peabody was sent as a member of a Red Cross Commission to Rumania to study the food and medical needs of that new ally of ours. While in Moscow arranging for shipments to Rumania, he was caught in the middle—literally—of the Bolshevik revolution which overthrew the Kerensky Government; his hotel, being in the direct line of fire, was almost shelled out. After a short period of army service in the United States and France, he returned to Boston, and, in 1919, took for his bride Virginia Chandler, a girl from the Midwest whom he had met on his trip to Europe with Dr. Christian. Their eight brief years of life together, from 1919 to 1927, were described as idyllic by all who knew them. Two sons came to round out the family.

In the next two years Francis Peabody, forty years old now, was offered as many outstanding positions in American medicine as any one person has probably ever been offered: the deanship of the new University of Chicago Medical School, the professorship of medicine at Johns Hopkins, Columbia, Yale, and Stanford Universities. But he chose to cast his lot with Boston medicine, and to take the opportunity offered him to build and direct the Thorndike Memorial Laboratories at the Boston City Hospital. At the same time he became Professor of Medicine at Harvard and Chief of the Harvard Services at the Boston City Hospital. Dr. Peabody saw here just the chance to try out what he had been thinking about ever since he was at the Rockefeller Institute ten years before— to do research as an integral part of a large hospital. Here at the City Hospital he could have a large and varied group of patients within easy reach of adequate research facilities and personnel; few hospitals could afford to have both the large number of beds and the good laboratories.

His conception went much further than this, however. He believed that the public had an " inherent right " to nothing less than the best possible medical care in their public hospitals. To give such good care the public hospital had to have money, research and teaching facilities the equal of any private hospital, so that the best physicians, teachers and students would be attracted.

Dr. Peabody wrote down these ideas of his in an excellent article called "The Functions of a Municipal Hospital." He also stressed here the importance of good nursing in the care of the patient and the place of social service in following up the patient outside of the hospital. High standards of nursing, he thought, could only be achieved by having a nursing school as a part of the hospital. And "the duty of the city towards the health of its citizens certainly extends beyond the wall of the hospital. . . . If a municipal hospital is to fulfill its functions it must support a well-staffed Social Service Department." [39]

In 1927 Dr. Peabody, writing to Dr. Pratt, whom he addresses as "my scientific godfather," gives perhaps the best summary of his conception of his clinic at the Boston City Hospital: "My great desire has been to have a medical clinic in which the highest type of scientific work was carried on in conjunction with the most human and sympathetic attitude towards the patients—a type of spiritual atmosphere that may be expressed by the word 'Christian.' " [40]

The Thorndike Memorial Laboratories were dedicated on November 15, 1923, with Mayor James Michael Curley, Dr. William J. Mayo of the Mayo Clinic, and others as speakers—the beginning of a new venture in which the City was accepting and fully supporting a research laboratory as a part of its hospital. During the five years that Dr. Peabody worked there, he devoted his time, with the singleness of purpose that was one of his greatest qualities, to making his clinic the equal of any, any place. He brought many other outstanding physicians there to work with him. He continued to do research himself, studying the physiology and pathology of the blood-forming organs, especially in pernicious anemia, where his work laid the foundation for Minot's discovery of liver therapy and its rationale. And, best of all, Dr. Peabody took an active part in teaching medicine. His rounds were famous for the wisdom and sympathy with which he approached each patient; he was followed around by students and visiting physicians from all over the world. He thought long and carefully about his teaching wards, and one of his last writings, in 1927, was a remarkable letter to Dr. Longcope at Johns Hopkins which was later published under the title, "The Soul of the Clinic." [41] After reciting with good humor the multitude of impossible qualities which a chief of medicine is expected to embody—"a man who has had

[39] Peabody, F. W., *Boston M. & S. J., 189*: 125, 1923.
[40] Pratt, Joseph H., *loc. cit.*
[41] Peabody, F. W., *Doctor and Patient*, New York: Macmillan Co., 1930, p. 72 *et seq.*

an intensive scientific training, has done important research, is a good administrator, is a competent teacher, and finally has had clinical experience "[42]—Peabody says that he thinks the " Chief " should be a clinician first of all, actively setting the standards of the ward's work, and stimulating, helping and advancing his assistants, rather than looking after his own research career. Dr. Peabody always had an " open door " for his staff and students.

Dr. Peabody, unlike Dr. Cabot, felt strongly that the general practitioner was more important today than ever. " Never," he says, " was the public in need of wise, broadly trained advisers so much as it needs them today to guide them through the complicated maze of modern medicine." [43] He was opposed to the kind of group practice where many different specialists see the patient but no one doctor understands or is responsible for the whole patient. " The practice of medicine is intensely personal," Peabody says, " and no system or machine can be substituted for the personal relationship." [44] On every important subject on which Dr. Peabody worked—typhoid, cardiac dyspnea, etc.—he wrote at least one paper especially to present the subject to the general practitioner.

It was in the Summer of 1926, over a year after the first, apparently benign gastric hemorrhage, that an exploratory operation revealed that Peabody had an inoperable malignancy. He was told the truth about his condition. With this knowledge he retreated to his summer cottage in Maine for a short convalescent period after the operation, and then returned to Boston, his father writes, " not with broken courage or spiritual depression, but with complete self-mastery and serenity, and began his laboratory and hospital service with undiminished fidelity and continuity." [45] And here began, for Francis Peabody's many friends, one of the most stirring experiences of their lives. For the next sixteen months, up to his last day, this young man, just at the beginning of the full flowering of his career, the loved and respected physician, lived in the daily company of death, as all knew, and yet lived a joyful, busy, peaceful life, supporting his family and friends even more than they supported him, teaching them by his own example the right way to live and to die.

His friends—Hans Zinsser, Longcope, many others—came from near and far for another visit with their friend in the pleasant garden of

[42] *Ibid.*, p. 74.
[43] *Ibid.*, p. 20.
[44] *Ibid.*, p. 23.
[45] *Francis Weld Peabody*, pp. 63-64.

William James's home in Cambridge, which the Peabodys had taken; and it seems as if almost every one was moved to write his own account of those remarkable visits. One of the best was written by Peabody's lifelong friend, Langdon Warner, and appeared in the *Boston Evening Transcript*:

You came hesitating, perhaps, and wondering how you could stand it. But you smoked, gossiped, and reported the news; discussed a marriage, a birth, or a death; told your troubles, took some of the invalid's grapes, and left. There had been no sad-eyed bravery about it, no attempt to ignore the obvious. His eye was as clear and familiar and merry as the day he graduated, or played on the school football team; and his voice, if not always strong, was as unshaken as ever. And all this time, when our hearts were standing still with the pity of it, his task was gently to show us that there was no need for horror. Above all, there was to be no fight. Those men who know most about such affairs tell us that this attitude of mind is indeed the only one which can properly overcome death. He himself needed no convincing on this point, nor did his companion. Those two together, in the words of a distinguished physician who travelled to see him, did more for the practice of healing than a whole course in the Medical School.[46]

It was in November, 1926, after he knew his diagnosis, that Dr. Peabody gave his simple and beautiful lecture on " The Care of the Patient." This little essay abounds in wisdom, taken from his own experience, particularly about practicing medicine within a hospital. His concluding lines, familiar to most of us, give us perhaps the best picture of the quality of his own spirit:

" The good physician knows his patients through and through, and his knowledge is bought dearly. Time, sympathy, and understanding must be lavishly dispensed, but the reward is to be found in that personal bond which forms the greatest satisfaction of the practice of medicine. One of the essential qualities of the clinician is interest in humanity, for the secret of the care of the patient is in caring for the patient."

[46] Warner, L., quoted in *Francis Weld Peabody*, pp. 69-70.